M000218736

Michigan Manual of
Neonatal
Intensive Care

3rd edition

Steven M. Donn, MD
Professor of Pediatrics
Director, Division of Neonatal-Perinatal Medicine
University of Michigan Health System
Ann Arbor, Michigan

HANLEY & BELFUS
An Imprint of Elsevier

HANLEY & BELFUS
An Imprint of Elsevier

The Curtis Center
Independence Square West
Philadelphia, Pennsylvania 19106

Library of Congress Control Number: 2003101724

MICHIGAN MANUAL OF NEONATAL INTENSIVE CARE
THIRD EDITION   ISBN 1-56053-564-4

Printed in the United States of America

Last digit is the print number: 9 8 7 6 5 4 3 2 1

CONTENTS

IV. Fluids, Electrolytes, and Nutrition

V. Neurologic Problems

CONTRIBUTORS

Janet C. Allen, M.S.W.
Clinical Social Worker, Department of Social Work, University of
Michigan Health System, Ann Arbor, Michigan

Mohammad A. Attar, M.D.
Clinical Instructor, Division of Neonatal-Perinatal Medicine, Department of
Pediatrics, University of Michigan Health System, Ann Arbor, Michigan

John D.E. Barks, M.D.
Associate Professor, Division of Neonatal-Perinatal Medicine, Department
of Pediatrics; Director, Neonatology Research Programs, University of
Michigan Health System, Ann Arbor, Michigan

Michael A. Becker, R.R.T.
Senior Allied Health Technical Specialist, Neonatal Respiratory Care,
Department of Critical Care Support Services, University of Michigan
Health System, Ann Arbor, Michigan

William M. Bellas, D.O.
Fellow, Division of Neonatal-Perinatal Medicine, Department of Pediatrics,
University of Michigan Health System, Ann Arbor, Michigan

Varsha Bhatt-Mehta, Pharm.D., FCCP
Clinical Assistant Professor of Pharmacy, Pediatrics, and Communicable
Diseases; Clinical Pharmacist, Pediatric and Neonatal Intensive Care,
University of Michigan Health System, Ann Arbor, Michigan

Peter Blos, Jr., M.D.
Lecturer in Child Psychiatry, Department of Psychiatry, University of
Michigan Health System, Ann Arbor, Michigan

Mary E.A. Bozynski, M.D., M.S.
Professor of Pediatrics, Associate Chair for Education, Division of
Neonatal-Perinatal Medicine, Department of Pediatrics, University of
Michigan Health System, Ann Arbor, Michigan

Suzanne H. Butch, M.A., M.T. (ASCP), S.B.B.
Chief Technologist, Clinical Pathology Laboratories, University of
Michigan Health System, Ann Arbor, Michigan

Steven M. Donn, M.D.
Professor, Department of Pediatrics; Director, Division of Neonatal-Perinatal Medicine, University of Michigan Health System, Ann Arbor, Michigan

Cyril Engmann, MBBS
Fellow, Division of Neonatal-Perinatal Medicine, Department of Pediatrics, University of Michigan Health System, Ann Arbor, Michigan

Molly R. Gates, M.S., R.N.C.
Clinical Nurse Specialist, Neonatal Outreach Coordinator, Department of Nursing, University of Michigan Health System, Ann Arbor, Michigan

Susan K. Gibney, R.N., M.S., L.L.P.
Clinical Nurse II, Holden Neonatal Intensive Care Unit, Bereavement Support Coordinator, University of Michigan Health System, Ann Arbor, Michigan

Jennifer L. Grow, M.D.
Fellow, Division of Neonatal-Perinatal Medicine, Department of Pediatrics, University of Michigan Health System, Ann Arbor, Michigan

Theresa Han-Markey, M.S., R.D.
Didactic Program Director and Lecturer, University of Michigan School of Public Health, Human Nutrition Program, Ann Arbor, Michigan

Robert H. Hayashi, M.D.
J. Robert Willson Professor of Obstetrics, Department of Obstetrics and Gynecology; Director, Division of Maternal-Fetal Medicine, University of Michigan Health System, Ann Arbor, Michigan

Ronald B. Hirschl, M.D.
Associate Professor, Division of Pediatric Surgery, Department of Surgery, University of Michigan Health System, Ann Arbor, Michigan

Wendy Kenyon, R.N., B.S.N.
Clinical Nurse II, Holden Neonatal Intensive Care Unit, Department of Nursing, University of Michigan Health System, Ann Arbor, Michigan

Mary E. Linton, R.N., M.S.N., N.N.P.
Formerly, Coordinator, Neonatal Nurse Practitioner Program, Holden Neonatal Intensive Care Unit; Department of Nursing, University of Michigan Health System, Ann Arbor, Michigan

Shobha Malviya, M.D.
Associate Professor, Section of Pediatric Anesthesiology, Department of Anesthesiology, University of Michigan Health System, Ann Arbor, Michigan

Nancy A. McIntosh, R.N., Ph.D.
Clinical Nurse Specialist, Division of Pediatric Pulmonology, Department of Nursing, University of Michigan Health System, Ann Arbor, Michigan

Charles R. Neal, Jr., M.D., Ph.D.
Assistant Professor, Division of Neonatal-Perinatal Medicine, Department of Pediatrics, University of Michigan Health System, Ann Arbor, Michigan

Clark E. Nugent, M.D.
Clinical Associate Professor, Department of Obstetrics and Gynecology, University of Michigan Health System, Ann Arbor, Michigan

Steven W. Pipe, M.D.
Assistant Professor, Division of Pediatric Hematology-Oncology, Department of Pediatrics, University of Michigan Health System, Ann Arbor, Michigan

Paul I. Reynolds, M.D.
Clinical Associate Professor, Department of Anesthesiology; Chief, Division of Pediatric Anesthesiology, University of Michigan Health System, Ann Arbor, Michigan

Lori Q. Riegger, M.D.
Assistant Professor, Section of Pediatric Anesthesiology, Department of Anesthesiology, University of Michigan Health System, Ann Arbor, Michigan

B. Jane Scheff, R.N.
Staff Nurse, Holden Neonatal Intensive Care Unit, Department of Nursing, University of Michigan Health System, Ann Arbor, Michigan

Robert E. Schumacher, M.D.
Associate Professor, Department of Pediatrics, Division of Neonatal-Perinatal Medicine, University of Michigan Health System, Ann Arbor, Michigan

William E. Smoyer, M.D.
Robert C. Kelsch Professor and Director, Division of Pediatric Nephrology, Department of Pediatrics, University of Michigan Health System, Ann Arbor, Michigan

Oliver S. Soldes, M.D.
Clinical Assistant Professor, Section of Pediatric Surgery, Department of Surgery, University of Michigan Health System, Ann Arbor, Michigan

Cosmas J. M. Van de Ven, M.D.
Clinical Associate Professor, Department of Obstetrics and Gynecology; Division of Maternal-Fetal Medicine, University of Michigan Health System, Ann Arbor, Michigan

Elizabeth L. Workman, R.N.
Staff Nurse, Holden Neonatal Intensive Care Unit, Department of Nursing, University of Michigan Health System, Ann Arbor, Michigan

Eileen G. Wright, R.N.
Clinical Nurse Specialist, Holden Neonatal Intensive Care Unit, Department of Nursing, University of Michigan Health System, Ann Arbor, Michigan

FOREWORD

Neonatology has been a medical specialty for a scant three decades. Advances in this arena have been remarkable. It is difficult enough for senior attending neonatologists to keep up with all the innovations, much less for trainees to do so. For the past decade, *The Michigan Manual* has been a resource that provides state-of-the-art information in a handy, easy-to-read resource that can be practically carried by the clinician.

This tome has evolved from a House Staff Manual produced at one of the premier academic neonatal intensive care units (NICUs) in the world. Both practical and wide-ranging, the third edition of *The Michigan Manual of Neonatal Intensive Care* remains a lab coat pocket–sized resource that can be readily accessible to clinicians, whether they are in training or are seasoned veterans. The book can easily be referred to on clinical rounds. The current edition emphasizes basic management of diverse disorders, as well as important technical skills, such as catheter placement. Of necessity, the scope of the latest edition has expanded. There are a number of new chapters that reflect the latest management of multiple conditions. The contents are in logical order, starting with prenatal diagnosis and fetal assessment. This edition includes wide-ranging topics that are not available in most neonatology textbooks, including perinatal outreach, medical record documentation, and the function of an ethics committee. Many chapters list suggested background material should the reader decide to further explore a particular area.

The vast majority of neonatal illnesses are discussed in *The Michigan Manual of Neonatal Intensive Care*. Moreover, management of these disorders are covered comprehensively. Standard therapies and "rescue therapies" (e.g., high-frequency ventilation and inhalational nitric oxide) are well-described. Of particular note are the descriptions of mechanical ventilation of various respiratory diseases as well as the use of extracorporeal membrane oxygenation (ECMO). The University of Michigan is internationally renowned for these areas of neonatology. The quality of the latter sections reflects the preeminence of this center and its clinicians.

I find the practical aspects of the manual to be quite well done. The standardized NICU admission template is easy to use and will ensure that key aspects of the history and physical examination will not be missed. A good description of a variety of technical procedures is present. Everyday issues of patient care are carefully addressed, including management of fluids, electrolytes, and enteral and parenteral nutrition; use of antibiotics; and ventilator assistance and strategies. Subjects that are of everyday importance yet are often neglected in standard neonatology textbooks are covered in this work, including the roles of the neonatal nurse practitioner and social worker, interaction with parents and dealing with the family's frequent problems with coping, and aspects of neonatal follow-up. Other posthospitalization topics also receive consideration: home apnea monitoring, risk for SIDS, and others.

The Michigan Manual of Neonatal Intensive Care is particularly useful for pediatric and neonatology trainees and neonatal nurse practitioners. The reader of this manual will find that, once again, Dr. Donn has superbly edited it to present complicated issues in a standardized format that is both comprehensive and useful.

> Thomas E. Wiswell, M.D.
> Professor of Pediatrics
> Director of Neonatal Research
> State University of New York
>   at Stony Brook
> Stony Brook, New York

PREFACE

Neonatal intensive care has undergone a technologic revolution since the first edition of this manual was published 11 years ago. Standard treatments for newborns with respiratory failure now include surfactant replacement therapy, patient-triggered and high-frequency ventilation, real-time pulmonary graphic monitoring, and inhaled nitric oxide. Antibiotic management of infectious diseases includes an expanded array of antimicrobials. Refinements in infant nutrition have improved both parenteral and enteral formulations. Imaging techniques have advanced to digital technology and give three-dimensional views of neonatal anatomy. Our colleagues in maternal-fetal medicine have also pioneered advances in fetal diagnosis and treatment. Doppler assessment, antenatal corticosteroids, and intrapartum chemoprophylaxis for group B streptococcal infection are but a few of these advances.

Keeping pace in this rapidly changing field can be quite challenging, even for the most experienced neonatologist. It can be especially daunting for the medical student, house officer, and fellow assigned to the neonatal intensive care unit (NICU). In addition, we have entered the era of evidence-based medicine, which can add another layer of confusion to the physician or trainee at the bedside of a critically ill baby in the middle of the night.

The purpose of this manual is to present a logical, step-by-step approach to the major problems in neonatal intensive care. It should not, however, be misconstrued to represent the only acceptable means of diagnosis and treatment. The intent of the first edition was to develop a consistent way to deal with a large, high-census, high-acuity population in a teaching hospital, given the substantial number of rotating personnel.

There are a number of changes in the third edition. Beyond revision of the text and suggested readings from the second edition, new chapters have been added. These include prenatal diagnosis, antepartum and intrapartum fetal assessment, multifetal gestation, grief and bereavement, and medical informatics. I am quite pleased that the production of the book has been assumed by Hanley & Belfus, Inc. It has been a pleasure to work with Bill Lamsback, Editorial Director, and Cecelia Bayruns, Production Editor. I am very grateful to Marcy Kroll, the copy editor, who painstakingly and meticulously brought consistency and readability to the outline format. I would also like to acknowledge the efforts of many individuals who made the third edition a reality: my colleagues, both past and present, who took the time to contribute, revise, and advise; the incredible staff of neonatal nurses and respiratory therapists with whom it is my good fortune to work every day; and my secretary, Susan Peterson, now a veteran of multiple medical texts, who prepared the entire manuscript and improved it along the way. I also appreciate the wonderful feedback I received from readers of the previous manuals, whose suggestions have been incorporated into this edition.

Finally, there is no reason to think that the advances we have witnessed are going to decelerate. Readers are urged to keep current through periodicals and continuing medical education. Still, it is my hope that the third edition of *The Michigan Manual of Neonatal Intensive Care* will make those nights in the NICU a little better for those who use it and a lot better for the babies who are served.

Steven M. Donn, M.D.

ABBREVIATIONS USED THROUGHOUT THIS BOOK

AA	amino acids
AAP	American Academy of Pediatrics
Ab	abortion
ABG	arterial blood gas
ABR	audiometric brainstem response
ACE	angiotensin-converting enzyme
ACh	acetylcholine
ACT	activated clotting time
AD	autosomal dominant
ADH	antidiuretic hormone
AFib	atrial fibrillation
AFl	atrial flutter
AGA	appropriate for gestational age
AGS	adrenogenital syndrome
AIDS	acquired immunodeficiency syndrome
ALTE	apparent life-threatening event
Ao	aortic
AOI	apnea of infancy
AOP	apnea of prematurity
AR	autosomal recessive
ARDS	adult respiratory distress syndrome
ASD	atrial septal defect
ATN	acute tubular necrosis
AV	atrioventricular
BAER	brainstem audiometric evoked response
BID	twice a day
BP	blood pressure
BPD	bronchopulmonary dysplasia
bpm	beats, breaths per minute
BT	Blalock-Taussig
BUN	blood urea nitrogen
BW	birthweight
C	cervical
CBC	complete blood count
CBG	capillary blood gas, capillary blood glucose
CCHB	congenital complete heart block
CDC	Centers for Disease Control and Prevention
CDH	congenital diaphragmatic hernia

CHD	congenital heart disease
CHF	congestive heart failure
CIE	counterimmunoelectrophoresis
cm	centimeter
CMV	cytomegalovirus
CNS	central nervous system
CPAP	continuous positive airway pressure
CPR	cardiopulmonary resuscitation
CSF	cerebrospinal fluid
CT	computed tomography
CVP	central venous pressure
CXR	chest radiograph (x-ray)
d	day
dL	deciliter
DBP	diastolic blood pressure
DC	direct current
D/C	discharge or discontinue
DIC	disseminated intravascular coagulopathy
dL	deciliter
DOL	days of life
DPT	diphtheria-pertussis-tetanus
DTR	deep tendon reflexes
DVT	deep vein thrombosis
Dx	diagnosis
$D_{2.5}W$	dextrose (2.5%) in water
$D_{10}W$	dextrose (10%) in water
E	energy
EA	esophageal atresia
ECG	electrocardiogram
ECMO	extracorporeal membrane oxygenation
EDC	estimated date of confinement
EEG	electroencephalogram
EFAD	essential fatty acid deficiency
ELBW	extremely low birthweight
EMG	electromyogram
EP	electrophysiologic
ESR	erythrocyte sedimentation rate
ET	endotracheal
$ETCO_2$	end-tidal carbon dioxide
ETCPAP	endotracheal continuous positive airway pressure
ETT	endotracheal tube
F	French

FDA	Food and Drug Administration
FE	fractional excretion
FFP	fresh frozen plasma
FHR	fetal heart rate
FiO$_2$	fraction of inspired oxygen
FRC	functional residual capacity
FSP	fibrin split products
FTT	failure to thrive
G	gravida
g	gram
GA	gestational age
GBS	group B streptococcus
GDM	gestational diabetes mellitus
GE	gastroesophageal
GFR	glomerular filtration rate
GI	gastrointestinal
GU	genitourinary
H	hour
HBIG	hepatitis B immune globulin
HCT	hematocrit
HFJV	high-frequency jet ventilation
HFO	high-frequency oscillation
HFPPV	high-frequency positive pressure ventilation
HFV	high-frequency ventilation
Hgb	hemoglobin
HIV	human immunodeficiency virus
HPF	high power field
HR	heart rate
hr	hour
HSM	hepatosplenomegaly
HSV	herpes simplex virus
Hz	hertz
IAP	intrapartum antibiotic prophylaxis
ICCRC	Infant and Child Care Review Committee
ICH	intracranial hemorrhage
ID	internal diameter
IDM	infant of diabetic mother
I:E	inspiratory to expiratory ratio
Ig	immunoglobulin
IM	intramuscular
IMV	intermittent mandatory ventilation
INR	international normalized ratio

IPV	inactivated polio vaccine
ITP	idiopathic thrombocytopenic purpura
IU	international unit
IUGR	intrauterine growth retardation
IV	intravenous
IVC	inferior vena cava
IVH	intraventricular hemorrhage
IVP	intravenous pyelogram
JEB	junctional epidermolysis bullosa
kcal	kilocalorie
kg	kilogram
L	liter
LA	left atrium
LC	living children
LGA	large for gestational age
LIP	lymphoid interstitial pneumonitis
LMP	last menstrual period
LP	lumbar puncture
LPM	liters per minute
L/S	lecithin/sphyngomyelin ratio
LV	left ventricle
L3–L4	third through fourth lumbar vertebrae
M	molar
m	meter
μ	micro
MAC	minimum alveolar concentration
MAP	mean arterial pressure
MAS	meconium aspiration syndrome
MBC	mean bactericidal concentration
MCS	multichannel study
MCT	medium-chain triglycerides
mEq	milliequivalent
MG	myasthenia gravis
MIC	mean inhibitory concentration
min	minute
mL	milliliter
mm	millimeter
MMR	measles, mumps, rubella vaccine
MRI	magnetic resonance imaging
MVI	multiple vitamin infusion
NEC	necrotizing enterocolitis
NG	nasogastric

NICU	neonatal intensive care unit
NP	nasopharyngeal
NPCPAP	nasopharyngeal continuous positive airway pressure
NPO	nothing by mouth
NST	nonstress test
NTB	necrotizing tracheobronchitis
OD	outer diameter
OFC	occipital frontal circumference
OG	orogastric
OI	oxygenation index
OPV	oral polio vaccine
osm	osmolality
oz	ounce
P	para
PAC	premature atrial contraction
$PaCO_2$	arterial carbon dioxide tension
PaO_2	arterial oxygen tension
Paw	mean airway pressure
PB	periodic breathing
PCA	postconceptional age
PCG	pneumocardiogram
pcpt	precipitation
PCR	polymerase chain reaction
PCVC	percutaneous central venous catheter
PDA	patent ductus arteriosus
PEEP	positive end-expiratory pressure
PFO	patent foramen ovale
PG	phosphatidyl glycerol
PIE	pulmonary interstitial emphysema
PIP	peak inspiratory pressure
PNA	postnatal age
pkt	packet
PKU	phenylketonuria
PL	pressure limit
PMI	point of maximal intensity
PO	by mouth (*per os*)
PPHN	persistent pulmonary hypertension of the newborn
PPV	positive pressure ventilation
PR	per rectum
PRBC	packed red blood cell
PRN	as needed
PROM	premature rupture of membranes

PS	pressure support
PT	prothrombin time
PTT	partial thromboplastin time
PUFA	polyunsaturated fatty acids
PVC	premature ventricular contraction
PVH	periventricular hemorrhage
PVL	periventricular leukomalacia
PVR	pulmonary vascular resistance
q	every
QID	four times daily
RA	right atrium
RBC	red blood cell
RDS	respiratory distress syndrome
RFI	renal failure index
ROP	retinopathy of prematurity
RSV	respiratory syncytial virus
RV	right ventricle
RVT	renal vein thrombosis
SAH	subarachnoid hemorrhage
SaO_2	arterial oxygen saturation
SBP	systolic blood pressure
SC	subcutaneous
S/D	systolic/diastolic ratio
SDH	subdural hemorrhage
SGA	small for gestational age
SIADH	syndrome of inappropriate secretion of antidiuretic hormone
SIMV	synchronized intermittent mandatory ventilation
SIDS	sudden infant death syndrome
SK	streptokinase
SLE	systemic lupus erythematosus
STD	sexually transmitted disease
SVC	superior vena cava
SvO_2	venous oxygen saturation
SVT	supraventricular tachycardia
T	thoracic
TAPVR	total anomalous pulmonary venous return
TAR	thrombocytopenia-absent radius
TBW	total body water
TCP	tribasic calcium phosphate
$TcPCO_2$	transcutaneous carbon dioxide tension
$TcPO_2$	transcutaneous oxygen tension
TEF	tracheoesophageal fistula

TEWL	transepidermal water loss
THAM	tris-hydroxy aminomethane
T_i	inspiratory time
TID	three times daily
TM	tympanic membrane
TPA	tissue plasminogen activator
TPN	total parenteral nutrition
TORCH	toxoplasmosis, other, rubella, cytomegalovirus, and herpes simplex
T8(10)	eighth (tenth) thoracic vertebra
U	unit(s)
U/A	urinalysis
UAC	umbilical artery catheter
UK	urokinase
UPJ	ureteropelvic junction
URI	upper respiratory infection
USN	ultrasound
UTI	urinary tract infection
UVC	umbilical vein catheter
UVJ	ureterovesical junction
VA	venoarterial
VCU	voiding cystourethrogram
VCUG	vesicoureterogram
VER	visual evoked response
Vfib	ventricular fibrillation
VLBW	very low birthweight
V/Q	ventilation-perfusion
VSD	ventricular septal defect
VT	ventricular tachycardia
V_t	tidal volume
VV	venovenous
vWF	von Willebrand factor
WBC	white blood cell
WPW	Wolff-Parkinson-White syndrome

Section I   MATERNAL-FETAL MEDICINE

Chapter 1

Prenatal Diagnosis

Clark E. Nugent, M.D.

I. **Amniocentesis**
 A. Indications
  1. Suspected fetal anomaly
   a. Chromosomal
    i. Karyotype
    ii. Fluorescence in situ hybridization (FISH)
     (a) Commercially available InSight chromosomes 13, 18, 21, X, Y
     (b) Looking for microdeletions, e.g., q22,11 in DiGeorge syndrome
   b. Alpha fetoprotein for neural tube defects
   c. DNA
   d. Enzyme analysis
  2. Infection
   a. Bacterial/viral cultures
   b. PCR
  3. Erythrocyte alloimmunization
   a. Delta OD 450
   b. Fetal blood type determination by DNA analysis of amniocytes
  4. Pulmonary maturity
   a. Fluorescence polarization
    i. ≥ 55 mature
    ii. 40–54 intermediate (2% risk of RDS)
    iii. ≤ 39 immature (42% risk of RDS)
   b. Lamellar body count
   c. Foam stability index no longer commercially available
   d. L/S ratio becoming less available
  5. Therapeutic "amnioreduction" for massive polyhydramnios
 B. Technique
  1. Genetic amniocentesis usually done at ≥ 15 weeks' gestation
  2. Ultrasound guidance
   a. Select pocket away from fetal face, umbilical cord insertion
   b. With oligohydramnios, be wary of umbilical vein

1

    masquerading as a pocket of fluid. Color Doppler useful in making this decision.

  3. 22- or 20-gauge spinal needle

  4. Typical volume 20–40 mL depending on which studies are being done

  5. Rh immune globulin administered to Rh-negative women

C. Complications

  1. Pregnancy loss rate 0.25–0.5%

  2. Ruptured membranes

  3. Onset of labor

  4. Infection (rare)

  5. Fetal injury (rare)

II. Chorionic Villus Sampling

A. Essentially a placental biopsy

B. Primary indication is suspected fetal anomaly

  1. Karyotype

  2. FISH

C. Technique

  1. Transcervical

    a. Uses a 1.9-mm catheter with a bendable stylet

    b. Optimal gestational age 10–12 weeks

      i. May not be able to reach placenta at later gestational ages

      ii. Increased risk of limb reduction defects at gestational ages < 10 weeks

  2. Transabdominal

    a. Uses a 20-gauge spinal needle

    b. Can be performed at ≥ 10 weeks if the placenta is accessible

    c. Samples tend to be smaller than with transcervical

    d. Considerably more patient discomfort than with transcervical

  3. Contraindications

    a. Active vaginal or cervical infection (transcervical approach)

    b. Erythrocyte alloimmunization

    c. Rh immune globulin administered to Rh-negative women

D. Complications

  1. Pregnancy loss 0.5–1%

  2. Bleeding 9.7%

  3. Cramping 0.6%

  4. Fluid leak 0.1%

  5. Limb reduction defects 0.03–0.1%

  6. Infection (rare)

7. Potential for significantly greater fetomaternal bleeding than with amniocentesis (thus, the relative contraindication with alloimmunization)

III. Fetal Blood Sampling (a.k.a. Percutaneous Umbilical Blood Sampling [PUBS], a.k.a. Funipuncture, a.k.a. Cordocentesis)

A. Indications
1. Alloimmunization
   a. Erythrocyte
   b. Platelet
2. Rapid karyotype
3. Congenital infection
4. Suspected fetal anemia

B. Technique
1. Access technically difficult prior to 18 weeks
2. Ultrasound visualization of cord
   a. Placental insertion preferred
   b. Free loop of cord more tenuous
   c. Fetal cord insertion problematic if fetal movement present
3. 22- or 20-gauge spinal needle
4. Umbilical vein preferred over artery
   a. Larger diameter
   b. Umbilical artery spasm leading to fetal bradycardia with arterial puncture
5. Verify fetal origin of blood
   a. Direct visualization of needle in umbilical vein
   b. Potential laboratory methods
      i. Mean corpuscular volume greater in fetal cells (provide reference range)
      ii. Antigen differences in fetal cells
   c. Blood collected into syringes coated with anticoagulant (heparin or EDTA)

C. Complications
1. Pregnancy loss 1.5%
2. Cord trauma
   a. Hematoma
   b. Bleeding from puncture site
      i. May last from seconds to minutes
      ii. Fetal exsanguinations reported in procedures done for fetal thrombocytopenia or platelet disorders. Recommended that washed maternal platelets be available for immediate transfusion in these cases.

3. Contamination of sample with maternal blood
4. Rupture of membranes
5. Premature labor
6. Infection (rare)

Suggested Reading

American College of Obstetricians and Gynecologists: Assessment of Fetal Lung Maturity. Washington, DC, ACOG, 1996, ACOG educational bulletin 230.

American College of Obstetricians and Gynecologists: Prenatal Diagnosis of Fetal Chromosomal Abnormalities. Washington, DC, ACOG, 2001, ACOG practice bulletin 27.

Centers for Disease Control and Prevention: Chorionic villus sampling and amniocentesis: Recommendations for prenatal counseling. MMWR Morb Mortal Wkly Rep 44:1–12, 1995.

Antepartum Fetal Assessment

Robert H. Hayashi, M.D.

I. Fetal Movement Counting

  A. Expectation

    1. In the second/third trimester, periods of fetal movements last for 40 minutes, with quiet periods of 20 minutes.

    2. Usually, mothers appreciate gross fetal movements 70–80% of the time. Decreased appreciation of fetal movements may occur with anterior placental location, hydramnios, obesity, and fetal anomalies.

    3. Peak fetal movement time is usually 9:00 P.M. to 1:00 A.M., secondary to relative hypoglycemia in mother.

  B. Evidence base

    1. Only descriptive studies. Rayburn reports that, of the 5% who reported decreased fetal movement (using the Cardiff "count to ten" method), there was a 60-fold increase in stillbirths, 2–3-fold increase in labor fetal distress, 10-fold increase in severe IUGR, and 10-fold increase in low Apgar scores compared to control group with adequate fetal movements.

    2. Method

      a. Use "count to ten" method in evening time when mother can be recumbent. Should get $\geq$ 10 fetal movements in 2 hours. Call the hospital or obstetrician if $\leq$ 10 fetal movements.

      b. Start the fetal movement counting at 28 weeks' gestation.

II. Contraction Stress Test (CST)

  A. Expectation—uterine contractions simulating labor will decrease placental blood flow during contractions. With a decrease of fetal energy reserves, secondary to uteroplacental insufficiency, a fetal heart rate pattern of a late deceleration will occur with uterine contractions.

  B. Evidence base

    1. Only descriptive studies

    2. Perinatal mortality of $< 1/1000$ birth within 1 week of a negative CST

    3. Likelihood of perinatal mortality after a positive test is 7–15%.

    4. The high false positive rate of the CST (30–50%) is the limitation of this test method.

C. Method
   1. Patient in semi-Fowler position with slight left tilt
   2. BP taken every 5–10 minutes
   3. External maternal-fetal monitor applied to evaluate fetal heart rate pattern and uterine contractions (UC)
   4. Administer oxytocin at 0.5 mU/min and double the infusion rate every 20 minutes until one gets 3 UCs per 10 minutes.
   5. This usually takes a dose of 10 mU/min and may take up to 90 min.
D. Interpretation (Table 1)

TABLE 1
Interpretation of the Contraction Stress Test

Interpretation	Description	Incidence (%)
Negative	No late decelerations appearing anywhere on the tracing with adequate uterine contractions (three in 10 min)	80
Positive	Late decelerations that are consistent and persistently present with the majority (> 50%) of contractions without excessive uterine activity; if persistent late decelerations seen before the frequency of contractions is adequate, test interpreted as positive	3–5
Suspicious	Inconsistent late decelerations	5
Hyperstimulation	Uterine contractions closer than every 2 min or lasting > 90 sec, or five uterine contractions in 10 min; if no late decelerations seen, test interpreted as negative	5
Unsatisfactory	Quality of the tracing inadequate for interpretation or adequate uterine activity cannot be achieved	5

III. Nonstress Test (NST)

A. Expectations
   1. Fetal heart rate accelerations reflect fetal well being.
   2. About 3–4 accelerations/hour are expected.
   3. Accelerations are associated with fetal movements 85% of the time at term, and fetal movements are associated with fetal heart rate acceleration 90% of the time.
   4. Decrease of acceleration with smoking, narcotics, and beta-blocker use in mother

B. Evidence base
  1. Descriptive studies only
  2. With reactive NST, perinatal mortality is 5/1000.
  3. With nonreactive NST, perinatal mortality is 30–40/1000.
C. Method
  1. Patient in semi-Fowler recumbency with slight left tilt
  2. BP taken every 10 minutes
  3. External fetal monitor
  4. Mother asked to press marker button attached to the monitor when she perceives fetal movement
  5. Criteria
      a. *Reactive* is two accelerations in a 20-minute window of the fetal heart rate.
          i. ≥ 32 weeks—15 bpm acceleration above baseline for 15 seconds
          ii. < 32 weeks—10 bpm acceleration above baseline for 10 seconds
      b. *Nonreactive* is the lack of a reactive pattern. This is expected about 15% of the time.
  6. Other issues
      a. Can use a vibro-acoustic stimulator (artificial larynx) for 3 seconds to stimulate a reaction within 3 minutes. Just as reliable as response to spontaneous fetal movement.
      b. A spontaneous episode of prolonged decelerations during NST has a higher positive predictive value for fetal compromise than a nonreactive NST.
      c. In high-risk pregnancies, increasing the frequency of testing to twice weekly can decrease the perinatal mortality from 6.1 to 1.9/1000 births.

IV. Biophysical Profile (BPP)
  A. Expectation
  1. Based on the fact that fetal biophysical activities that are present earliest in development are the last to disappear with progressive fetal hypoxia. The NST becomes nonreactive first, then fetal breathing movement disappears, next is fetal movement, then fetal tone is last to disappear. The amniotic volume decrease reflects chronic hypoxia. The BPP evaluates all five parameters.
  2. The BPP evaluation has been validated as early as 26 weeks' gestation.
      a. Evidence base

      i. Manning did a prospective blinded study in 216 high-risk pregnant patients. No perinatal deaths when all five activities were normal and 60% perinatal mortality when all parameters were not normal. He also reported a descriptive study of 26,780 high-risk pregnancies.

      ii. False positive rate was 20%.

      iii. False negative rate (all parameters normal) was 6.9/1000 births.

      iv. Corrected perinatal mortality rate with a normal BPP was 1.9/1000 births and 0.77/1000 births within 1 week.

  b. Method (Table 2)

  c. Management (Table 3)

      i. BPP of $\leq$ 6 occurs 3% of the time.

      ii. Use of antenatal steroids has increased the false-positive

TABLE 2
Technique of Biophysical Profile Scoring

Biophysical Variable	Normal (Score = 2)	Abnormal (Score = 0)
Fetal breathing movements	At least one episode of > 30 sec in 30 min observation	Absent or no episode of ≥ 30 sec in 30 min
Gross body movement	At least three discrete body/limb movements in 30 min (episodes of active continuous movement considered a single movement)	Up to two episodes of body/limb movements in 30 min
Fetal tone	At least one episode of active extension with flexion or full fetal flexion of fetal limb(s) or trunk; movement of limb in opening and closing of hand considered normal tone	Either slow extension with return to partial extension or absent movement
Reactive fetal heart rate	At least two episodes of acceleration of ≥ 15 bpm and 15-sec duration associated with fetal movement in 30 min	Fewer than two accelerations < 15 bpm in 30 min
Qualitative amniotic fluid	Volume fluid measuring 2 cm in two perpendicular planes	Either no amniotic fluid pockets or a pocket < 2 cm in two perpendicular planes

TABLE 3
Management Based on Biophysical Profile Score

Score	Interpretation	Management
10	Normal infant; low risk of chronic asphyxia	Repeat testing weekly; repeat twice weekly in diabetic patients and patients at ≥ 41 wks' gestation.
8	Normal infant; low risk of chronic asphyxia	Repeat testing at weekly intervals; repeat testing twice weekly in diabetics and patients at ≥ 41 wks' gestation; oligohydramnios is an indication for delivery.
6	Suspect chronic asphyxia	If ≥ 36 wks' gestation and conditions are favorable, deliver; if at > 36 wks and L/S < 2.0, repeat test in 4–6 hr; deliver if oligohydramnios is present.
4	Suspect chronic asphyxia	If ≥ 36 wks' gestation, deliver; if < 32 wks' gestation, repeat score.
0–2	Strongly suspect chronic asphyxia	Extend testing time to 120 min; if persistent score ≤ 4, deliver, regardless of gestational age.

rate (lowered the BPP score). The effect is on the NST and fetal breathing movement for a 48-hour period.

V. Doppler Flow Studies

A. Expectation

1. Systolic velocity reflects fetal cardiac contractions, whereas diastolic velocity reflects interaction between peak flows and vessel wall compliance, heart rate, and vascular impedance of the site perfused downstream.

2. Umbilical artery Doppler study reflects fetal placental perfusion. With increased impedance of placental blood flow, one gets an increase of the S/D ratio, which can lead to absence or reversal of diastolic flow velocity.

3. Used clinically in IUGR pregnancies.

   a. Method

   i. Commonly used is the S/D velocity ratio.

   ii. The Doppler ultrasound probe should be aimed at the mid-umbilical cord portion during fetal quiet time, as fetal breathing movements will alter the S/D ratios.

B. Management

1. Absent or reversal of diastolic flow indicates intense ongoing fetal surveillance, not emergent delivery.

2. Reversal of diastolic flow is even more predictive of poor perinatal outcome than absent flow.

VI. Strategy of Antenatal Testing in the Perinatal Assessment Center, University of Michigan Health System

   A. In low-risk pregnancies, testing is upon indication e.g., decreased fetal movement, and repeated weekly if necessary.

   B. In high-risk pregnancy (e.g., diabetes, IUGR, prolonged pregnancy, hypertension or history of stillbirth), the testing is twice weekly.

   C. We tend to use the "modified BPP," which is an NST and amniotic fluid index (AFI).

   D. If the NST is nonreactive and/or AFI is decreased, a BPP is done.

Chapter 3

Electronic Fetal–Maternal Surveillance

Robert H. Hayashi, M.D.

I. **Expectation**

    A. Electronic fetal heart rate (FHR) monitoring has become the standard means for evaluating fetal oxygenation in labor.

    B. The basis of FHR monitoring is fetal brain monitoring. Control of the FHR is a response to baroreceptors, chemoreceptors and metabolic change. Although hypoxia is the major concern effecting these changes, many other stimuli can alter FHR patterns.

    C. The goal of FHR monitoring is to detect hypoxia in labor and allow the clinician to implement nonoperative interventions.

II. **Methods**

    A. The methodology of FHR monitoring by external means using the Doppler technology is quite sophisticated and nearly equivalent to the fetal scalp electrode.

    B. However, care must be taken not to mistake a maternal heart rate recording inter-mixed with FHR recording (especially with maternal tachycardia in labor).

    C. Pattern definitions

        1. Normal FHR 110–160 bpm

            a. Tachycardia is baseline > 160 bpm

            b. Bradycardia is baseline < 110 bpm

        2. Variability—short-term or beat-to-beat

            a. Absent: amplitude undetected, a flat line

            b. Minimal: amplitude ≤ 5 bpm

            c. Moderate: amplitude 6–25 bpm (normal)

            d. Marked: amplitude > 25 bpm

        3. Periodic decelerations (in relation to uterine contractions)

            a. Early—shallow, uniform with onset and end, reflecting uterine contractions. Vagal response to head compression.

            b. Late—similar in appearance as early deceleration, but onset and end are delayed relative to uterine contraction response to hypoxia. Onset is usually 30 seconds after onset of contraction, or even the peak of contraction.

            c. Variable—rapid deceleration and return to baseline occurring at variable relationships to contraction; vagal response to cord compression. It is the most common periodic deceleration.

    i. Mild: < 30-second duration and < 80 bpm depth
    ii. Moderate: depth < 80 bpm
    iii. Severe: depth < 70 bpm for > 60 seconds
   d. Prolonged bradycardia: FHR deceleration for 2–10 minutes. If > 10 minutes, it is considered a change of baseline.

III. Evidence Base

A. Only five randomized, controlled trials have been done. Efficacy is not supported in low-risk pregnancy. In high-risk pregnancy it decreased the incidence of neonatal seizures. It has a high specificity and a false positive rate of 50%.

B. FHR acceleration in labor has the same reassuring status as in the nonstress test.

C. Loss of beat-to-beat variability is highly correlated to fetal hypoxia, and late deceleration and loss of variability is most highly correlated to fetal hypoxia.

D. ACOG has requested that the term *perinatal asphyxia* be eliminated in relationship to FHR pattern changes and the term *nonreassuring fetal status* (NRFS) be used.

IV. Management (Intervention)

A. For NRFS, nonsurgical interventions include: maternal oxygen administration, maternal lateral position, and increased hydration. Also, if oxytocin infusion is running, discontinue or decrease it.

B. Fetal scalp pH is a method to determine fetal acid/base status at the moment of sampling. This methodology is not used in most centers, including the author's.

C. Fetal pulse oximetry. The FDA recently approved this approach. A flat probe is applied to the fetal cheek area with ruptured membranes and a nearly engaged head. Using infrared technology, the fetal oxygen saturation can be continuously determined. A normal range of 30–70% saturation is utilized. A reading below the 30% threshold for 10 minutes requires an expedited delivery. Otherwise, labor is allowed to continue even with NRFS.

Suggested Reading

Druzin ML, Gabbe SE, Reed KL: Antepartum fetal evaluation. In Gabbe SE, Niebyl JR, Simpson JL (eds): Obstetrics: Normal and Problem Pregnancies, 4th ed. New York, Churchill Livingston, 2002, pp 313–349.

Garite TJ: Intrapartum fetal evaluation. In Gabbe SG, Niebyl JR, Simpson JL (eds): Obstetrics: Normal and Problem Pregnancies, 4th ed. New York, Churchill Livingston, 2002, pp 313–349.

Chapter 4

Multifetal Gestation

Cosmas J. M. Van de Ven, M.D.

I. Epidemiology

A. Incidence of multifetal gestation in the USA:
Twins: 23/1000 births or 1:43 births
Triplets: 0.9/1000 births or 1:1143 births

B. In the USA between 1973 and 1990, the birth rates increased by:
Singletons   32%
Twins   65%
Triplets   221%

C. Incidence of twin gestation:
6/1000 births in Japan
53/1000 births in Nigeria
15/1000 births worldwide

D. Variation in incidence results from variation in dizygotic twins.

E. Monozygotic twin rates are similar across the world at 4/1000 births.

F. Twins:
1. 30% are monozygotic, i.e., originate from one ovum, also called *identical*.
2. 70% are dizygotic, i.e., originate from two separate ova, also called *fraternal*.
3. Twin births constitute 96% of all multiple births.

II. Etiology

A. Etiology of multiple gestation remains unknown.

B. Associations
1. Increased serum gonadotropins
2. Abnormal fertilization
3. Polar body twinning
4. Two ova in one follicle

C. Monozygous twins
1. 0.4% incidence throughout the world
2. No environmental factors known
3. Increased rates in reproductive technology

D. Dizygous twins
1. Increased with advanced maternal age

2. Increased with higher parity
3. Increased with reproductive technology
   a. 10% with clomiphene citrate
   b. 40% with gonadotropins
4. Familial trends (maternal), increased serum gonadotropin levels
5. Racial trends: Asian < Caucasian < African-American

III. Chorionicity

A. Di-Di: diamniotic, dichorionic. Each twin is in its amniotic sac and has its own placenta.
B. Di-Mo: diamniotic, monochorionic. Each twin is in its own amniotic sac, but they share one placenta.
C. Mo-Mo: monoamniotic, monochorionic. Both twins are in one amniotic sac and share one placenta.
D. Of all twin pregnancies, 20% are monochorionic (all are monozygotic) and 80% are dichorionic (75% are dizygotic, and 25% are monozygotic).
E. Of the monozygotic twins, the chorionicity is: Di-Di in 33%, split in first 2–3 days after fertilization; Di-Mo in 66%, split between 3rd and 8th day; Mo-Mo in 1%, split between 8th and 13th day (split between 13th and 15th day will result in conjoined twins).
F. Determination of zygosity is important because of increased risk of congenital anomalies and monochorionicity in monozygous twins.
G. Determination of chorionicity is important because of marked increase in obstetric complications in monochorionic pregnancies.
H. The diagnosis of twins and the chorionicity are determined by ultrasound in early second trimester.
I. Determination of zygosity at birth
   1. 35% are different sex, therefore dizygous.
   2. 20% will have a monochorionic placenta, therefore monozygous.
   3. 45% will be same sex with a dichorionic placenta and will need blood group or genetic analysis. Of these, 37% will be dizygous and 8% will be monozygous.
   4. Perinatal mortality, i.e., intrauterine demise and neonatal death, is closely associated with the chorionicity of the placentas.
      a. Mo-Mo twins: 50% perinatal mortality
      b. Di-Mo twins: 25% perinatal mortality
      c. Di-Di twins: 9% perinatal mortality
   5. Summary
      a. Of all twins
         i. 70% dizygous (fraternal), all are diamniotic-dichorionic
         ii. 30% monozygous (identical), 1/3 diamniotic-

dichorionic, 2/3 diamniotic-monochorionic, 1% monoamniotic-monochorionic
  b. Of all twins
     i. 80% diamniotic, dichorionic; 7/8 dizygous, 1/8 monozygous
     ii. 20% diamniotic, monochorionic; all are monozygous

IV. Morbidity and Mortality
  A. Overall perinatal mortality
     1. Twins: 48/1000
     2. Triplets: 123/1000
     3. Quadruplets: 175/1000
  B. Infant mortality
     1. Singletons: 8.6/1000
     2. Twins: 56.6/1000
     3. Triplets: 166.7/1000
  C. Severe handicap
     1. Singletons: 20/1000
     2. Twins: 34/1000
     3. Triplets: 58/1000
  D. In twins, more than 80% of perinatal mortality occurs before 30 weeks' gestation.

V. Complications during Pregnancy
  A. Preterm delivery
     1. Overall preterm delivery in the USA = 11% of all deliveries or 440,000 infants per year.
        a. 10% of preterm infants are twins.
        b. 25% of perinatal deaths are twins.
     2. More than 50% of twins and more than 90% of triplets are born before 37 weeks' gestation.
     3. Prophylaxis
        a. Bed rest, no proven benefit
        b. Cerclage, no benefit, may actualy increase preterm delivery
        c. Steroids, proven benefit
        d. Tocolytics, no proven benefit
     4. Triplets
        a. Average gestational age: 34 weeks
        b. 90% < 37 weeks
        c. 20% < 32 weeks
  B. Intrauterine growth restriction
     1. 60–70% of all twins are born small for gestational age (SGA).

  2. Growth of twins follows a pattern similar to singletons until approximately 32 weeks' gestation. After 32 weeks, the biparietal diameter and femur length continue to follow the singleton curve; however, weight gain drops.

  3. Growth discordance between twins is defined as a discrepancy of the estimated fetal weight (by ultrasound) of $> 20\%$.

  4. Growth discrepancy of $> 25\%$ is associated with differences in height, weight, and developmental delay into adult life.

C. Twin-twin transfusion syndrome (TTTS)

  1. Occurs only in monochorionic placentation

  2. Incidence of TTTS

   a. 15% of monochorionic pregnancies

   b. Perinatal mortality 60–90%

  3. Almost all monochorionic placentas have vascular anastomoses.

   a. Most common are arterioarterial anastomoses (high resistance).

   b. Venovenous anastomoses are rare (low resistance).

   c. Of concern are arteriovenous anastomoses, where a cotelydon receives blood from one twin but the blood returns to the other twin.

  4. TTTS is thought to occur in those with arteriovenous anastomoses.

  5. Acute TTTS

   a. In regard to the arterioarterial and venovenous anastomoses, there will be free exchange between these anastomoses with quick equilibration in pressure; therefore, minimal transfusion occurs from one twin to the other.

   b. However, when fetal demise of one twin occurs, there will be rapid exsanguination of the other twin from loss of perfusion pressure; this may lead to hypotension, CNS necrosis, and demise. In addition, thrombotic or coagulopathic events may occur.

   c. Acute TTTS may occur in any trimester with the demise of one twin. In addition, it may occur at time of delivery.

  6. Chronic TTTS

   a. Chronic TTTS represents the more classic presentation.

    i. Growth discrepancy

    ii. Hypovolemic, anemic donor with oligohydramnios

    iii. Hypervolemic, cardiac hypertrophy, congestive heart failure in the recipient, with polyhydramnios

  7. Neonatal criteria

     a. Weight discrepancy > 20%

     b. Hemoglobin difference > 5 g/dL

  8. Differential diagnosis of discordant twins with poly/ oligohydramnios

     a. Etiology

       i. TTTS

       ii. Congenital or chromosomal anomalies

       iii. Placental insufficiency

       iv. Cord insertion anomalies

     b. Diagnosis

       i. Detailed fetal survey

       ii. Consider obtaining karyotype of both twins

  9. Doppler velocimetry has not been helpful in the diagnosis; high S/D ratios can be seen in both twins. Absent or reversed diastolic flow has a high correlation with poor neonatal outcome. The appearance of a biphasic waveform in the umbilical vein may be indicative of cardiac failure.

 10. Therapeutic options

     a. Most studied and promising management involves serial amniocentesis of the polyhydramnios.

     b. Other therapeutic options

       i. Intrauterine laser ablation of vascular communications

       ii. Maternal digitalization (experimental)

       iii. Maternal indomethacin (experimental)

       iv. Selective removal of twin (abandoned)

       v. Selective feticide

       vi. Umbilical cord banding

     c. Whether or not to intervene is mainly determined by gestational age; 90–100% mortality at < 20 weeks.

D. Intrauterine demise of one twin

  1. Only 50% of twin pregnancies identified in *first* trimester will result in delivery of two live infants.

  2. Intrauterine demise of one twin occurs in 2–5% of twin pregancies *after* 12 weeks' gestation and in 14–17% of triplets.

  3. Morbidity and mortality of remaining twin depends on chorionicity and gestational age. In dichorionic twins there is no evidence of increased neurologic morbidity.

  4. Proposed mechanisms include embolization of tissue thromboplastin through placental anastomoses and hypotension secondary to transfusion into dead fetus.

  5. 50–80% of twin pregnancies with one fetal demise will result in preterm delivery.

      6. The incidence of maternal disseminated intravascular coagulation was initially reported as 25% after 4–5 weeks of fetal demise. Newer data suggest that this is rare.

E. Cord insertion anomalies
    1. Velamentous cord insertion
      a. 2% of singletons
      b. 14% of dichorionic twins
      c. 27% of monochorionic twins
    2. Risk for vasa previa
    3. Abnormal fetal heart rate tracings in labor

F. Acardia
    1. 1% of monozygotic twins
    2. 1:35,000 births
    3. Perinatal morbidity appears associated with the weight discrepancy between the normal and the acardiac twin.
      a. If weight ratio > 70%:
        i. 90% preterm delivery
        ii. 40% polyhydramnis
        iii. 30% congestive heart failure
      b. If weight ratio < 70%:
        i. 75% preterm delivery
        ii. 30% polyhydramnios
        iii. 10% congestive heart failure
    4. Therapeutic options
      a. Maternal digitalization
      b. Indomethacin
      c. Umblical cord ligation (most promising)

G. Additional obstetric complications in multifetal gestations
    1. Maternal anemia (> 30%)
    2. Placenta previa
    3. Abruptio placentae
    4. Preeclampsia (40–60%)
    5. Malpresentations
    6. Postpartum hemorrhage from uterine atony

H. Other less common complications
    1. Fetus papyraceus, early fetal demise, amniotic fluid absorbed, fetus in membranes
    2. Vanishing twin
    3. Aplasia cutis. Fetal demise of twin causes diffuse, patchy skin lesions on survivor.
    4. Conjoined twins: 1:50,000 births
    5. Chimerism (two genetically dissimilar cell lines)

       a. Twinning in only part of the original cell lines

       b. Very early twin–twin transfusion with establishment of two blood cell lines

   6. Spontaneous abortions, risk at least twofold higher (30%)

   7. Congenital anomalies

       a. Singleton: 4%

       b. Dizygotic twins: 8%

       c. Monozygotic twins: 16%

VI. Multifetal Pregnancy Reduction and Selective Termination

A. Very few data are available on natural course of multifetal gestations, specifically < 20 weeks.

B. Loss rates estimates prior to 20 weeks for twins are 10%, for triplets 13%, and for quadruplets 20%.

C. Natural history for triplets

   1. Premature delivery: 90% < 37 weeks, 20% < 32 weeks, 9% < 28 weeks.

   2. Perinatal mortality: 123/1000 births

   3. Associated morbidity for triplets

       a. 21% mild developmental problems

       b. 11% severe neurologic disabilities

   4. Natural history for quadruplets

       a. Premature delivery: 100% < 37 weeks, 75% < 34 weeks, 47% < 32 weeks, 13% < 28 weeks.

       b. Associated mortality and morbidity for quadruplets

          i. Perinatal mortality 175/1000

         ii. Neonatal mortality 120/1000

   5. Average gestational age at delivery

       a. Twins: 36 weeks, average BW 2473 g

       b. Triplets: 33 weeks, average BW 1666 g

       c. Quadruplets: 30 weeks, average BW 1414 g

   6. Because the major morbidity and mortality of multifetal gestations are secondary to prematurity and intrauterine growth restriction, multifetal pregnancy reduction was introduced to improve outcome.

   7. Multifetal pregnancy reduction (MPR) techniques

       a. Transvaginal aspiration

       b. Transvaginal intrathoracic KCl injection

       c. Transabdominal intrathoracic KCl injection

   8. It appears that MPR from triplets–to–twins may have an increased early (< 24 weeks) loss rate, but an improved gestational age and BW at time of delivery.

9. Current literature suggests an improved outcome after MPR for quadruplets and higher order multifetal pregnancies. The benefit in triplet gestations is less clear.

VII. Genetic Diagnosis in Multiple Pregnancies

A. Aneuploidy increases with maternal age.

B. Multiple gestation increases with maternal age, secondary to both the natural dizygotic rate and the need for reproductive technology.

C. For monozygotic twins, the age-related risk for aneuploidy applies, since both have the same karyotype.

D. There is some evidence of an increased incidence in chromosomal anomalies associated with monozygotic twins.

E. Genetic risk in dizygotic twins
1. Risk that one fetus is affected is the sum of the age-related aneuploidy incidence.
2. Risk that both fetuses are affected is the multiplication of the individual risks.
3. Difficult ethical dilemmas may occur when one twin carries a chromosomal abnormality.

F. Amniocentesis in twins (ultrasound guidance)
1. Visualization of two clearly separated sacs
2. Transmembrane aspiration of both sacs
3. Installation of 1 mL of 1:10 mL diluted indigo carmine
4. Methylene blue is not used; it may oxidize reduced hemoglobin to methemoglobin leading to hemolytic anemia and hyperbilirubinemia. In addition, use in early second trimester is associated with intestinal atresia.

G. Chorionic villus sampling in twins
1. Increased difficulty in assuring aspiration of different chorion frondosum
2. Contamination with villi from the other twin occurs in 4% of samples.
3. Procedure-induced loss rates appear similar to singletons, but baseline loss rate is significantly higher, i.e., 3%.

H. Alpha-fetoprotein screening
1. Singletons
   a. 2.5 MOM (multiples of the mean)
      i. 75% sensitivity for open neural tube defects
      ii. 2–3% false-positive rate
2. Twins
   a. 2.5 MOM
      i. 89% sensitivity

  ii. 30% false-positive rate
 b. 3.5 MOM
  i. 75% sensitivity
  ii. 15% false-positive rate
 c. 5.0 MOM
  i. 40% sensitivity
  ii. 3% false-positive rate

VIII. Intrapartum Management

A. Vertex–vertex
 1. 40% of twin pregnancies
 2. Recommend vaginal delivery
 3. 80% will succesfully deliver vaginally

B. Vertex–nonvertex
 1. 40% of twin pregnancies
 2. Recommend vaginal delivery
 3. 50–70% success rate of external podalic version of second twin to vertex
 4. Epidural anesthesia recommended
 5. Delivery of second twin in breech presentation (for infants > 1500 g) carries same morbidity compared with cesarean delivery.
 6. Delivery of second twin can also be accomplished by total breech extraction; again morbidity rates are similar to those delivered by CS.

C. Nonvertex first-presenting twin
 1. 20% of twin pregnancies
 2. Cesarean section is recommended mode of delivery.
 3. When presenting twin is breech and second twin vertex, incidence of interlocking is 0.1%.

D. Delivery of second twin
 1. Clamp cord immediately, risk for exsanguination of remaining twin if monochorionic placenta.
 2. Ultrasound in delivery room, oxytocin, external or internal version spontaneous breech or breech extraction

Suggested Reading

Benirschke K: Multiple gestation: Incidence, etiology and inheritance. In Creasy RK, Resnick R (eds): Maternal-Fetal Medicine, 4th ed. Philadelphia, W.B. Saunders, 1999, pp 585–597.

Chitkara V, Berkowitz RL: Multiple gestations. In Gabbe SG, Niebyl JR,

Simpson JL (eds): Obstetrics: Normal and Problem Pregnancies, 4th ed. New York, Churchill Livingstone, 2002, pp 827–867.

Crowther CA: Multiple pregnancy. In James DK, Steer PJ, Weiner CP, Gonik B (eds): High-Risk Pregnancy Management Options, 2nd ed. Philadelphia, W.B. Saunders, 1999, pp 127–151.

Keith LG, Papiernik E, Keith DM, Luke B: Multiple Pregnancy Epidemiology, Gestation, and Perinatal Outcome. New York, Parthenon, 1995.

Malone FD, D'Alton ME: Multiple gestation: Clinical characteristics and management. In Creasy RK, Resnick R (eds): Maternal-Fetal Medicine, 4th ed. Philadelphia, W.B. Saunders, 1999, pp 598–615.

Section II NEONATOLOGY BASICS

Chapter 5

Neonatal Admission Work-up

Steven M. Donn, M.D.

I. Identifying Statements (replaces chief complaint):
"1100 g 30-week AGA male delivered by $1°$ cesarean section to a 22-year-old $G_1 P_{0-1}$ mother for progressive preeclampsia."

II. Maternal Obstetrical History
Include significant past history especially pregnancy losses, complications, or infertility problems, e.g.:
"$G_5 P_1 Ab_3 LC_0$
1987 spontaneous Ab 8 weeks
1988 spontaneous Ab 12 weeks
1990 1250 g term female trisomy 18, died 12 hours
1991 spontaneous Ab 11 weeks"

III. History of Pregnancy
   A. Last menstrual period
   B. Estimated date of confinement
   C. Prenatal care
   D. Weight gain
   E. Medications or drugs, including OTC preparations, substance abuse
   F. Illnesses or infections
   G. Alcohol or tobacco use
   H. Blood type/antibody screen
   I. Serology and cultures
   J. Gestational age dating (quickening, ultrasound, fundal height)
   K. Complications (e.g., bleeding or spotting, edema, abdominal pain)

IV. Labor
   A. Onset of uterine activity (spontaneous, induced)
   B. Duration
   C. Intensity of contractions
   D. Membrane status (intact, ruptured spontaneously or artificially, and before/after labor)
   E. Amniotic fluid (volume, color, character)
   F. Presentation (e.g., vertex, breech, transverse) and position (e.g., occiput anterior)

G. Augmentation (oxytocin)
H. Monitoring (auscultation, electronic)
I. Analgesia (type, route)

V. Delivery
A. Mode (vaginal, abdominal)
B. Assistance (forceps, vacuum extraction)
C. Anesthesia or analgesia
D. Complications

VI. Immediate Neonatal Period
A. Apgar scores (include breakdown)
B. Resuscitation provided (e.g., ventilation, drugs)
C. Neonatal course (include procedures, tests)

VII. Transport Data (for Outborns)
Include information regarding treatment(s) rendered, complications, and how infant tolerated transport.

VIII. Family History
Include *pertinent* information regarding heritable and familial conditions.

IX. Social History
A. Parents' marital status
B. Planned versus unplanned pregnancy
C. Legal custody of infant
D. Religious preference (especially Jehovah's Witness)
E. Adoption
F. Socioeconomic status

X. Physical Examination
General observation: weight, length, head circumference. Include growth percentiles.
Vital signs: include blood pressure
Head: shape, molding, trauma if present, anterior fontanel, sutures
Eyes: pupils, red reflex, conjunctivas, extra-ocular motion
Ears: canals, TMs
Nose: patency of nares, septum, flaring
Pharynx: palate, gums, uvula, tongue
Neck: trachea, masses, webbing

Chest: retractions, grunting, respiratory rate and effort, chest excursions, lung sounds, symmetry, anteroposterior diameter

Heart: rate, rhythm, murmurs, precordial activity, pulses, and perfusion

Abdomen: liver span, spleen, masses, hernias, umbilicus, number of vessels, distention, tenderness

Genitourinary: kidneys, genitalia, urethra

Anus: patency

Extremities: range of motion, number of digits, hand or foot anomalies, hip examination

Skin: rashes or lesions, maturity

Neurologic: tone, activity and reactivity, primitive responses, DTRs, sensory function

XI. Gestational Age Assessment (e.g., Ballard or Dubowitz Examination)

XII. Laboratory Data
List results of studies thus far completed or pending.

XIII. Impression
List all working diagnoses, in order of importance.
1. 3.75 kg, 43-week, post-term AGA male
2. Meconium aspiration syndrome
3. Persistent pulmonary hypertension secondary to #2
   a. Hypoxemia
   b. Acidosis
4. Pneumomediastinum secondary to #2
5. Suspected sepsis
6. Polydactyly right hand

XIV. Plan
List all appropriate diagnostic procedures and therapeutic interventions that are indicated.

XV. Additional Documentation
   A. Procedure notes (for all procedures done by you to date)
   B. Informed consent(s)
   C. Parents have seen/touched infant
   D. Staff consultation
   E. Notification of referring physician, mother's obstetrician

Chapter 6

Neonatal Resuscitation: General Principles

Cyril Engmann, MBBS, and Steven M. Donn, M.D.

I. **Introduction**

Over 90% of newborns make the transition from intrauterine to extrauterine life with little or no assistance. The remaining 10% require some assistance, with 10% of these requiring intensive resuscitative measures to restore cardiopulmonary function. It is estimated that, worldwide, more than 1 million newborns per year may benefit from adequate resuscitation.

II. **Normal Fetal Cardiopulmonary State (Figure 1)**

A. Oxygenation of blood occurs at the placenta, not the lungs.

B. Alveoli are filled with fluid.

C. Oxygenated blood from the placenta goes through the umbilical vein to the inferior vena cava—50% via the ductus venosus and 50% through the hepatic circulation. From the inferior vena cava, blood goes to the right atrium where it is directed preferentially across the foramen ovale to the left atrium. This facilitates oxygen delivery to the heart and brain.

D. Blood that passes from the right atrium to the right ventricle is ejected into the pulmonary artery, then across the patent ductus arteriosus into the aorta.

E. Relatively little blood reaches the pulmonary parenchyma/alveoli because of high pulmonary vascular resistance.

F. Decreased pulmonary blood flow results in low pulmonary venous return with consequent low left atrial pressure, which permits patency of the foramen ovale.

III. **Normal Physiologic Events at Birth**

A. Fluid in the alveoli is absorbed into lung tissues during first and subsequent breaths of the infant.

B. Clamping of umbilical vessels removes the low resistance placental circulation and raises systemic blood pressure.

C. Pulmonary vascular resistance (PVR) falls dramatically, stimulated by lung expansion and increased oxygenation.

D. The net results of these changes are increased pulmonary blood

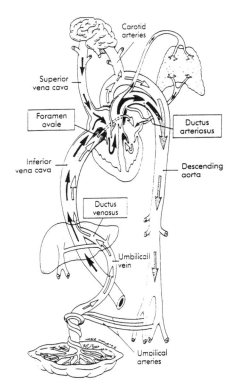

Figure 1. Key elements of fetal circulation. Low-resistance placental circuit and high-resistance pulmonary circuit result in shunting of oxygenated blood returning from the placenta away from the lungs to other systemic organs via the ductus arteriosus and foramen ovale. (From Bloom RS: Delivery room resuscitation of the newborn. In Fanaroff AA, Martin RJ (eds): Neonatal-Perinatal Medicine. Diseases of the Fetus and Infant, 7th ed. St. Louis, Mosby, 2002, p 417, with permission.)

flow, increased pulmonary venous return, increased left atrial pressure, closure of the PFO, and PDA blood flow reversal.

IV. Abnormal Physiologic Events at Birth

These may result in failure of the infant to expand the lungs and establish spontaneous respirations after delivery, resulting in:

A. Residual alveolar fluid

B. Hypoxemia and acidosis

C. Hypercapnia

D. Pulmonary vasoconstriction with consequent increased PVR, decreased pulmonary blood flow, and large right–to–left shunting through the PDA and PFO

E. Clinically, respiratory effort is first affected, manifested by rapid breathing, followed by primary apnea. If further resuscitation is not instituted, the heart rate may begin to fall at this time, and irregular gasping may ensue, followed by secondary apnea. Blood pressure is usually maintained until the onset of secondary apnea.

F. Even vigorous assisted ventilation may be inadequate if earlier hypoxemia/acidosis impaired myocardial function and vital organ blood flow, and contributed to the positive feedback loop of shock, or if significant cardiopulmonary anomalies are present.

V. Anticipation/Identification of High-Risk Pregnancies

A. Good communication is essential. Frequently those attending the delivery are the last people to be informed of impending problems. Approximately one third of infants who require resuscitation will have no identifiable risk factors.

B. Planning/preparation. Mental review of neonatal resuscitation protocols prior to the arrival of the infant is a helpful practice.

C. Personnel. If a high-risk delivery is suspected, at least two people are needed whose sole responsibility is the infant. Prior to the delivery, the specific role to be played by each resuscitator should be clarified.

D. Basic equipment
1. Radiant warmer/prewarmed blankets
2. Oxygen with flowmeter and tubing
3. Adjustable suction source, catheters, bulb syringe
4. Stethoscope
5. Self-inflating bag with infant masks and 100% O_2 reservoir. (An anesthesia bag is acceptable if the user is skilled and comfortable with its use.)
6. Oro/nasogastric tubes
7. Laryngoscope with #0,1 blades and spare bulbs and batteries
8. Endotracheal tubes, 2.5- to 4.0-mm internal diameter
9. Umbilical catheters, forceps, tape
10. Syringes, needles
11. Three-way stopcock
12. Medications and fluids—$NaHCO_3$, epinephrine, naloxone, dextrose, volume expanders
13. Clock

VI. Conduct of Resuscitation (Figure 2)

A. Coordination between resuscitation personnel is vital (e.g., count out loud or tap out heart rate upon auscultation of heart).

B. Specify/designate specifically who in the delivery room should do what if extra help is needed.

C. Continuous reappraisal of resuscitative efforts is critical.

D. At least one person should keep track of the "big picture," or overall conduct of the resuscitation.

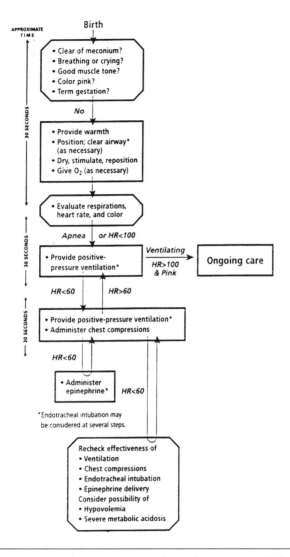

Figure 2. Conduct of neonatal resuscitation. (From Kattwinkel J (ed): Textbook of Neonatal Resuscitation, 4th ed. Dallas, American Academy of Pediatrics–American Heart Asssociation, 2000, p 6–2, with permission.)

    E. Thermoregulation
        1. Radiant warmer
        2. Rapidly dry the infant and remove wet towels.
    F. Assure airway patency.
        1. Position infant properly while supine, with neck slightly

extended. Elevate shoulders 1–2 cm with shoulder roll. The head may be turned to the side if secretions are profuse.

2. Suction the mouth, then the nose.
3. If amniotic fluid was meconium-stained:
    a. An infant with depressed respirations, should have the trachea immediately intubated and suctioned under direct vision. Use an endotracheal tube attached to an adapter and regulated suction. Repeat until efflux is clear, or until risk of continuing outweighs potential benefits (typically around the third passage).
    b. After tracheal toilet, aspirate the gastric contents when the infant is stable.
    c. If the infant is vigorous, no intubation and suctioning is required. Vigorous is defined as strong respiratory efforts, good muscle tone, and a heart rate greater than 100 bpm.

G. Gentle but firm stimulation—gently flick the soles, or rub the back. If there is poor or absent respiratory effort after two attempts at stimulation, further stimulation attempts are unlikely to be successful.

H. Sequential assessments
    1. Is the infant making respiratory effort?
        a. If yes, go to 2.
        b. If no, initiate positive pressure ventilation (PPV) with 90–100% oxygen at 40–60 bpm. Assess efficacy by breath sounds and chest excursions. Endotracheal intubation is necessary at this point only if a diaphragmatic hernia is suspected, bag and mask is ineffective despite proper technique, or rapid access for administration of selected resuscitation medications is necessary.
    2. Is the heart rate > 100 bpm?
        a. If yes, go to 3.
        b. If no, but > 60 bpm, initiate positive pressure ventilation (PPV).
        c. If no and < 60 bpm, initiate PPV, cardiac massage, and administer epinephrine intravenously or endotracheally (0.1–0.3 mL/kg of 1:10,000 formulation).
    2. Is central cyanosis present?
        a. If no, observe.
        b. If yes, administer free-flow oxygen 90–100% (accomplished with flow at 5–8 L/min with tubing 0.5 cm from nares) and gradually wean.

I. If PPV is necessary, reassess after 20 seconds while delivering 90–100% O_2 free-flow.

1. If spontaneous respiratory effort and heart rate > 100 bpm, observe for cyanosis and attempt to wean free-flow oxygen.
2. If no spontaneous respiratory effort, or heart rate < 100 bpm, resume PPV:
   a. If heart rate < 60 bpm, institute cardiac massage. Assess efficacy by palpating brachial pulses.
   b. If heart rate > 60 bpm, continue PPV alone.
   c. If no spontaneous respiratory effort and heart rate > 100 bpm, continue PPV; if maternal opiate use within 4 hours of delivery, consider naloxone (0.1 mg/kg) (unless the mother is a known opiate user).

J. If continued PPV with or without cardiac massage is necessary, reassess after 30 seconds.
1. If there is spontaneous respiratory effort and heart rate > 100 bpm, observe for cyanosis and attempt to wean free-flow oxygen.
2. If no spontaneous respiratory effort, or heart rate < 100 bpm, resume PPV.
   a. If heart rate < 60 bpm, resume cardiac massage and administer epinephrine (0.1–0.3 mL/kg of 1:10,000 formulation intravenously or endotracheally).
   b. If heart rate > 60 bpm, use PPV alone.

K. Serial reassessment is done every 30 seconds during PPV with or without cardiac massage. Continue PPV/cardiac massage as needed. Epinephrine may be repeated every 5 minutes. If no response to 1:10,000 formulation of epinephrine, give same volume of 1:1,000 formulation.

L. Place an orogastric tube after 2 minutes and tape it in place. Aspirate the stomach contents and place the tube to "chimney."

M. Establish vascular access (the umbilical vein is the preferred route for rapid access).
1. Obtain a blood gas measurement, hematocrit, and other necessary laboratory tests. A venous gas may be most useful for assessing tissue oxygenation and acid-base balance; arterial gas is more reflective of lung function.
2. Initiate glucose infusion to establish and/or maintain normoglycemia.

N. If blood gas evaluation reveals metabolic acidosis *and* adequate ventilation, you may treat with $NaHCO_3$ (2 mEq/kg); THAM (tris-hydroxyaminomethane) (4–8 mL/kg of 0.3M) may be given even if ventilation is inadequate or unknown.

O. Document all events carefully.

P. Call for additional help as needed.

Q. Common problems interfering with effective resuscitation:
1. Improper performance
   a. Head and neck position?
   b. Airway patency?
   c. Mask size and application?
   d. Adequacy of bag compression?
   e. Sternal placement of fingers?
   f. Firm surface under infant?
   g. Adequacy of sternal compression?
2. Mechanical difficulties
   a. Oxygen turned on?
   b. Airway connectors loose or unconnected?
   c. Oxygen tubing misrouted or unconnected?
   d. Suction not turned on at the wall?
   e. Suction connectors loose or unconnected?
3. Endotracheal tube problems
   a. Right main bronchus?
   b. Esophagus?
   c. Occlusion?
4. Hypovolemia?
5. Pneumothorax or other intrathoracic air leak?
6. Maternal medication (e.g., opiate, anesthetic)?
7. Congenital anomaly of cardiopulmonary system or airway?
8. Birth trauma?

R. Call referral or tertiary center for advice and/or transport.

S. When to stop? Termination of resuscitation is a difficult issue, which should have guidelines. Noninitiation of resuscitation may be appropriate in infants with confirmed gestation < 23 weeks, birthweight < 400 g, anencephaly, or trisomy 13 or 18. Remember that prenatal records may be incomplete and/or unreliable and there is more to be gained by attending the delivery and, if in doubt, initiating resuscitation. After more information is available, withdrawal of support may be initiated if the outcome is clearly going to be unfavorable. Ongoing counseling with the family is imperative. If full resuscitative measures, i.e., PPV, cardiac compressions, and repeated epinephrine administration, continue for more than 15–20 minutes with asystole still present, discontinuation may be appropriate. Consultation with a tertiary center may be invaluable.

Chapter 7

Neonatal Resuscitation: Special Procedures

Steven M. Donn, M.D., and Cyril Engmann, MBBS

I. **Orotracheal Intubation**
  A. Equipment
    1. Laryngoscope—check bulb, batteries, blades
    2. Endotracheal tube (ETT)—see Table 4 for guidelines for selection of appropriate size. A small air leak is acceptable.
    3. Metal stylet may be helpful—assure that tip does not protrude beyond end of ETT or through sidehole.
    4. Adjustable suction with appropriate catheters, bulbs
    5. Pre-cut tape, tincture of benzoin, or other adhesive
    6. Bag and mask with 100% O_2 adapter
    7. Oxygen source with flowmeter and tubing
  B. Preparation
    1. Place infant in supine position with shoulders elevated, head slightly extended, jaw forward.
    2. Oxygen flow to infant's airway should be maintained.
    3. Suction as necessary.
  C. Visualization
    1. Hold the laryngoscope in your *left* hand, low down on the handle.
    2. Insert the blade into the right side of mouth. As the blade is moved to the midline, the tongue will be pushed to the left to allow visualization.
    3. The blade tip is inserted into the vallecula (space between base of tongue and epiglottis).
    4. The handle of the laryngoscope is then picked *straight up.* This moves the epiglottis anteriorly and reveals the vocal cords. The handle should not be pulled back (as if it were a lever) since this may damage the alveolar ridge and/or glottic area. Gentle external pressure on the cricoid cartilage or larynx may be helpful to better visualize the epiglottis and vocal cords.
  D. Insertion
    1. The grooved portion of the blade is for visualization, *not* tube passage.
    2. Suctioning may be required for optimal visualization.
    3. The ETT is inserted through the right side of the mouth along

TABLE 4
Guidelines for Endotracheal Intubation

Birthweight (kg)	Tube Size (mm ID)	Depth of Insertion (cm at lip)
≤ 1.0	2.5	7
1.0–2.0	3.0	8
2.0–3.0	3.5	9
≥ 3.0	3.5 or 4.0	10

the right edge of the blade, and with curvature from left to right. Visualize the epiglottis and vocal cords throughout the insertion and advancement of the ETT.

4. Place the tip of the tube between the vocal cords and rotate its curve into the proper plane as it is guided down the trachea.

5. Insert the tube until the black marker line above the tip of the ETT is at the vocal cords or its tip is palpated in the suprasternal notch. See Table 4 for guidelines for depth of insertion (for oral tubes).

6. Remove the blade and stylet while securing the endotracheal tube in place.

7. Ventilate the infant and assess for the presence and equality of breath sounds and absence of gastric ventilation. Adjust the tube position as needed. Note tube markings at the lip for landmark of desired insertion depth.

E. Fixation

1. Once positioned properly, secure tube adequately with tape and tincture of benzoin.

2. Check final position radiographically with the head in *neutral* position. (This may be unnecessary after reintubation if good breath sounds and chest excursions and a prior chest radiograph demonstrated good position at same insertion depth.)

3. Trim excess tube length.

II. External Cardiac Massage

A. Provide a firm surface under the infant. Placing your hands around the infant so that your fingertips are beneath the thoracic spine is effective.

B. Place thumbs in parallel or crossover position over the lower third of sternum, avoiding the xiphoid if possible. An alternative technique is to place fingertips perpendicular to the lower third of the sternum while sliding your other hand under the back to assure a firm surface.

C. Depress the sternum 0.5–1.0 cm and release it without removing thumbs/fingertips from the sternum.

D. Coordinate PPV and chest compression, 30 breaths and 90 compressions per minute.

E. Assess efficacy of compressions by palpation of brachial pulses.

III. Umbilical Vein Catheterization (*see* page 48)

IV. Establishment of Intraosseous Access

A. This is useful when other vascular access is unavailable and the endotracheal route alone is inadequate or inappropriate.

B. The flat, medial aspect of the proximal tibia below the tibial tuberosity is commonly used.

C. Prepare area with iodophor.

D. A needle with a stylet (bone marrow needle or 18- to 20-gauge spinal needle) is used.

E. The needle is advanced perpendicular to the skin until the periosteum is reached.

F. The needle is then angled and advanced 60° caudally to avoid the epiphyseal plate. A screwing to–and–fro motion is used to penetrate the cortex. An abrupt change in resistance is noted when the marrow space is entered and the needle can then support itself upright.

G. Bone marrow or blood should be aspirated to assure placement. Saline is then infused and should meet little resistance.

H. Administer medications in intravenous doses.

I. Fluid should be infused constantly to avoid clotting of the needle by marrow.

J. Complications
   1. Epiphyseal injury
   2. Infection
   3. Inappropriate placement with extravasation
   4. Fat embolism

V. Intracardiac Administration of Medications

A. Rarely necessary, but usually used when no vascular access available or endotracheal and/or intravenous administration is unsuccessful (even with highest doses of medication), or as a "last ditch" maneuver.

B. Establish the position of heart. If there is dextrocardia, tension pneumothorax, etc., the location may be altered.

C. Prepare chest area with iodophor.

D. Palpate the xiphoid process.

E. Insert 22-gauge, 1.0- to 1.5-inch needle immediately subxiphoid and aim for tip of left shoulder; an approach may also be made through the fourth intercostal space midway between the left sternal border and the midclavicular line.

F. Gently aspirate as the needle is slowly advanced.

G. Entry into the ventricle is apparent with blood return.

H. Inject the drug and remove the needle.

I. Continue cardiac massage after injection to distribute the drug.

J. Potential complications
  1. Coronary artery damage
  2. Hemopericardium
  3. Pneumothorax/pneumopericardium
  4. Myocardial injury
  5. Infection
  6. Injection into inappropriate space

VI. Pneumothorax Evacuation by Thoracentesis

A. The diagnosis is suspected by suggestive changes in breath sounds and chest excursions, transillumination, or chest radiograph. In emergent situations during resuscitation, empiric thoracentesis may occasionally be necessary.

B. Assemble equipment.
  1. Scalp vein needle (usually 21 or 23 gauge)
  2. Three-way stopcock
  3. 30-mL syringe (or larger)
  4. Iodophor

C. Prepare the insertion site with iodophor. Free air in the chest rises and, for a supine infant, anterior placement in the midclavicular line in the most anterior intercostal space is appropriate.

D. Connect needle, stopcock, and syringe with stopcock turned off to infant.

E. Using sterile technique, pull skin above insertion site cephalad to use Z-technique. (When needle is later withdrawn from pleural space and skin is released, tissues will slide over the track and prevent leakage of air into inappropriate sites.)

F. Insert the needle below the skin over the body of a rib. Turn the stopcock on toward the baby. Apply gentle suction once the needle is below the skin.

G. Direct the needle above the rib to avoid neurovascular structures that course on the inferior surface of the rib.

H. Advance the needle until the pleural cavity is entered as evidenced

by a sudden change in resistance. Suction is accompanied by evacuation of pleural air.

I. Aspirate pleural air and expel into the atmosphere by turning the
stopcock as needed until no more air comes or there is continuous
airflow.

   1. If there is no more airflow, examine the infant for normalization
of breath sounds and chest excursions, or use transillumination
to assess whether the pneumothorax was sufficiently evacuated
or the needle was displaced from the appropriate site and needs
to be repositioned. If sufficiently evacuated, withdraw the needle. Recheck later to assess for reaccumulation of the air leak.

   2. If there is continuous airflow, either place a chest tube, or have
someone continuously aspirate the syringe, or put the end of the
butterfly tubing under a water seal (at level below infant) until a
chest tube can be placed.

VII. Chest Tube Insertion

A. Indication—to drain air or fluids that accumulate in the pleural
space

   1. Tension pneumothorax

   2. Pneumothorax not under tension, but causing respiratory or circulatory compromise

   3. Bronchopleural fistula

   4. Pleural effusion

   5. Hemothorax

   6. Empyema

   7. Chylothorax

B. Procedural technique

   1. Needle aspiration of a pneumothorax should be performed
while preparations are made for chest tube insertion.

   2. Take care to provide adequate oxygen during the procedure. An
assistant should monitor the infant's status. Oximetry or transcutaneous monitoring is suggested.

   3. The site is prepped and draped in a sterile manner. If time permits, a sterile gown should be worn.

   4. The use of local anesthetic (1% lidocaine) and/or systemic
analgesic is mandatory; pain accentuates vagal tone. Raise a
small wheal over the incision site.

   5. For a pneumothorax, a small incision is made with a scalpel
blade in the third to fifth intercostal space in the anterior axillary or midclavicular line. Avoid the nipple, breast, and inferior
rib margin.

6. The proper site for insertion will allow the chest tube to be as efficient as possible.
   a. Anterior for the removal of gas
   b. Posterior for the removal of fluid
7. A 10–12 F tube is inserted into the pleural space. This may be accomplished either with a trocar or by blunt perforation with a hemostat. The hemostat technique is strongly recommended for infants < 1000 g. To avoid lacerating the intercostal vessels, stay close to the superior border of the rib.
   a. Technique without trocar
      i. Make an incision through the skin approximately the same size as the chest tube.
      ii. Use a curved mosquito hemostat to dissect the subcutaneous tissue, making a passageway only the size of the chest tube.
      iii. Close the hemostat and perforate the pleura, directing pressure above the rib (to avoid the vascular and neural structures).
      iv. Be careful not to damage the lung parenchyma by inserting the closed hemostat too aggressively.
      v. Listen for the release of air as the indication that the space has been entered.
      vi. Open the tips of the hemostat, and insert the chest tube between the ends.
      vii. Insert the tube until the side holes are within the pleural space.
      viii. After attaching to a drainage system, secure the chest tube either by suturing (using the "purse-string" technique) or tape.
   b. Technique using a trocar
      i. To assure ease of removal, pull out the trocar and lubricate the tube with normal saline, then replace the trocar.
      ii. Follow directions in a (i–v) above.
      iii. Using a straight hemostat, guide the chest tube (with trocar) into the pleural space.
      iv. To avoid entering too far, place a clamp about 1.5 cm from tip of tube and insert it up to this point; be sure the side holes are within the pleural space.
      v. Remove the trocar, advance the tube to a parasternal position, then secure it. The incision may be sealed with an iodine-containing ointment or a topical antibiotic.
8. The thoracostomy tube is placed to underwater seal and/or

continuous drainage at -10 to -20 cm H_2O. Observe the bubbling and/or fluctuation with respirations.
9. If transillumination was positive initially, transilluminate to assess resolution of the pneumothorax. Repeat the transillumination periodically while chest tube(s) is (are) in place.
10. Confirm position of the tube radiographically.
11. If pneumothorax recurs, consider:
   a. Tube occlusion
   b. Tube malposition or slippage
   c. Pleural loculation, necessitating additional drainage
   d. Reposition the patient.
12. Removal of the chest tube
   a. Clinically and radiologically determine when the chest tube is no longer needed.
   b. Place the chest tube to water seal without suction for 6–12 hours.
   c. Evaluate for the reaccumulation of the fluid or gas by physical examination, chest radiography, and/or transillumination.
   d. Cleanse the area with an antiseptic solution.
   e. Remove tape/sutures.
   f. Place petroleum jelly dressing over insertion site and/or cinch purse-string suture as the chest tube is being removed to prevent air reentry.
   g. Apply clean, dry dressing to the site.
13. Complications
   a. Infection
   b. Blood loss
   c. Equipment malfunction
   d. Chest tube displacement
   e. Trauma
      i. Lung perforation
      ii. Phrenic nerve injury
      iii. Thoracic duct disruption
      iv. Vascular injury

VIII. Defibrillation and Cardioversion
   A. Introduction
   1. The DC cardioverter and defibrillator delivers a single electric shock at a preset energy level (joule, watt-sec) when discharged.
   2. The cardioverter mode synchronizes the discharge with the R wave of the QRS after pressing discharge button.

3. The defibrillator mode delivers the discharge at the instant of button depression.
4. Since the need for emergent defibrillation or cardioversion occurs infrequently, it is important for each institution to be familiar with its own equipment.

B. Paddle positions
1. It is important to separate paddles to avoid "arcing" of discharge in air rather than through myocardium. Paddles should be well coated with conducting jelly to prevent skin burns.
2. Infants—anterior paddle: midline of chest, slightly to the left; posterior paddle: posterior chest wall.

C. Defibrillation
Used to reverse ventricular fibrillation. Energy dosage across external chest wall: patients < 50 kg: 2–6 watt-sec/kg body weight.

D. Cardioversion
1. Supraventricular tachyarrhythmia is the most common abnormal tachyarrhythmia in infants. Direct current cardioversion should not be used until other means such as manipulation of vagal tone, or pharmacologic remedies such as adenosine, digoxin, propranolol, verapamil, or transesophageal pacing have been tried. Very few infants should require direct current cardioversion. Because many infants tolerate tachyarrhythmias well, cardioversion seldom is required emergently, and consultation with a pediatric cardiologist can be obtained. Energy dose: 0.5–2.0 watt-sec/kg
2. Requires the synchronization mode. In general, ventricular tachycardia and atrial flutter require more low-energy discharge for cardioversion. Atrial fibrillation may require more energy. Be prepared to go to immediate defibrillation. Patients should be sedated properly. Levels to initiate cardioversion should be low and are increased stepwise until capture of the heart is achieved. Once capture, but not a stable sinus rhythm has been achieved, further escalation of energy is futile. Electrolyte status, acid-base balance, ventilation, and possibility of digoxin toxicity should be evaluated prior to cardioversion.

Suggested Reading

Chameides L, Brown GE, Raye JR, et al: Guidelines for defibrillation in infants and children. Report of the American Heart Association target activity group: Cardiopulmonary resuscitation in the young. Circulation 56:502A–503A, 1977.

Dick M, Scott WA, Serwer GS, et al: Acute termination of supraventricular tachyarrhythmias in children by transesophageal pacing. Am J Cardiol 61:925–927, 1988.

Donn SM, Faix RG: Delivery room resuscitation. In Spitzer AR (ed): Intensive Care of the Fetus and Neonate, 2nd ed. Philadelphia, Hanley & Belfus, 2003.

American Heart Association, Emergency Cardiac Care Committee and Subcommittees: Guidelines for cardiopulmonary resuscitation and emergency cardiac care. Part VI. Pediatric advanced life support. JAMA 268:2262–2275, 1992.

Faix RG: Neonatal resuscitation. In Donn SM, Faix RG (eds): Neonatal Emergencies. Mt. Kisco, NY, Futura Publishing, 1991, pp 15–30.

Fletcher MA, MacDonald MG, Avery GB: Atlas of Procedures in Neonatology, 2nd ed. Philadelphia, Lippincott Williams & Wilkins, 1993, pp 253–269, 309–333.

Jacobs MM, Phibbs RH: Prevention, recognition and treatment of perinatal asphyxia. Clin Perinatol 16:785–807, 1989.

Kattwinkel J (ed): Textbook of Neonatal Resuscitation. Dallas, American Heart Association–American Academy of Pediatrics, 2000.

Nelson NM: Respiration and circulation before birth. In Smith CA, Nelson NM (eds): The Physiology of the Newborn Infant. Springfield, IL, Charles C. Thomas, 1976, pp 15–17.

Niermeyer S: Evidence-based guidelines for neonatal resuscitation. Neoreviews 2:E38–E44, 2001.

Rosenfeld LE: The diagnosis and management of cardiac arrhythmias in the neonatal period. Semin Perinatol 17:135–148, 1993.

Wu T, Waldemar AC: Pulmonary physiology of neonatal resuscitation. Neoreviews 2:E45–E50, 2001.

Zak LK, Donn SM: Thoracic air leaks. In Donn SM, Faix RG (eds): Neonatal Emergencies. Mt. Kisco, NY, Futura Publishing, 1991, pp 311–326.

Chapter 8

Neonatal Airway

Paul I. Reynolds, M.D.

I. **Differences between Neonatal and Adult Airway**

A. Infants are obligate nasal breathers. Nasal obstruction for prolonged periods of time (e.g., choanal atresia) can be fatal. Newborns also have much more narrow nares compared to adults. This can make passage of nasotracheal tube more difficult.

B. Unlike an adult, the newborn's tongue rests at the roof of the mouth during quiet respiration. The tongue is also large in relation to the mouth, making both mask ventilation and oral intubation more difficult.

C. The newborn's head is large in relation to the body. During mask ventilation or laryngoscopy, the goal is to align the oral, tracheal, and pharyngeal axis (sniffing position). In an adult, this is accomplished by placing a pillow behind the head. However, in the newborn or infant, because of relatively large head, the pillow should be placed behind the shoulders (Figure 3).

D. The larynx is higher in the neck of an infant (C3–4) when compared to an adult (C4–5). This, in combination with a shorter neonatal neck can lead to more difficult laryngeal visualization during direct laryngoscopy.

E. The epiglottis in adults is broad, with its axis parallel to the trachea, whereas an infant's epiglottis is long, narrow, and floppy, angulated away from the axis of the trachea. During laryngoscopy, the tip of the newborn's epiglottis is lifted by the laryngoscope for glottic visualization.

F. Adults' vocal folds are perpendicular to the axis of the trachea, whereas the vocal folds of an infant have a lower anterior attachment to the glottis than posteriorly. This can sometimes lead to difficulty in passing the ETT through the newborn's glottis.

G. The narrowest portion of adult larynx is at the level of the vocal folds, while the narrowest portion of neonatal larynx is at the level of the cricoid ring, the only complete ring in the trachea. This has implications with ETT size. (See below.)

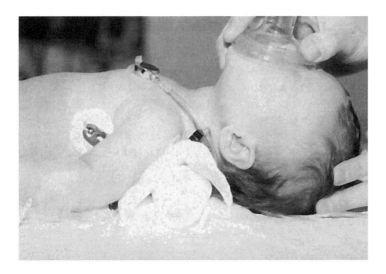

Figure 3. Optimal positioning of the infant for mask ventilation or laryngoscopy.

II. History

A. One should suspect a difficult airway in a neonate if any of the following history is elicited:

1. Noisy breathing or stridor
2. Variable airway related to position
3. Problems with feeding leading to severe coughing and cyanosis
4. Infant or child who has airway problems associated with either URI or feeding will probably have the same problems when given sedatives or narcotics.
5. History of difficult intubation in the past

III. Physical Examination

A. The following should be included in the routine neonatal exam prior to intubation:

1. Look at facies; abnormal facies or ears may be associated with difficult airway.
2. Check patency of nares bilaterally.
3. Mouth opening, size of tongue
4. Mandibular size and mobility
5. Check full flexion, extension, and rotation of neck.
6. Goal of laryngoscopy is to displace the soft tissues of the mandible (tongue) into an incomplete bony ring formed by the mentum, mandibular rami, and the hyoid bones. Any restriction

in this incomplete boney ring, or increase in the soft tissue mass to be displaced, can lead to a difficult airway.

IV. Airway Management

A. All formulas are rough guides only. *Choose the right size and length for each particular patient.*

    1. Diameter

        a. By convention, ETTs are sized by internal diameter.(However, it is the outside diameter that fits the patient!)

        b. Different brands of tubes have different outside diameters for same internal diameter. If there is no leak, then the pressure against the submucosa may exceed capillary perfusion pressure, leading to postextubation edema, croup, or subglottic stenosis.

B. Length

    1. If too short, accidental extubation may occur

    2. If too long, endobronchial, or carinal stimulation induces bronchospasm. Look to see length of tube needed to reach cords, then pass correct amount through (thick black line just visible) (Table 5).

C. Common problems with intubation

    1. Esophageal intubation—***look*** to see if ETT is going through cords.

        a. Breath sounds can be confusing, especially with bronchospasm.

        b. If in doubt, take it out.

    2. Endobronchial intubation—take care with length of ETT.

TABLE 5
Nasotracheal Tube Length for Preterm Infants

Weight (g)	Gestation (wks)	Length (cm)
750	25	7
1000	27	7.5
1500	31	8
1700	32	8.5
2000	34	9
2200	35	9.5
2500	36	10
2800	37	10.5
3200	39	11
3500	40	11

     a. If left uncorrected, complete lung collapse is possible.
3. Bronchospasm—especially when carina stimulated
     a. Check ETT length, consider sedation.
4. Postextubation stridor—excessive ETT diameter causes mucosal ischemia.
     a. A swelling at level of cricoid when tube removed
     b. Prevent by *always* checking for leak.
     c. Treat with nebulized epinephrine.
5. "Unable to pass nasal ETT"—remember, adenoids are large in children.
     a. It is *not* our job to remove them!
     b. Definite twist is needed to turn ETT bevel through cords or it will get caught on anterior wall of trachea.

Suggested Reading

Cote CJ, Todres ID: The pediatric airway. In Cote CJ, Ryan JF, Todres ID, Goudsouzian NG (eds): A Practice of Anesthesia for Infants and Children, 2nd ed. Philadelphia, W.B. Saunders, 1993, pp 55–85.

Donn SM, Kuhns LR: Mechanism of endotracheal tube movement with change of head position in the neonate. Pediatr Radiol 9:37–40, 1980.

Reynolds P: Pediatric difficult airways. In Norton ML (ed): Atlas of the Difficult Airway, 2nd ed. St. Louis, Mosby, 1996, pp 245–266.

Chapter 9

Vascular Catheters

Steven M. Donn, M.D.

I. Umbilical Artery Catheters (UAC)

A. Indications
1. $FiO_2 > 0.4$
2. Infant < 1000 g who needs central catheter
3. Need for continuous intravascular blood pressure monitoring

B. Removal
1. Assess the need for UAC when FiO_2 decreases to 0.35–0.4. Discuss with attending staff the advisability of removal.
2. When infant's condition is chronic and/or stable, periodically review the continued need for the UAC.
3. Any sign of vascular or embolic complication (e.g., leg blanching or cyanosis, loss of pulses, bloody stool) that is not relieved by 10 minutes of warming contralateral leg

C. Complications
1. Vasospasm
2. Embolization, thrombosis
3. Hypertension
4. Hemorrhage
5. NEC
6. Infection
7. Vascular damage
8. Paresis or paraplegia (spinal cord injury)

D. UAC insertion technique
1. This should be performed as a sterile, elective surgical procedure using sterile gown, mask, cap, and gloves.
2. Check tray for necessary equipment—e.g., scalpel, forceps, stopcocks, scissors, umbilical tape.
3. Assemble stopcocks, catheter, flush syringe. Use heparinized solution. Catheter size—3.5 for small premature infants (< 1500 g); 5.0 for larger infants.
4. Estimate length of insertion. High (T8–T10) is equal to shoulder–umbilicus length plus an additional length equal to the birthweight (to nearest 0.5 kg). Example: shoulder–umbilical length = 10 cm. Weight = 1.25 kg, insert catheter 10 cm + 1.5 cm = 11.5 cm. Alternative for high placement: one-third of

body length (vertex to heel) and 1 cm for umbilical stump. Low (L3–L4 interspace) is twice the distance from symphysis pubis to umbilicus plus height of umbilical stump.

5. Thoroughly prep with iodine solution; do *not* use alcohol. Drape abdomen.
6. Secure base of stump with umbilical tape for hemostasis.
7. Using straight hemostat, clamp cord 0.5–1.0 cm above skin. Cut cord just below hemostat (using it as a guide) in a caudal–to–cephalad direction. ***Do not*** "saw." Tighten tape if bleeding occurs.
8. Identify vessels.
9. Dilate artery *very* gently using Iris forceps *without* teeth.
10. Insert catheter and apply continuous but gentle pressure until catheter begins to advance; do ***not*** stop once catheter is advancing as this may induce vasospasm. If catheter will not advance to desired depth, do ***not*** force it, because vascular rupture and significant bleeding may ensue.
11. If unable to pass "curve" at 5 cm, retract stump in cephalad direction and attempt to advance gently.
12. Once positioned, check for blood return and pulsations.
13. Optional purse string suture may be placed around base *in jelly,* but it is not necessary to tie in catheter. Do ***not*** damage umbilical vein with this suture.
14. Tape bridge is constructed. Be sure all connections are tightly joined.
15. Double stopcock method is used.
16. If blanching or excessive mottling of extremity occurs, warm *contralateral* leg with soaks. If no improvement in 10 minutes, pull catheter. Circulation should be assessed by Doppler auscultation of pulse.
17. Position of catheter *must* be confirmed radiographically immediately after placement. *A misplaced arterial line can have life-threatening sequelae.*
18. Remove or loosen umbilical tape after correct position is ascertained to avoid cord necrosis.
19. If unable to catheterize artery easily, *call for attending or fellow help.*

E. UAC removal technique
  1. May be done by physician or certified nurse
  2. Discontinue heparin infusion.
  3. Catheter may be withdrawn to 50% of its inserted length acutely, then stop.

4. Reminder should be withdrawn at rate of 1 cm/min to allow vasospasm. If pulsations are present, further withdrawal should be delayed.
5. Post-withdrawal bleeding may be stopped by direct pressure, or if stump is present, application of umbilical tape may be necessary.
6. Stump should be dressed with triple dye or iodine ointment, but gauze and tape are to be avoided.

F. Miscellaneous
1. Vasoconstrictive agents (epinephrine, dobutamine, dopamine, and norepinephrine) are ***not*** to be infused via UAC.
2. If difficulty is encountered either in drawing blood or infusing fluids, consider removing UAC.
3. *Infraumbilical cutdown should not be attempted without direct supervision by an experienced individual.*
4. Infants of diabetic mothers or infants with erythroblastosis fetalis should have low UAC placement. Infants with suspected congenital heart disease should have high UAC placement.

II. Umbilical Vein Catheter (UVC)

A. Indications
1. Need for immediate vascular access (e.g., severe hypoglycemia, resuscitation)
2. Exchange transfusion
3. Central venous pressure monitoring

B. Removal
1. If placed for acute resuscitation, as soon as adequate alternate parenteral access is established
2. When exchange transfusion is finished, unless imminent need for repeat exchange is anticipated
3. May be pulled out directly; use pressure to control bleeding.
4. Consider triple dye or other antiseptic treatment of umbilical stump after catheter removal.

C. Technique
1. Sterile gown, gloves, mask, cap
2. Prep abdomen with iodine solution—do not use alcohol.
3. Fill catheter with flush—remove all air bubbles.
4. Insert to where there is a good blood return (usually 3–5 cm). With this position radiographic confirmation is unnecessary. For CVP monitoring, or for use as a central line, catheter should be advanced to the inferior vena cava at junction with right atrium (level approximated by measuring umbilical-

xiphoid distance). Position should be confirmed radiographically to assure placement above the diaphragm.

D. Complications

1. Hepatic necrosis if hypertonic solution is inadvertently run into portal system
2. Cerebral emboli via persistent ductus venous—foramen ovale shunt
3. NEC
4. Cirrhosis with varices
5. Embolization (air, clots)
6. Infection
7. Bleeding

Suggested Reading

Edwards MS, Fletcher MA: Exchange transfusions. In Fletcher MA, MacDonald MG, Avery GB (eds): Atlas of Procedures in Neonatology. Philadelphia, J.B. Lippincott, 1983, pp 363–372.

Feick HJ, Donn SM: Vascular access. In Donn SM, Faix RG (eds): Neonatal Emergencies. Mt. Kisco, NY, Futura Publishing, 1991, pp 31–49.

Workman EL, Donn SM: Intravascular catheters. In Donn SM, Fisher CW (eds): Risk Management Techniques in Perinatal and Neonatal Practice. Armonk, NY, Futura Publishing, 1996, pp 531–549.

Chapter 10

Percutaneous Intravenous Central Catheters

Elizabeth L. Workman, R.N.

I. Introduction

Percutaneous intravenous central catheter (PICC) placement is an elective procedure, but should be anticipated before appropriate IV access sites are exhausted.

II. Indications

A. Central access for TPN administration

B. Long-term IV antibiotic/antifungal administration access

C. Stable access for vasoactive drug administration

III. Techniques

A. Assemble the necessary equipment

    1. Catheter placement tray and appropriate size catheter

        a. L-cath system—polyurethane 24- and 28-gauge single lumen, 20-gauge double lumen

        b. Gesco system—silastic 23-gauge single lumen

    2. Add extra sterile towel drapes, if desired.

    3. Add sterile T-connector.

    4. Heparinized normal saline flush (1.0 units/mL)

    5. Tape measure

    6. Povidone–iodine solution

B. The procedure should be performed using sterile gown, mask, cap, and gloves.

C. Select vein for cannulation. Commonly used veins:

    1. Posterior auricular

    2. External jugular

    3. Antecubital

    4. Saphenous

D. Measure the approximate distance from the insertion site to the right atrium. The catheter should be inserted slightly less than this length to avoid tip placement in the right atrium.

E. Prepare the area thoroughly using povidone-iodine solution. Drape with sterile towels.

F. Before handling catheter, remove any powder from sterile gloves using damp sterile towel. This is necessary to prevent possible entry of powder into the vascular space with subsequent phlebitis.

G. Prepare for venipuncture by cleaning off solution with alcohol, and if desired, use tourniquet to locate vein.

H. Puncture vein with introducer needle and thread catheter the premeasured distance using forceps. Never pull the catheter back into the introducer needle, as the catheter may be inadvertently sheared by the needle tip. If using an upper extremity, keep the head turned to face the cannulated side to temporarily "occlude" the jugular vein allowing the catheter to pass into the SVC.

I. If using the L-cath catheter, remove the stylet, attached a heparinized flush to hub, and gently aspirate before flushing. Blood return must be achieved before flushing. If no blood return, pull back catheter until blood returns on aspiration. The catheter may be advanced without the wire stylet in place with small amounts of flush. Always reconfirm blood return when final position is achieved.

J. Secure catheter with adhesive strips.

K. Confirm placement with radiograph—reposition as necessary. Tip should not terminate in right atrium, contralateral subclavian, or internal jugular veins.

L. Loop excess length of catheter, secure with adhesive strips entire site with transparent sterile dressing.

M. Add prefilled T-connector to hub. Secure to extremity in a manner that will protect the hub–catheter connection from breaking.

N. Blood should not be withdrawn or transfused through the catheter because of the high risk of clotting.

O. Solutions running through the PICC should be heparinized (1.0 unit/mL).

IV. Removal

A. The catheter should be removed as soon as it is no longer required or if complications occur.

B. It may be pulled out directly using local pressure to assure hemostasis.

V. Complications

A. Phlebitis

B. Excessive clotting

C. Breakage at level of hub

D. Edema of cannulated arm (usually resolves with elevation and loosening of occlusive tape)

Suggested Reading

Feick HJ, Donn SM: Vascular access and blood Sampling. In Donn SM, Faix RG (eds): Neonatal Emergencies. Mt. Kisco, NY, Futura Publishing, 1990, p 29.

Workman EL, Donn SM: Intravascular catheters. In Donn SM, Fisher CW (eds): Risk Management Techniques in Perinatal and Neonatal Practice. Armonk, NY, Futura Publishing, 1996, pp 531–549.

Chapter 11

Transillumination

Steven M. Donn, M.D.

I. Definition

A. Use of a high-intensity light to help define normal or abnormal structure or function. Diffusion of light is a function of density and composition of tissue.

B. Chun gun — incandescent light source with published standard lucencies for skull

C. Mini light — fiber-optic light source

D. RMI, Omni light, Welch-Allyn — bright fiber-optic light sources

II. Conditions Generally Associated with Positive Transillumination (Wide Rim of Lucency or Abnormal Dark Area)

A. Skull
1. Hydrocephaly
2. Hydranencephaly
3. Anencephaly
4. Porencephaly
5. Encephalocele

B. Chest
1. Pneumothorax
2. Pneumomediastinum
3. Pneumopericardium

C. Abdomen
1. Distended bladder
2. Pneumoperitoneum (falciform ligament may be seen)
3. Distended bowel loops
4. Hydrocele
5. Cystic kidneys
6. Hydronephrosis
7. Scrotal masses (cystic)

III. Miscellaneous

A. Transillumination may be helpful in distinguishing cystic from solid masses (e.g., cystic hygroma).

B. Transillumination is useful for finding veins and arteries for sampling or catheter insertion.

C. The procedure is more effective in a darkened room after time for visual adaptation to darkness.

D. If a high-intensity light source is used, care must be taken to avoid burning the patient. To do this, a red filter is inserted in front of the light source and contact with the skin is limited.

E. Cellophane should be used to cover the light head to prevent cross-contamination between babies.

Suggested Reading

Donn SM, Kuhns LR: Pediatric Transillumination. Chicago, Year Book, 1983.

Chapter 12

Shock and Hypotension

Charles R. Neal, Jr., M.D., Ph.D., and Steven M. Donn, M.D.

I. **Definition**

Shock comprises a syndrome in which there is insufficient organ perfusion to meet tissue metabolic needs.

A. Hypovolemia, secondary to acute blood loss, is the most common cause of shock in the newborn.

B. Consequences of severe shock include alterations in cellular metabolism, energy production, and waste product excretion, which result in cellular dysfunction and eventually cell death.

C. All organ systems are potentially affected.

II. **Determinants of Organ Perfusion**

A. The *delivery of oxygen to the periphery* depends on the functional capability of three organ systems.

1. Circulatory system
   a. Adequate cardiac output
   b. Integrity of local vascular beds and appropriate regulation of regional blood flows

2. Hematologic system
   a. Ability to carry oxygen
   b. Ability to deliver oxygen to tissues

3. Pulmonary system
   a. Reoxygenation of venous blood
   b. Elimination of carbon dioxide

B. *Cardiac output* is defined as stroke volume × heart rate.

1. Stroke volume is the amount of blood ejected by the right or left ventricle during systole; it is influenced by several factors.
   a. Preload is the amount of blood filling the ventricles during diastole.
      i. Determines ventricular end-diastolic fiber length
      ii. Starling's law states that an increase in preload results in an increase in the force of myocardial contraction and a greater stroke volume, up to the threshold of overload.
      iii. When the optimal level of preload is exceeded, myocardial fibers overstretch, resulting in incomplete emptying and decreased stroke volume.

       b. Afterload is the resistance against which the ventricle ejects during systole.

       c. Myocardial contractility

    2. Cardiac output in the newborn is much more dependent on *heart rate* than stroke volume, and acute bradycardia may be poorly tolerated.

C. *Blood flow to organs and tissues* is dependent on central and local vasoregulation.

D. *Oxygen-carrying capacity* is the maximal amount of oxygen that can be taken up by hemoglobin in blood.

    1. 1 g of hemoglobin binds 1.36 mL of dissolved O_2.

    2. Fetal hemoglobin has a greater affinity for oxygen than adult hemoglobin.

       a. This is reflected by a shift in the O_2 dissociation curve to the left, resulting in decreased oxygen delivery to tissues.

       b. Hypothermia, hypocarbia, and alkalosis also shift the curve to the left, with consequent decreased unloading of oxygen to the tissues.

E. *Adequate lung ventilation and perfusion* are critical factors in maintaining oxygen delivery.

F. *Oxygen extraction by tissues* may be inappropriate, despite adequate oxygen delivery in such clinical settings as sepsis and prolonged antecedent hypoxic-ischemic injury.

III. Etiologies of Shock

A. Functional hypovolemia

    1. Acute blood loss (external or internal)

    2. Vasodilating drugs such as tolazoline and phentolamine

    3. Analgesic agents such as morphine more commonly cause hypotension when used in conjunction with sedatives.

    4. Postoperative third spacing

    5. Fluid and electrolyte losses, such as those observed during high output renal failure and overaggressive diuretic use

B. Distributive hypovolemia

    1. Observed secondary to aberrant regulation of local and regional vascular beds

    2. Often seen during fulminant sepsis

C. Cardiogenic shock

    1. Congenital heart disease, such as hypoplastic left heart syndrome

    2. Arrhythmias, particularly supraventricular tachycardia

    3. Myocardial dysfunction following asphyxia and with metabolic derangements

4. Impaired venous return
   a. Seen with pericardial tamponade, pneumothorax, and abdominal distention
   b. High intrathoracic pressure from positive pressure ventilation
5. Drug toxicity

IV. Stages of Shock

A. During *compensated shock* perfusion is maintained to vital organs by intrinsic compensatory mechanisms, including the release of endogenous catecholamines and aldosterone, and peripheral vasoconstriction.
   1. Clinically, the infant will display mottling, with a mildly elevated heart rate.
   2. The newborn will also have body positioning and limited spontaneous activity to reduce insensible water loss and minimize oxygen consumption.

B. During *uncompensated shock* intrinsic mechanisms fail to meet the metabolic demands of the organs and tissues.
   1. Toxic materials are released from damaged tissues inducing cellular injury and vasomotor dysfunction.
   2. Stagnant microcirculation, hypoxemia, and acidosis have a further impact on the coagulation system leading to DIC and local thrombosis.
   3. The clinical appearance in the uncompensated newborn is much more indicative of a shock state.
      a. Extreme hypoperfusion with pallor and/or cyanosis
      b. Persistent hypotension
      c. Poor capillary refill
      d. Lethargy or obtundation

C. In *irreversible shock,* vital organs, such as the brain and heart sustain terminal injury, and death is inevitable.

V. Evaluation and Management of Shock

A. It is important to identify high-risk situations in anticipation of potential problems.
   1. Umbilical cord accidents, such as prolapse or avulsion
   2. Placental abnormalities, including placenta previa and abruptio placentae
   3. Severe hemolysis, as is observed with maternal blood group incompatibility
   4. Severe hemorrhage from any source
      a. In utero fetomaternal hemorrhage or twin-to-twin transfusion syndrome

   b. Postnatally, an intraventricular or other intracranial hemor-
      rhage, or subgaleal bleed
5. Severe systemic asphyxia
6. Infection/sepsis
7. Congenital heart disease, such as a severe arrhythmia, or structural abnormality
8. Maternal factors that may affect the newborn infant, including
   infection, hypotension, or recent exposure to anesthetic agents
   or vasoactive medications
9. Severe intrathoracic air leak

B. It is important to be proficient in recognizing a clinical picture indicative of shock or impending shock.
1. Lethargy
2. Pallor, observed in presence of acute hemorrhage
3. Prolonged capillary refill (> 3 seconds).
4. Weak peripheral pulses
5. Apnea, abnormal respiratory effort, or cyanosis
6. Anuria or oliguria (< 0.5 mL/kg/hr)
7. Metabolic and/or respiratory acidosis
8. Heart rate abnormalities, especially bradycardia
9. Hypotension (Figure 4)—may be a late sign
   a. It should be noted that several different reference ranges
      based on "healthy" infants have been published, with vari-
      able assessments of the influence of birthweight and/or ges-
      tational age.
   b. Initial clinical studies in small groups correlated blood pres-
      sure with death and adverse neurologic outcome in prema-
      ture infants.
      i. Some authors advocated that such sequelae in very low
         birthweight (VLBW) infants were observed almost ex-
         clusively with persistent mean arterial pressure < 30
         mmHg (see Miall-Allen, 1987).
      ii. Preliminary studies such as these brought about a con-
          servative approach to management of what may be nor-
          mal blood pressure in VLBW infants.
   c. More recent clinical studies in VLBW infants have provided
      remarkably consistent normative data for blood pressure.
      i. These studies have demonstrated that *many preterm in-
         fants maintain their normal blood pressure in the 20–25
         mmHg range.*
      ii. These studies indicate that *careful consideration should
          be made before initiating volume and/or pressor therapy*

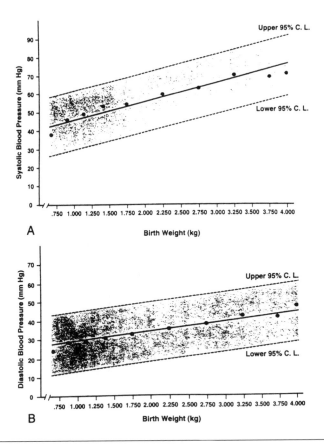

Figure 4. Linear regression of mean systolic blood pressure (*A*) and diastolic blood pressure (*B*) on birthweight in 329 infants admitted to NICU on day 1 of life. (From Zubrow AB, Hulman S, Kushner H, et al: Determinants of blood pressure in infants admitted to neonatal intensive care units: A prospective study. J Perinatol 15:470–479,1995, with permission of Nature Publishing Group.)

to raise blood pressure in the otherwise well-appearing VLBW infant (for review, see Engle, 2001).

C. Initial supportive measures (Figure 5)
  1. Maintain adequate gas exchange.
    a. Provide supplemental oxygen.
    b. Provide mechanical ventilation with minimal pressures needed for adequate oxygenation and ventilation.
    c. Treat any air leak or abdominal distention.
  2. Establish adequate cardiac output as necessary.
    a. Cardiac massage

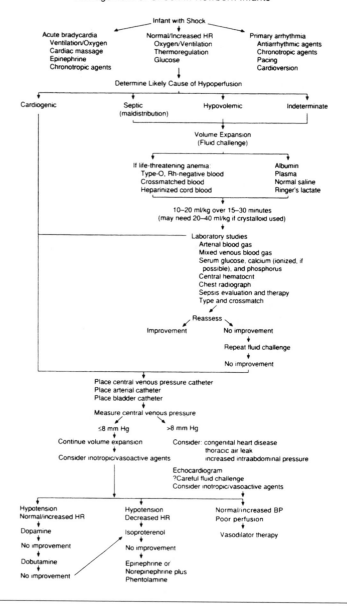

Figure 5. Management of shock in newborn infants. (Modified from Faix RG, Pryce CJE: Shock and hypotension. In Donn SM, Faix RG (eds): Neonatal Emergencies. Mount Kisco, NY, Futura Publishing, 1991, p 383, with permission.)

      b. Epinephrine
      c. Treatment of primary arrhythmias (*see* Chapter 60)
      d. Chronotropic and/or inotropic agents as necessary to provide adequate tissue perfusion and urine output
   3. Maintain adequate core temperature.
   4. Avoid hypoglycemia, hypocalcemia, and hypophosphatemia.
D. Determine likely cause of hypoperfusion.
   1. Hypovolemic shock in the newborn most commonly results from *acute* blood loss.
      a. Cord accidents, significant maternal hemorrhage, and severe fetomaternal hemorrhage.
      b. Suggestive physical findings include pallor and prolonged capillary refill.
   2. Distributive (septic) shock may be suspected in cases of maternal fever, fetal tachycardia, or evidence of chorioamnionitis.
      a. These findings are all high-risk factors for sepsis.
      b. Suggestive physical findings include temperature instability, tachycardia, and prolonged capillary refill.
   3. Cardiogenic shock may accompany severe intrapartum asphyxia, congenital heart disease, or dysrhythmias.
      a. Suggestive physical findings in this group include cardiomegaly and hepatomegaly.
      b. Abnormal precordial activity is observed on examination.
E. Volume expansion (Table 6) can be first line of therapy if the newborn is not in cardiogenic shock.
   1. The most important therapeutic goal is to restore the circulating blood volume and provide adequate organ perfusion to minimize ischemic sequelae.
   2. The choice of fluid depends upon the etiologic process as well as availability.
      a. If there was acute hemorrhage, compatible whole blood or reconstituted packed red blood cells may be used.
      b. Crystalloid may be used as a first choice for volume expansion in the hypovolemic infant.
         i. Colloid theoretically remains in the intravascular space, facilitating increased preload and stroke volume, but clinical studies comparing 5% albumin to normal saline for hypovolemic hypotension have demonstrated no difference between solutions.
        ii. Crystalloid is preferred in cases where capillary leak is present, as colloid may diffuse across injured endothelial barriers, increasing extravascular oncotic forces and persistent edema.

TABLE 6
Recommended Solutions for the Treatment of Hypovolemic Shock

Solution	Amount	Comments
Whole blood or reconstituted packed red blood	10–20 mL/kg	Expansion of intravascular volume; increases oxygen carrying capacity
Uncrossmatched type O, Rh-negative blood	10–20 mL/kg	As above; indicated in unusual circumstances; subsequent typing may be difficult
Heparinized cord blood	10–20 mL/kg	Readily available; risk of anticoagulation of infant and subsequent hemorrhage; less favorable oxygen delivery characteristics than products containing adult hemoglobin
Colloid (5% albumin, plasmanate)	10–20 mL/kg	Expansion of intravascular volume; maintains colloid osmotic pressure; may minimize pulmonary and peripheral edema
Fresh frozen plasma	10–20 mL/kg	Expansion of intravascular volume; principle indication is replacement of clotting factors; expensive even compared to other colloids
Normal saline, lactated Ringer's or isotonic glucose	20–40 mL/kg	Eventual expansion of extracellular volume (interstitial > intravascular space); readily available; large amounts may cause hemodilution and decrease oxygen-carrying capacity

Adapted from Faix RG, Pryce CJE: Shock and hypotension. In Donn SM, Faix RG (eds): Neonatal Emergencies. Mt. Kisco, NY, Futura Publishing, 1991, p 379, with permission.

   iii. Colloid is unnecessary and expensive.
  3. Remember that rapid volume expansion can increase the risk of intracranial hemorrhage.
 F. Laboratory studies
  1. Arterial blood gases to assess lung function
  2. Mixed venous blood gases to assess tissue metabolism and oxygen extraction
   a. Only possible if there is vascular access to the right atrium, right ventricle or pulmonary artery
   b. Appropriate and accessible on patients receiving ECMO
  3. Follow glucose, calcium, and phosphorus levels, especially after fluid adjustments are made.
  4. The central hematocrit may be misleading in assessing blood volume immediately after acute blood loss, so serial hematocrits should be obtained.
  5. Blood cultures and other indicated tests for infection

6. Type and crossmatch for possible transfusion
7. Chest radiograph if respiratory distress or cyanosis
8. Consider an echocardiogram.

G. Assess the response to volume expansion, and correct sources of shock/hypotension.

1. If metabolic acidosis is present, if there is poor urine output, or if other evidence of hypoperfusion persists, repeat careful volume expansion, unless cardiogenic shock is present.
2. Consider buffer therapy only if the acidosis (metabolic and/or respiratory) is severe.
   a. Sodium bicarbonate ($NaHCO_3$), 4.2%, 1–2 mEq/kg.
      i. Do not administer in presence of hypercarbia.
      ii. Do not administer in presence of hypernatremia or hypercapnia.
   b. THAM (0.3 M) may be used in the presence of either hypercarbia or hypernatremia.
      i. Administer 4–8 mL/kg.
      ii. Be aware of potential for hypoglycemia and decreased respiratory effort.
   c. Aspirate pneumothorax, if present.
   d. Consider initiation of antibiotic therapy.
   e. Correct metabolic disturbances.

H. Monitoring (if not already in place)

1. Place an arterial catheter to monitor serial arterial blood gases and blood pressure.
   a. If arterial access cannot be obtained, cuff pressures may be used but must be verified from multiple sites.
   b. It has been suggested that the cuff pressure at which pulse oximetric waveform disappears more accurately reflects systolic pressure than pressure obtained using an oscillometric technique.
2. Place a bladder catheter to monitor urine output as an indicator of renal perfusion.
3. Central venous pressure (CVP) can be measured if a central venous catheter has been placed.
   a. This provides and excellent index of right ventricular preload and intravascular volume.
      i. Be certain catheter tip is at junction of vena cava and right atrium and that transducer is at same level as tip.
      ii. Briefly discontinue positive airway pressure for more accurate measurement of CVP.
      iii. Abdominal distention and intrathoracic air leak should

be alleviated, since they may cause alterations in CVP independent of preload and intravascular volume.

    iv. If the absolute CVP is $\leq$ 8 mmHg ($\leq$ 10 cm H_2O) and the infant still manifests signs of hypoperfusion and no evidence of cardiogenic shock, gradually administer volume expanders until CVP reaches this threshold.

  b. One can also measure mixed venous blood gases if cardiogenic shock is suspected.

  c. If one is unable to fulfill above caveats for measuring CVP, or if uncertain if they have been addressed, an alternative approach is to use CVP as a trend indicator to reflect changes in the elastic state of the vascular bed.

    i. As intravascular volume increases, the elastic limits of the bed are reached and CVP rises much more rapidly.

    ii. If a fluid challenge causes CVP to rise $\geq$ 4 mmHg ($\geq$ 5 cm H_2O), then the infant is fluid replete and further volume expansion is unlikely to help.

    iii. In this setting or that of cardiogenic shock, vasoactive therapy is the logical next step.

I. Vasoactive drug therapy (Table 7)

TABLE 7
Inotropic and Vasoactive Agents Commonly Used in Shock

Drug	Dose (μg/kg/min)	Hemodynamic Effect	Comment
Dopamine	1–5 5–15 15–20	Splanchnic, renal and cerebral vasodilatation. Increased contractility and heart rate Peripheral and renal vasoconstriction	Stimulates beta receptors by direct and indirect mechanisms; may cause tachy-dysrhythmias; may increase pulmonary vascular resistance; doses > 20 μg/kg/min occasionally required for normotension, but may result in severe tissue ischemia
Dobutamine	1–20	Increased contractility	Minimal effect on heart rate; no selective renal effect

(Table continues on following page)

TABLE 7
Inotropic and Vasoactive Agents Commonly
Used in Shock (*Continued*)

Drug	Dose (μg/kg/min)	Hemodynamic Effect	Comment
Isoproterenol	0.05–0.5	Increased contractility and heart rate; peripheral vasodilatation	May cause tachy-dysrhythmias; increases myocardial oxygen consumption
Epinephrine	0.05–1.0	Increased contractility and heart rate; marked peripheral, renal and mesenteric vasoconstriction	May cause tachy-dysrhythmias; increases myocardial oxygen consumption; increases glucose levels; increased risk of severe tissue ischemia
Norepinephrine	0.05–1.0	Marked peripheral vasoconstriction	May cause severe tissue and organ ischemia; use in combination with vasodilator
Nitroprusside	0.05–8.0	Peripheral arterial and venous vasodilatation	Risk of cyanide toxicity
Phentolamine	1–20	Alpha antagonist: arterial and venous dilation	May produce reflex tachycardia; expensive
Hydralazine	0.1–0.5 (mg/kg) q3–6h	Peripheral arterial vasodilatation	May produce reflex tachycardia

Adapted from Faix RG, Pryce CJE: Shock and hypotension. In Donn SM, Faix RG (eds): Neonatal Emergencies. Mt. Kisco, NY, Futura Publishing, 1991, p 381, with permission.

1. Choice of agent depends on hemodynamic needs.
   a. Chronotrope
   b. Inotrope
   c. Vasoconstriction/afterload augmentation
   d. Vasodilatation/afterload reduction
2. Most of these agents do not act purely on one of the above categories, but have variable (often dose-dependent) effects on each of them.
   a. An awareness of the differential effects of each agent is important in selection of vasoactive drugs.
   b. Unfortunately, data are limited in human newborns, and

judgments must often be based on extrapolation from adult or animal data.

3. At least one randomized, blinded trial found dopamine to be superior to dobutamine for treatment of hypotension in preterm infants with RDS who had already undergone volume expansion, although dobutamine was still frequently effective.

J. Glucocorticoid therapy

1. Often effective in circumstances where volume expansion and vasoactive agents have been unsuccessful.

2. Hydrocortisone may be used at 3–5 times maintenance dose.

   a. Maintenance hydrocortisone dosing is 15 mg/m^2/day, *divided* every 6 hr

   b. A simplified method for calculating body surface area (BSA) in m^2 is below:

   $$\frac{[\text{weight (kg)} \times 4] + 7}{\text{weight (kg)} + 90}$$

   i. Example: if the weight is 950 g, BSA would be:

   $$\frac{[\text{weight (kg)} \times 4] + 7}{\text{weight (kg)} + 90}$$

   $$\frac{[0.95 \times 4] + 7}{0.95 + 90}$$

   $$\frac{[3.8] + 7}{90.95}$$

   $$0.12 \text{ M}^2$$

   ii. For a hydrocortisone *burst* (*3X maintenance*), the dose would be $(45) \times (0.12) = 5.4$ mg/day.

   iii. Divided by 4 for dosing every 6 hr = 1.35 mg/dose.

   iv. *Maintenance* dose would be 1.8 mg/day = 0.45 mg/dose.

3. Dexamethasone is dosed in the range of 0.25–0.50 mg/kg per dose, given every 12 hr.

4. *Dosing guidelines* (hydrocortisone burst):

   a. Once a decision has been made to provide steroid therapy, and a cortisol level has been obtained, administer a hydrocortisone burst as *3X* maintenance dosing (i.e., 45 mg/m^2/d) divided every 6 hr for 8 doses (48 hours).

   b. Dexamethasone can be administered in place of hydrocortisone. May be given in doses of 0.25–0.5 mg/kg every 12 hr, over 24 hours (2 doses) or 48 hours (4 doses).

Suggested Reading

Engle WD: Blood pressure in the very low birth weight neonate. Early Hum Dev 62:97–130, 2001.

Faix RG, Pryce CJ: Shock and hypotension. In Donn SM, Faix RG (eds): Neonatal Emergencies. Mt. Kisco, NY, Futura Publishing, 1991, pp 371–386.

Fauser A, Pohlandt F, Bartmann P, Gortner L: Rapid increase of blood pressure in extremely low birth weight infants after a single dose of dexamethasone. Eur J Pediatr 152:354–356, 1993.

Hegyi T, Carbone MT, Anwar M, et al: Blood pressure ranges in premature infants. I. The first hours of life. J Pediatr 124:627–633, 1994.

Helbock HJ, Insoft RM, Conte FA: Glucocorticoid-responsive hypotension in extremely low birth weight newborns. Pediatrics 92:715–717, 1993.

Keeley SR, Bohn DJ: The use of inotropic and afterload-reducing agents in neonates. Clin Perinatol 15:467–489, 1988.

Kitterman JA, Bland RD: Shock in the newborn infant. In Thibeault DW, Gregory GA (eds): Neonatal Pulmonary Care, 2nd ed. Norwalk, CT, Appleton-Century-Crofts, 1986, p 413.

Klarr JM, Faix RG, Pryce CJE, Bhatt-Mehta V: Randomized, blind trial of dopamine versus dobutamine for treatment of hypotension in preterm infants with respiratory distress syndrome. J Pediatr 125:117–122, 1994.

Langbaum J, Eyal FG: A practical and reliable method of measuring blood pressure in the neonate by pulse oximetry. J Pediatr 125:591, 1994.

Miall-Allen VM, deVries L, Whitelaw AG: Mean arterial blood pressure and neonatal cerebral lesions. Arch Dis Child 62:1068–1069, 1987.

Skinner JR, Milligan DWA, Hunter S, Hey EN: Central venous pressure in the ventilated neonate. Arch Dis Child 67:374–377, 1992.

Seri I, Evans J: Controversies in the diagnosis and management of hypotension in the newborn infant. Curr Opin Pediatr 13:116–123, 2001.

Versmold HT, Kitterman J, Phibbs R, et al: Aortic blood pressure during the first twelve hours of life in infants with birth weight 610 to 4,220 grams. Pediatrics 67:607–613, 1981.

Zubrow AB, Hulman S, Kushner H, Falkner B: Determinants of blood pressure in infants admitted to neonatal intensive care units: A prospective multicenter study. Philadelphia Neonatal Blood Pressure Study Group. J Perinatol 15:470–479, 1995.

Chapter 13

Dopamine and Dobutamine Drips

Steven M. Donn, M.D., and Charles R. Neal, Jr., M.D., Ph.D.

I. **To formulate a solution where 1.0 mL/hr delivers 5 μg/kg/min:**
   A. Multiply patient weight (in kg) × 30
   B. Take this number (in milligrams) of dopamine or dobutamine and add to 100 mL fluid
   Example: Baby weighs 2.1 kg
   2.1 × 30 mg = 63 mg
   63 mg Dopamine in 100 mL D_5W yields:

   1.0 mL/hr =   5 μg/kg/min
   2.0 mL/hr = 10 μg/kg/min
   3.0 mL/hr = 15 μg/kg/min
   4.0 mL/hr = 20 μg/kg/min

II. **To determine the amount of pressor in milligrams to be added to 100 mL of IV fluid, if fluid administration must be limited:**

$$6 \times \text{weight (kg)} \times \frac{\text{desired pressor infusion rate (μg/kg/min)}}{\text{desired fluid infusion rate(mL/hr)}}$$

Example: Baby weighs 2.1 kg
A. For 1.0 mL/hr to deliver 5.0 μg/kg/min:

$$6 \times 2.1 \times \frac{5.0}{1.0} = 63$$

thus, add 63 mg to 100 mL fluid.
B. For 1.0 mL/hr to deliver 10.0 μg/kg/min:

$$6 \times 2.1 \times \frac{10.0}{1.0} = 126$$

thus, add 126 mg to 100 mL fluid.

Section III. PHARMACOLOGY

Chapter 14

Neonatal Pharmacokinetics

Varsha Bhatt-Mehta, Pharm.D., and Steven M. Donn, M.D.

I. Introduction

A. This chapter is intended as a neonatal drug dosing and monitoring guide, derived from current literature.

B. It includes pharmacologic agents used in the NICU that have a narrow therapeutic index.

C. Entries include recommendations for:

1. Loading dose
2. Maintenance dose and interval
3. Desired serum/plasma concentration
4. Timing of sampling
5. Examples of available products

D. Although each drug included is optimally dosed with the aid of drug concentration measurements, not all patients require this. Need for serum concentrations is assessed according to:

1. Drug used
2. Length of therapy
3. Condition of patient

II. Choosing Optimal Sampling Times

A. Monitoring of serum/plasma drug concentration presumes a definite relationship between drug concentration and subtherapeutic, therapeutic, and toxic responses.

B. Relationship is best examined when:

1. Samples are drawn during postdistribution phase for loading and maintenance doses.
2. Samples are drawn at steady state for maintenance doses.

C. Time to reach steady state concentration

1. Depends on half-life (time required for concentration of the drug to decline by 50%)
2. Substantial variation in the half-life of various drugs in the neonatal population occurs because of immature hepatic and renal function.
3. In general, a duration of 3–5 half-lives predicts attainment of steady state.
4. Because maintenance doses are given approximately every one

   half-life, steady state can be assumed following at least three
   maintenance doses for most drugs.
   5. Obtaining steady state concentrations is important, since it is
      the most reliable indicator of tissue drug concentration.
D. Loading dose
   1. Administered to rapidly achieve and sustain steady state con-
      centration while maintenance doses are accumulating
   2. It is not necessary to wait until accumulation is complete to
      sample.
   3. Sampling interval may be selected during postdistribution
      phase following the loading dose.
E. Reloading
   1. If it becomes necessary to provide loading doses to existing
      maintenance dose regimens (e.g., following exchange transfu-
      sion; appearance of additional seizures, requiring higher anti-
      convulsant blood concentration), drug concentrations should be
      monitored at least once in the postdistribution phase of the
      loading dose.
   2. Continue maintenance dose schedule as before, though dose
      may need to be increased, depending on serum/plasma concen-
      trations achieved by reloading. If so, check concentration fol-
      lowing third new maintenance dose.
F. Sampling after dosage adjustment
   1. Usual adjustments include:
      a. Increase or decrease of dose
      b. Increase or decrease of interval
   2. Determination of concentration may be necessary if therapy
      continues beyond 72 hours after changes are made.
   3. Sampling should be done at new steady state level, following
      three doses.
G. Sampling following change in drug dosage form
   1. When form of drug changes (e.g., injectable to oral), drug con-
      centration should be determined at least once following attain-
      ment of steady state on the new regimen to ensure therapeutic
      levels.
   2. Thereafter, it may not be necessary to reevaluate unless there is a
      change in hepatic or renal function or the patient's clinical status.

III. Anticonvulsants
   A. Phenobarbital
      1. Loading dose
         a. IVH prophylaxis

Loading dose: 20 mg/kg
Begin first maintenance dose 12 hours after the loading dose.
   b. Seizure control
      Loading dose:* 20–30 mg/kg
      Spontaneously breathing infants: give by slow IV push over
      15–30 minutes. May give in 2–3 divided doses 20 minutes
      apart (use an infusion pump to control drug delivery). In-
      fants on assisted ventilation: may receive up to 30 mg/kg by
      slow IV push over 15–20 minutes.
      *1 mg/kg will, on average, increase level by 1 μg/mL.
2. Initial maintenance dose

Age Group/Disease State	Dose*	Interval[†]
Newborns (all groups)	5 mg/kg	q24h[‡]

*Some premature infants may require a decrease in dose from
   drug accumulation. Maintenance dose may be decreased to 3
   mg/kg/d if necessary (check serum concentration 1 week after
   starting phenobarbital treatment).
[†]Serum concentrations will not fluctuate much with once daily
   dosing since phenobarbital has a long half-life (> 100 hr) in
   newborns.
[‡]For IVH prophylaxis, 5 mg/kg every 24 hrs $\times$ 4 doses.
3. Desired serum concentrations (Table 8)

TABLE 8
Desired Phenobarbital Levels

Patient/Disease	Peak	Trough
Sedation	—	10–20 μg/mL
Seizure control	—	20–50 μg/mL (or higher)

4. Timing of blood samples for drug levels (Table 9)

TABLE 9
Timing of Blood Sampling

Route of Administration	Peak	Trough*
IV	—	Immediately prior to next dose
PO	—	Immediately prior to next dose

*Trough levels generally provide the most useful information for dosage adjustment.

5. Examples:
   Phenobarbital injection 10 mg/mL, 30 mg/mL, 60 mg/mL
   Phenobarbital oral solution 4 mg/mL

B. Phenytoin
    1. Loading dose for status epilepticus or seizures unresponsive to phenobarbital alone: 15–20 mg/kg. Should be administered by slow IV push in incremental doses of 5–10 mg/kg up to a maximum of 20 mg/kg.
        a. 1 mg/kg will increase the serum phenytoin level by approximately 1.2 μg/mL.

        b. *Rate of administration should not exceed 0.5 mg/kg/min.*
    2. Initial *intravenous* maintenance dose (Table 10)

TABLE 10
Intravenous Phenytoin Maintenance Dose*

Age Group/Disease State	Dose	Interval
Newborns < 10 days old	5 mg/kg/d	Divided q12h
Newborns > 10 days old	8–10 mg/kg/d	Divided q6h

*Oral phenytoin administration is not advisable in newborns because absorption is poor. However, if it does become necessary to use the oral route of administration, the maintenance dose should be 5–10 mg/kg/d divided every 4–6 hours. Maintenance therapy should be guided by closely monitored drug levels.

    3. Desired serum concentrations (Table 11)

TABLE 11
Desired Phenytoin Levels

Patient/Disease State	Peak	Trough
Newborns and infants	—	10–20 μg/mL total phenytoin
Altered phenytoin protein binding (newborns, hyperbilirubinemia, renal failure)	—	1–2 μg/mL free phenytoin*

*Free phenytoin plasma concentration measurement is desirable for certain patient populations.

    4. Timing of blood samples for drug levels (Table 12)

TABLE 12
Timing of Blood Sampling

Route of Administration	Peak	Trough*
IV	1 hr after injection	Immediately prior to next dose
PO	Midway in dosing interval	Immediately prior to next dose

*Trough levels provide the most useful information for dosage adjustments.

5. Examples:

Phenytoin sodium injection   50 mg/mL*

*For infusion dilute only in 0.9% sodium chloride for injection. The concentration should not exceed 1 mg/mL. Diluted injection should be used up (including infusion time) within 1 hour of diluting.

Phenytoin oral suspension   25 mg/mL

IV. Digoxin

1. Loading (total digitalizing) dose for CHF (Table 13)

TABLE 13
Digoxin Loading Dose*

Patient Population	PO	IM/IV (80% of PO Dose)
Premature infants	20 μg/kg	15 μg/kg
Term infants (up to 2 mos of age)	30–40 μg/kg	25–30 μg/kg
2–24 mos	40 μg/kg	30 μg/kg

*Total loading dose is administered in three unequally divided doses (½, ¼, ¼) given at 12 hr intervals in patients < 2 months of age and 8-hr intervals in patients > 2 months of age.

2. Maintenance dose (Table 14)

TABLE 14
Digoxin Maintenance Dose*

Age Group/Disease State	Dose/Route/Interval[†]	IM/IV
Premature infants	5 μg/kg/d	4 μg/kg/d
Term infants (up to 2 mos of age)	8–10 μg/kg/d	6–8 μg/kg/d
2–24 mos	10–12 μg/kg/d	8–10 μg/kg/d

*Titrate dose to obtain therapeutic effect as well as serum concentrations in a safe range.
[†]q24h for newborns and divided q12h in infants and children. Begin first maintenance dose 12 hours after last loading dose.

3. Desired serum concentrations (Table 15)

TABLE 15
Desired Digoxin Level

Patient/Disease State	Peak	Trough
All age groups*	—	1–2 ng/mL

*Children may tolerate higher serum concentrations, but there is no evidence that these higher levels offer any additional therapeutic benefit. Possible presence of digoxin-like immunoreactive substances which cross-react with the immunoassay for digoxin must be kept in mind when interpreting digoxin serum concentrations.

4. Timing of blood samples from drug levels (Table 16)

TABLE 16
Digoxin Blood Sampling

Route of Administration	Peak	Trough*
IM, IV, PO	6–8 hr after a dose	Immediately prior to next dose

*Trough concentrations provide the most useful information. Peak concentrations may be useful following a loading dose.

5. Examples:
   Digoxin injection   250 μg/mL
   Digoxin oral solution   50 μg/mL

V.   Methylxanthines
   A. Caffeine
   1. Loading dose: 10 mg/kg caffeine base*
      *On average, for every 1 mg/kg loading dose administered,
       serum concentrations will increase by 1.0 μg/mL.
   2. Initial maintenance dose (Table 17)

TABLE 17
Caffeine Maintenance Dose*

Age Group/Disease State	Dose	Interval
Newborns (for neonatal apnea)	2.5 mg/kg IV/PO	q24h

*Serum concentrations will not fluctuate excessively with once daily dosing because of the long half-life (60–100 hr) in newborns. Adult half-lives (nearly 4 hr) are achieved by approximately 3–5 mos of age.

3. Desired serum concentrations (Table 18)

TABLE 18
Desired Caffeine Levels

Condition	Peak	Trough
Neonatal apnea	—	5–20 μg/mL

4. Timing of blood samples for drug levels (Table 19)

TABLE 19
Caffeine Blood Sampling

Route of Administration	Peak	Trough
PO, IV	—	Immediately prior to next dose

5. Examples:
   a. Caffeine citrate (Cafcit) injection 20 mg/mL (equivalent to caffeine 10 mg/mL caffeine base)
   b. Caffeine citrate (Cafcit) oral solution 20 mg/mL (equivalent to 10 mg/mL caffeine base)
B. Theophylline/aminophylline
   1. Loading dose*
      a. 6 mg/kg of theophylline (7 mg/kg aminophylline) if no theophylline has been administered in the last 24 hr
      b. 2.5 mg/kg of theophylline (3 mg/kg aminophylline) can be given in emergencies if a *stat level cannot be obtained.*
      *On average, for every 1 mg/kg theophylline loading dose administered, serum theophylline concentrations will increase by 2 μg/mL.
   2. Initial maintenance dose (Table 20)

TABLE 20
Theophylline Maintenance Dose

Age Group	Theophylline Dose
27–30 wks GA	mg/kg/d = 5.81 − (0.02 × PNA in wks)
31–34 wks GA	mg/kg/d = 4.82 − (0.28 × PNA in wks)
35–40 wks GA	10 mg/kg/d ÷ q8h
Infants 6–52 wks	18–20 mg/kg/d ÷ q6–8h

GA = gestational age; PNA = postnatal age.

      a. The recommended doses are for achieving serum theophylline concentrations of 8 μg/mL in afebrile patients with normal renal, hepatic, and cardiac function not receiving drugs such as erythromycin or cimetidine (which may impair theophylline metabolism). Many patients will achieve concentrations less than 8–10 μg/mL and will require serum concentrations measurements to guide dosage increases.
      b. Asphyxia decreases theophylline clearance by approximately 50% and the dose may need to be decreased.
   3. Desired serum concentrations (Table 21)

TABLE 21
Desired Theophylline Levels

Patient/Disease State	Peak	Trough
Neonatal apnea	—	6–12 μg/mL

4. Timing of blood samples for drug levels (Table 22)

TABLE 22
Theophylline Blood Sampling

Route of Administration	Peak	Trough
Intermittent injection*	30 min after a 20 min infusion	Immediately prior to next dose
PO rapid release* (aquaphylline elixir)	2 hr after a dose	Immediately prior to next dose
PR	2 hr after a dose	Immediately prior to dose

*Obtain at steady state (3–5 × expected half-life). For newborns half-life ranges from 13–29 hr.

5. Examples:

Aminophylline injection	2 mg/mL theophylline
Aminophylline injection	25 mg/mL theophylline
Theophylline oral solution	5.3 mg/mL theophylline (nonalcoholic)

Suggested Reading

Aranda JV, Cook CE, Gorman W, et al: Pharmacokinetic profile of caffeine in the premature newborn infant with apnea. J Pediatr 94:663–668, 1979.

Benitz WE, Tatro DS: The Pediatric Drug Handbook. Chicago, Year Book, 1983.

Bhatt-Mehta V, Donn SM, Schork MA, et al: Prospective evaluation of two dosing equations for theophylline in premature infants. Pharmacotherapy 16:769–776, 1996.

Donn SM, Grasela TH, Goldstein GW: Safety of a higher loading dose of phenobarbital in the term newborn. Pediatrics 75:1061–1064, 1985.

Gal P, Boer HR, Tobach J, et al: Effect of asphyxia on theophylline clearance in newborns. South Med J 75:836–838, 1982.

Grasela TH, Donn SM: Neonatal population pharmacokinetics of phenobarbital derived from routine clinical data. Dev Pharmacol Ther 8:374–383, 1985.

Painter MJ, Pippenger C, MacDonald H, Pitlick W: Phenobarbital and diphenylhydantoin levels in neonates with seizures. J Pediatr 92:315–319, 1978.

Roberts RJ: Drug Therapy in Infants. Philadelphia, W.B. Saunders, 1984.

Chapter 15

Neonatal Drug Formulary

Varsha Bhatt-Mehta, Pharm.D., and Steven M. Donn, M.D.

I.   The following formulary (Table 23) lists pharmacologic agents commonly used in the newborn, with the exception of antimicrobials, which are listed separately in the following chapter.

II.   Drug names are listed generically. Occasionally, trade names are listed in parentheses.

III.   "Category or Class" of drug refers to its most common application.

IV.   "Indication for Use" refers to clinically recognized situations.

V.   "Dose and Interval" refers primarily to individual doses except where specified.

VI.   "Route" refers to the route of administration. If there are different doses for different routes, it will be specified.

VII.   "Side Effects" are those most commonly encountered.

VIII.   "Comments" are included to make specific recommendations or emphasize specific warnings.

TABLE 23
Neonatal Drug Formulary

Drug Generic (Trade)	Category or Class	Indications for Use	Dose and Interval	Route	Side Effects	Comments
Acetazolamide (Diamox)	Carbonic anhydrase inhibitor	Posthemorrhagic hydrocephalus	5–25 mg/kg/d div. q8h (max 100 mg/kg/d)	PO/IV	Metabolic acidosis	Start with lower dose. Titrate to effect, follow pH.
Acetylcysteine (Mucomyst)	Mucolytic	Tenacious pulmonary secretions	1–2 mL of 20% nebulized q6–8h	ET	Possible tachycardia	Aerosolized bronchodilator given 10–15 min prior to acetylcysteine improves efficacy
Adenosine (Adenocard)	Antiarrhythmic	SVT	Initial 0.05 mg/kg. Increase by 0.05 mg/kg every 2 min to a max of 0.25 mg/kg or termination of SVT	IV	Bradycardia, dyspnea	Dilute 1:10 in normal saline. Give by rapid IV push.
Albuterol (Proventil)	Bronchodilator	Bronchospasm	2 puffs q4–6h by MDI	ET	Tachycardia, hypertension, CNS stimulation	Document response (e.g., pulmonary mechanics testing) before continuing treatment.
Aminophylline	Methylxanthine	Apnea	Load: 6 mg/kg	IV	Tachycardia, vomiting, CNS stimulation Periextubation support	Follow serum levels closely. Withhold if HR >160 Maintenance: see Theophylline

Drug	Class	Indication	Dose	Route	Adverse effects	Comments
Arginine-HCl	Amino acid	Urea cycle defects	750 mg/kg/d	IV	Metabolic acidosis, hyperglycemia, hyperkalemia	Becomes essential amino acid if urea cycle not intact.
Atropine	Vagolytic	Bradycardia, excessive secretions	0.01–0.02 mg/kg/dose. Repeat if necessary.	IV	Thickened secretions	Unproven efficacy in resuscitation. Avoid during high-frequency ventilation.
Caffeine (base)	Methylxanthine	Apnea	Load: 10 mg/kg Maintenance: 2.5 mg/kg/d q24h	PO	Tachycardia, GI irritation, CNS stimulation	Double dose for caffeine citrate (1 mg base = 2 mg citrate)
Calcium chloride 10%	Electrolyte	Hypocalcemia	Symptomatic: 35–70 mg/kg/dose (0.35–0.7 mL/kg/dose) Maintenance: 75–300 mg/kg/d (0.75–3.0 mL/kg/d) div. q6–8h	IV	Bradycardia (give slowly), damage to subcutaneous tissues if infiltrated	Incompatible with sodium bicarbonate. Titrate to effect, follow serum level, especially ionized.
Calcium gluconate 10%	Electrolyte	Hypocalcemia	Symptomatic: 100–200 mg/kg/dose (1–2 mL/kg/dose) Maintenance: 200–800 mg/kg/d (2–8 mL/kg/d) div. q6–8h	IV/PO	Bradycardia (give slowly), damage to subcutaneous tissues if infiltrated	Incompatible with sodium bicarbonate. Titrate to effect, follow serum level, especially ionized.

(Table continues on following page)

TABLE 23
Neonatal Drug Formulary (*Continued*)

Drug Generic (Trade)	Category or Class	Indications for Use	Dose and Interval	Route	Side Effects	Comments
Captopril (Capoten)	ACE inhibitor	Hypertension	0.01–0.05 mg/kg/dose q8–24h Max: 0.5 mg/kg/dose q6–24h	PO	Cardiopulmonary compromise, hyperkalemia, agranulocytosis	Decrease dose in renal failure.
Carnitine (Carnitor)	Fatty acid transport	Carnitine deficiency	IV: 50 mg/kg load followed by 50 mg/kg/d infusion or 50 mg/kg/d div. q4–6h. Max: 300 mg/kg/d PO: 50–100 mg/kg/d div. q8–12h	IV/PO	Nausea, vomiting, abdominal cramps	Use when primary or secondary carnitine deficiency is suspected or confirmed. Plasma-free carnitine level 35–60 μmol/L.
Chloralhydrate	Hypnotic-sedative	Sedation	50 mg/kg/dose	PO/PR	Respiratory, CNS depression	Onset of action 30–60 min; habituating; pulmonary excretion; some paradoxical responders.
Chlorothiazide (Diuril)	Diuretic	Oliguria, edema (esp. pulmonary), hypertension	PO 20–50 mg/kg/d div. q12h IV 10–20 mg/kg/d div. q12h	IV/PO	Hypokalemia, alkalosis, hyperglycemia	Follow electrolytes, pH, glucose. Pharmacy will make suspension.

Drug	Classification	Indication	Dose	Route	Adverse Effects	Comments
Colloid (albumin, Plasmanate, FFP)	Blood volume expander	Hypovolemia, hypotension	10–20 mL/kg/dose	IV	Hypervolemia, pulmonary edema, congestive heart failure	Can be 5% Albumin, Plasmanate, or fresh frozen plasma; very expensive. Not proven to be better than crystalloid.
Crystalloid (0.9 NS, D5LR, LR)	Blood volume expander	Hypovolemia, hypotension	10–20 mL/kg/dose	IV	Hypervolemia, pulmonary edema, congestive heart failure	Can be normal saline, lactated Ringer's solution, or electrolyte and dextrose solution. Inexpensive
Dexamethasone (Decadron)	Corticosteroid	Adrenal insufficiency (physiologic replacement) Bronchopulmonary dysplasia Subglottic edema	0.03–0.15 mg/kg/d div. q12h 0.3–0.5 mg/kg/d div. q12h 1–2 mg/kg/dose q12h × 4–6 doses	IV/PO	Hyperglycemia, hypertension, hypertrophic cardiomyopathy, immunosuppression, adrenal suppression (with chronic use)	Wide dosage range. Treated infants may need stress doses for surgery, during infection, etc. Higher doses (up to 2 mg/kg/d) have been used for severe respiratory failure.
Dextrose 25% 10%	Carbohydrate	Hypoglycemia	2–4 mL/kg (25%) 2 mL/kg, then 5–8 mg/kg/min (10%)	IV IV	Hyperglycemia, rebound hypoglycemia	Do not exceed 12.5% concentration in peripheral IV. "Mini-bolus" (10%) may be better tolerated.

(Table continues on following page)

TABLE 23
Neonatal Drug Formulary (Continued)

Drug Generic (Trade)	Category or Class	Indications for Use	Dose and Interval	Route	Side Effects	Comments
Diazepam (Valium)	Benzodiazepine	Sedation	IV: 0.1 mg/kg q6–8h prn	IV	Potentiation with other depressants Use with caution in hyperbilirubinemia (displaces from albumin)	Use to stop status epilepticus. Do not give in or with dextrose (precipitates).
			PO: 0.1–0.8 mg/ kg/d div. q8h	PO		
		Seizures	IV: 0.1–0.2 mg/ kg prn (max. total 2 mg)	IV		
			PR: 0.5 mg/kg prn	PR		
Diazoxide (Hyperstat)	Antihypertensive	Severe hypertension	1–5 mg/kg/dose	IV	Hyperglycemia, salt and water retention, fever, blood dyscrasias	Give by rapid IV push; may repeat q5–15 min until BP controlled, then q2–4h. Used when other measures have failed.
		Refractory hypoglycemia	10–25 mg/kg/d div. q8h	PO		
Digoxin (Lanoxin, Digibind)	Cardiotonic	Congestive heart failure Tachyarrhythmias	*Load:* Preterm: PO: 20 µg/kg IV/IM: 15 µg/kg Term: PO: 30 µg/kg IV/IM: 22.5 µg/kg *Maintenance:* Preterm: PO: 5 µg/kg/day	PO IV/IM PO IV/IM PO	Arrhythmias	Be sure serum potassium is normal. Always double check dosage calculations. Monitor serum concentrations.

Drug	Classification	Indication	Dose	Route	Adverse effects	Comments
Dobutamine (Dobutrex)	Pressor	Hypotension	IV/IM: 4 μg/kg/day; Term: PO: 8–10 μg/kg/day; IV/IM: 6–8 μg/kg/day q12h; 2.5–20 μg/kg/min	IV/IM; PO; IV/IM; IV	Tachycardia, hypertension	Titrate to effect; higher doses may cause renal vasoconstriction. Do not infuse via arterial line.
Dopamine (Intropin)	Pressor	Hypotension	2.5–20 μg/kg/min	IV	Tachycardia, hypertension	Titrate to effect; higher doses may cause renal vasoconstriction. Do not infuse via arterial line.
Dornase alpha (Pulmozyme)	Proteolytic enzyme	Tenacious pulmonary secretions	2–5 mg q12–24h, using manufacturer recommended nebulizer	ET	Pharyngitis, laryngitis, chest pain, conjunctivitis	Unproven efficacy for meconium aspiration, pneumonia, chronic lung disease
Edrophonium (Tensilon)	Antiarrhythmic, anticholinesterase	SVT; Myasthenia gravis	0.05–0.1 mg/kg; 0.05–0.15 mg/kg	IV; SC/IM	Bradycardia, arrhythmias	May block bradycardia by pretreatment with atropine.
Enalapril (Vasotec)	ACE inhibitor	Hypertension	IV: 0.005–0.01 mg/kg/dose q8–24h depending on blood pressure.	IV	Cardiopulmonary compromise, hyperkalemia, agranulocytosis	Do not use in patients with renal artery stenosis. Decrease dose in renal failure.

(Table continues on following page)

TABLE 23
Neonatal Drug Formulary (Continued)

Drug Generic (Trade)	Category or Class	Indications for Use	Dose and Interval	Route	Side Effects	Comments
Enalaprilat			PO: 0.1 mg/kg/d q24h. Increase dose depending on blood pressure.	PO		
Epinephrine 1:10,000	Pressor	Bradycardia Hypotension	0.01 mg/kg (0.1 mL/kg) dose 0.05–1.0 μg/kg/min	IV IV	Tachyarrhythmias, increased myocardial oxygen consumption, hyperglycemia, risk of severe tissue ischemia	Never give via arterial line.
Epinephrine 1:1000	Pressor	Bradycardia	0.1 mg/kg (0.1 mL/kg)	ET		
Erythropoietin (Epogen, Procrit)	RBC stimulant	Anemia, chronic renal disease	50–100 units/kg 3 times per week	IV/SC	Many side effects which may be related to underlying diseases, but include hypertension, seizures, thrombotic events, and allergic reactions	Delayed onset of action (weeks), thus not suitable for acute anemia. Suspended in human serum albumin. Multidose vial contains benzyl alcohol.
Fentanyl (Sublimaze)	Sedative-analgesic	Pain, need for sedation	Bolus: 1–5 μg/kg q1–2h Infusion: 0.5–5 μg/kg/h	IV	CNS depression, chest wall rigidity	Can be reversed by naloxone. Tolerance develops quickly.

Drug	Class	Indication	Dose	Route	Side Effects	Comments
Flumazenil (Romazicon)	Benzodiazepine antagonist	Benzodiazepine-induced depression	8–15 µg/kg (max single dose 200 µg) repeated every minute to a maximum total accumulative dose of 0.5 mg/kg or 1000 µg, whichever is lower	IV	Seizures, agitation and CNS stimulation, flushing, vomiting	Avoid in patients receiving benzodiazepines for seizure control.
Furosemide (Lasix)	Diuretic	Oliguria, edema (especially pulmonary), hypertension, posthemorrhagic hydrocephalus	1–5 mg/kg	IV/PO	Hyponatremia, volume depletion, hypokalemia, hypercalciuria, nephrolithiasis and nephrocalcinosis (long-term use), hypochloremic alkalosis, ototoxicity.	Not recommended for long-term use. Follow electrolytes, calcium, pH. Oral dose is twice the parenteral.
Glucagon	Glucoregulatory hormone	Hypoglycemia	0.025–0.1 mg/kg/ dose q20–30 min prn	IM	Hyperglycemia	Do not use in SGA baby
Heparin	Anticoagulant	Anticoagulation, thrombolysis	Load: 50–100 units/kg Maintenance: 20–40 units/kg/h	IV	Bleeding	Titrate to effect. Use activated clotting time (ACT) of 180–200 sec as goal. Central catheters generally have heparin added to prevent clotting. Use 1.0 unit/mL if ≥1000 g.

(Table continues on following page)

TABLE 23
Neonatal Drug Formulary (Continued)

Drug Generic (Trade)	Category or Class	Indications for Use	Dose and Interval	Route	Side Effects	Comments
						Use 0.5 unit/mL if <1000 g. Avoid over-heparinization as infusion rates increase.
Hyaluronidase (Wydase)	Proteolytic enzyme	IV infiltration	Reconstitute and dilute to 15 units per mL. Then use 1.0 mL as 5 separate 0.2 mL injections around infiltration site.	SC	Tachycardia, hypotension	Administer promptly by injecting into site of infiltration.
Hydralazine (Apresoline)	Antihypertensive (vasodilator)	Hypertension	0.1–0.5 mg/kg/dose and 4–6h prn 0.5–1.0 mg/kg/d div. q6h	IV PO	Tachycardia, salt and water retention, blood dyscrasias	Use in situations where hypertension is not life-threatening and not related to fluid overload or unresponsive to diuretics alone.
Hydrocortisone (Cortef)	Corticosteroid	Physiologic replacement Adrenal insufficiency Stress dose	25 mg/m²/24h, div. q8h 5–150 mg/kg/24h div. q6–8h 50–100 mg/m²/	PO/IV IV/PO	Hyperglycemia, hypertension, growth retardation, immunosuppression, osteoporosis, electrolyte imbalances,	With adrenal suppression, anticipate need for stress doses (e.g., infection, surgery, etc.)

Drug	Classification	Indication	Dose	Route	Adverse effects	Comments
			24h. Start 48h before surgery, continue until 48h after surgery. Wean by 50% each day to physiologic dose of 25 mg/m²/day, then discontinue.	IV/IM	cataracts, myopathy, adrenal suppression	
		Hypoglycemia	5 mg/kg/d div. q12h			
Indomethacin (Indocin)	Prostaglandin synthesis inhibitor	Patent ductus arteriosus	<10 days: 0.2 mg/kg × 3 doses q12h >10 days: initial 0.2 mg/kg followed by 0.25 mg/kg q12h × 2 doses	IV	Oliguria, decreased mesenteric flow, platelet dysfunction, rapid infusions associated with decreased cerebral blood flow, hyponatremia	Do not give if platelets < 50,000/mm³ or if active bleeding, or if serum creatinine >1.8 mg/dL. Avoid arterial administration.
Insulin, regular	Glucoregulatory hormone	Hyperglycemia, hyperkalemia	0.01–0.1 unit/kg/h or 0.1–0.2 units/kg/dose q6–12h	IV SC	Hypoglycemia, hypokalemia	Follow serum glucose and potassium levels frequently during administration
Ipratropium (Atrovent)	Anticholinergic bronchodilator	Bronchospasm	2 puffs by MDI q6h	ET	Tachycardia, GI upset, CNS stimulation	Document effect before continuing treatment (e.g., pulmonary mechanics)

(Table continues on following page)

TABLE 23
Neonatal Drug Formulary (Continued)

Drug Generic (Trade)	Category or Class	Indications for Use	Dose and Interval	Route	Side Effects	Comments
Isoproterenol (Isuprel)	Pressor	Hypotension	0.1–0.4 μg/ kg/min	IV	Arrhythmias, hypoglycemia	Correct acidosis first. Titrate dose to heart rate. Follow serum glucose.
Kayexalate	Ion exchange resin	Hyperkalemia	0.5–1.0 g/kg, q2–6h prn	PR/PO	Electrolyte disturbances, alkalosis	Delayed onset; use other acute treatment concomitantly.
Lidocaine	Antiarrhythmic	Ventricular arrhythmias	Load: 0.5–1.0 mg/kg repeat q10 min to max of 5 mg/ kg Infusion: 0.01– 0.05 mg/kg/ min	IV	CNS toxicity (depression followed by stimulation), bradycardia, hypotension, heart block, cardiovascular collapse	Use preservative-free preparation *without* epinephrine. Toxic level > 6 μg/mL.
Lidocaine/ prilocaine cream (EMLA Cream)	Local anesthetic	Pain	2–5 g/site for painful procedures 60 min prior to procedure	Topical	None known	Eutectic mixture of local anesthetics, prilocaine and lidocaine. Apply 30–60 min prior to procedure.
Lorazepam (Ativan)	Benzodiazepine	Sedation	0.05–0.1 mg/ kg/dose q6– 8h prn	IV	CNS depression, "gasping syndrome"	Half-life 10–20 hours. Can be antagonized by flumazenil.
		Anticonvulsant	0.1 mg/kg/dose. Repeat as necessary.			

Drug	Category	Indication	Dose	Route	Toxicity	Comments
Magnesium sulfate 50%	Mineral	Hypomagnesemia	25–50 mg/kg/dose. Repeat q8–12h as necessary. (0.125–0.25 mL of a 20% solution.)	IV/IM	Neuromuscular and respiratory depression	Renal excretion. Must dilute to 20% concentration prior to administration.
Mannitol	Osmotic diuretic	Oliguria, edema	0.5–2.0 g/kg	IV	Hyperosmolality	Check serum osmolality first. Usually given as 12.5–20% solution.
Methadone	Synthetic narcotic	Neonatal abstinence syndrome	0.2–0.4 mg/kg/d div. q12h	PO/IV	Dependency, CNS and respiratory depression, bradycardia, hypotension	Difficult to titrate; long acting
		Narcotic dependence	0.2 mg/kg/d div. q12h, if previous narcotic history unknown. If converting from another narcotic, calculate equivalent dose and administer as q12h dose.	PO/IV IV/PO		
Metoclopramide (Reglan)	GI prokinetic agent	Feeding intolerance	0.1 mg/kg/dose q6–8h	PO/IV	Dystonic reactions, extrapyramidal signs, irritability, vomiting	Use to facilitate gastric emptying. Efficacy in reflux is unproven.

(Table continues on following page)

TABLE 23
Neonatal Drug Formulary (Continued)

Drug Generic (Trade)	Category or Class	Indications for Use	Dose and Interval	Route	Side Effects	Comments
Midazolam (Versed)	Benzodiazepine	Sedation	Load: 0.1 mg/kg Maintenance: 0.02–0.25 mg/kg/h	IV	Hypotension, possible lowering of seizure threshold	Provides no analgesia. Wean slowly (10–15%/day) for all infusions lasting longer than 3 days.
Morphine sulfate	Narcotic analgesic	Pain and/or sedation	0.05–0.1 mg/kg/dose q2–6h or 0.01–0.04 mg/kg/h	IV/SC	CNS and respiratory depression, hypotension, urinary retention, decreased GI motility	Habituating; can be reversed by naloxone. Wean all continuous infusions lasting more than 5–7 days (wean rate 10–20%/day).
Naloxone neonatal (Narcan)	Narcotic antagonist	Narcotic-induced depression	0.01 mg–0.1 mg/kg/dose. Repeat every 2–3 min as needed.	IV/IM/SC/ET		Avoid use in infant of substance-abusing mother. May need to repeat dose several times. For ET dilute to 1–2 mL with NS.
Nifedipine (Adalat)	Calcium channel blocker	Hypertension	0.05–0.5 mg/kg/dose q1–2h	PO	Fluid retention, calcium and magnesium disturbances	Not for use in life-threatening hypertension.

Drug	Category	Indication	Dose	Route	Toxicity	Comments
Nitroprusside, (Nitropress)	Sodium vasodilator	Hypertension	0.05–5.0 μg/kg/min	IV	Thiocyanate toxicity, hypotension, metabolic acidosis	Use in life-threatening hypertension. Use cautiously with renal disease.
Norepinephrine (Levophed)	Pressor	Hypotension	0.01–2.0 μg/kg/min	IV	Tachycardia, hypertension	Avoid arterial infusion. Monitor BP.
Pancuronium (Pavulon)	Skeletal muscle relaxant	Need for paralysis	0.05–0.1 mg/kg/dose q1–2h prn	IV	Edema, skeletal muscle atrophy (long-term use)	Do not use without concomitant sedation. Also decreases oxygen consumption.
Paraldehyde	Anticonvulsant	Seizures	0.15 mL/kg q4–6h	IM/PR	CNS depression	Excreted by lung, assure adequate ventilation. Administer by glass syringe (it melts plastic). Can be given IV if diluted to 5% solution.
Pentobarbital (Nembutal)	Barbiturate	Intractable seizures Pentobarbital coma	4 mg/kg (may repeat once) *Load:* 10–15 mg/kg slow IV over 1–2 h *Maintenance:* 1–3 mg/kg/h (maintain burst-suppression on EEG)	IV IV	CNS and cardiorespiratory depression	Used only in refractory status epilepticus. Infant must be receiving assisted ventilation and blood pressure monitoring before receiving dose.

(Table continues on following page)

TABLE 23
Neonatal Drug Formulary (Continued)

Drug Generic (Trade)	Category or Class	Indications for Use	Dose and Interval	Route	Side Effects	Comments
Phenobarbital	Barbiturate	Seizures, sedation, IV prophylaxis	*Load:* Term: 30 mg/kg Preterm: 20 mg/kg *Maintenance:* 3–5 mg/kg/d	IV IV/IM/PO	Sedation, respiratory depression (at extremely high serum levels)	Very long (100–200 h) half-life; may be given once daily. Maintenance dosage may be useful in treating cholestatic jaundice. Therapeutic level 20–50 μg/mL
Phentolamine (Regitine)	Alpha-adrenergic blocker (vasodilator)	Infiltration of IV solutions containing vasoconstrictive agents	0.1 mg/kg (2–5 mg max total dose). Prepare solution by diluting 2.5–5 mg in 10 mL NS.	SC	Hypotension possible with extremely large doses	Inject solution SC into affected area. Monitor blood pressure. Use within 12 hours of infiltration.
Phenytoin (Dilantin)	Anticonvulsant	Seizures	Load: 15–20 mg/kg Maintenance: 5 mg/kg/d div. q12h	IV	CNS depression, arrhythmias, hyperglycemia	Very poor oral absorption in newborn. If IM, drug crystallizes in muscle. Therapeutic level 10–20 μg/mL.
Potassium chloride	Electrolyte	Hypokalemia	2–3 mEq/kg/day	IV/PO	Arrhythmias, thrombophlebitis (IV) GI irritation (PO)	Maximum concentration 40 mEq/L. Give slowly IV.

Drug	Classification	Indication	Route	Dose	Side effects	Comments
Propranolol (Inderal)	Beta-adrenergic blocker	Tachyarrhythmias, hypertension, hypertrophic cardiomyopathy, neonatal thyrotoxicosis	IV PO	0.01 mg/kg/dose q6h, increase prn to max of 0.15 mg/kg/dose q6h 0.25 mg/kg/dose q6h, increase prn to max of 5 mg/kg/d	Bradycardia, hypotension, bronchospasm, hypoglycemia	Wide individual variability in response. Monitor HR, BP, serum glucose.
Prostaglandin E_1 (Prostin)	Vasodilator	Need to maintain patency of ductus arteriosus	IV	0.05–0.1 µg/kg/min (max 0.4 µg/kg/min)	Apnea, fever, seizures, flushing, bradycardia, hypotension	Can be given via UAC.
Ranitidine (Zantac)	H_2 receptor antagonist	Decrease gastric acidity	PO IV	2 mg/kg/dose q8h 2 mg/kg/d div. q8h or 2 mg/kg/d as continuous infusion.	None known	Consider use concomitantly with corticosteroid therapy. Adjust dose in renal failure.
Sodium bicarbonate (4.2%, 0.5 mEq/mL)	Buffer	Metabolic acidosis	IV	1–3 mEq/kg/dose. Repeat as needed.	Hypernatremia, hyperosmolality, hypercarbia	Assure adequate ventilation, do not give if $PaCO_2$ >50 torr ("closed flask phenomenon"). Do not give faster than 1 mL/min. Follow serum sodium.

(Table continues on following page)

TABLE 23
Neonatal Drug Formulary (Continued)

Drug Generic (Trade)	Category or Class	Indications for Use	Dose and Interval	Route	Side Effects	Comments
Spironolactone (Aldactone)	Diuretic	Oliguria, edema (especially pulmonary), hypertension	1.7–4.0 mg/kg/d div. q12h	PO	Rash, GI upset, lethargy	Potassium-sparing. Delayed onset of action. Pharmacy makes suspension.
Surfactants (Exosurf, Survanta)	Exogenous pulmonary surfactants	Respiratory distress syndrome	Exosurf: 5 mL/kg/dose, 2–3 doses Survanta: 4 mL/kg/dose, 2–3 doses	ET	Hypoxia, desaturation if given too rapidly. Increased incidence of IVH, pulmonary hemorrhage, and PDA have been reported with various preparations.	Watch for sudden compliance changes after administration and respond appropriately.
Susphrine	Adrenergic	Hypoglycemia	0.005 mL/kg/dose q8h	IM/SC	Tachycardia, hypertension, local reaction	Works best in term AGA or LGA infant
THAM (Tris, Tromethamine) 0.3M	Buffer	Metabolic/mixed acidosis	4–8 mL/kg/dose	IV	Hyperkalemia, hypoglycemia, respiratory depression	Give slowly
Theophylline	Methylxanthine	Apnea, periextubation support	Load: 5 mg/kg Maintenance: 27–30 wks GA: mg/kg/d theophylline = 5.81 – (0.02 × PNA in wks)	PO	Tachycardia, vomiting, CNS stimulation	Wide pharmacokinetic variability, follow serum concentration. Withhold if HR >160/min.

Drug	Class	Indication	Dose	Route	Adverse effects	Comments
			31–34 wks GA: mg/kg/d theophylline = 4.82 + (0.28 × PNA in wks) *Term:* [0.3(age in weeks)+8] mg/kg/d div. q8–12h. Divide 24h calculated dose to be given as TID. PNA = postnatal age. For aminophylline, increase calculated theophylline dose by 20%.			
Tincture of opium (1:25 dilution)	Opiate	Neonatal abstinence syndrome	0.8–2.0 mL/kg/day div. q4h	PO	Sedation, respiratory depression	Decrease 10% per day as tolerated.
Tissue plasminogen activator (TPA)	Thrombolytic	Major vessel thrombosis	Bolus: 0.5 mg/kg over 10 min. Maintenance: 0.1–0.5 mg/kg/h	IV	Nausea, vomiting, hypotension, fever, bleeding from IV access sites.	Monitor PT, PTT; high doses may cause bleeding.

(Table continues on following page)

TABLE 23
Neonatal Drug Formulary (*Continued*)

Drug Generic (Trade)	Category or Class	Indications for Use	Dose and Interval	Route	Side Effects	Comments
Zidovudine (Retrovir)	Antiviral	Neonatal AIDS	2 mg/kg/dose q6h × 6 wks 1.5 mg/kg/dose q6h × 6 wks	PO IV	Severe anemia and neutropenia, GI upset	May also be given IV, 1–3 mg/kg per dose, infused over 60 min. Give within first 8–12 h of life. Best drug for CNS disease.

Chapter 16

Antimicrobial Agents

Varsha Bhatt-Mehta, Pharm.D., and Jennifer L. Grow, M.D.

I. **Acyclovir**

   A. Dosage regimen: HSV infection

   1. For > 33 weeks and normal renal function, 30–60 mg/kg/d divided every 8 hr for 14–21 d

   2. For < 33 weeks *or* serum creatinine 0.8–1.1 mg/dL with urine output > 1.0 mL/kg/hr, 40 mg/kg/d divided every 12 hr for 14–21 d

   3. For serum creatinine 1.2–1.5 mg/dL *or* urine output < 0.5 mL/kg/hr, 10 mg/kg/d every 24 hr.

   4. For serum creatinine > 1.5 mg/dL *or* urine output < 0.5 mL/kg/hr renal failure, 5 mg/kg/d every 24 hr

   B. Route

   IV as 1-hr infusion

   C. Comments/cautions

   Much more water soluble than adenine arabinoside and equally effective for treatment of serious neonatal herpes simplex infection. Monitor renal, hepatic, hematopoietic function during therapy. *Must consult with attending physician before use.* Resistant strains of herpes simplex have been reported. Recipients reportedly less likely to develop herpes-specific antibodies than those treated with adenine arabinoside, with attendant theoretical increased risk of recurrences, although supporting clinical data are sparse. Treatment of varicella-zoster infection may require double above dose occasionally.

II. **Amikacin Sulfate**

   A. Dosage regimen

   1. If < 1200 g and 0–4 wks: 7.5 mg/kg/dose every 18–24 hr

   2. If 1200–2000 g and ≤ 7 d: 15 mg/kg/dose every 12 hr

   3. If 1200–2000 g and > 7 d: 22.5 mg/kg/dose every 8–12 hr

   4. If > 2000 g and ≤ 7 d: 7.5–10 mg/kg/dose every 12 hr

   5. If > 2000 g and > 7 d: 30 mg/kg/dose every 8 hr

   6. If significant renal dysfunction, may load with 10 mg/kg and then follow serum concentration for subsequent dosing

B. Route

IV as 20-min infusion or IM

C. Comments/cautions

Consult with attending physician before use. Dose modification may be necessary in presence of renal dysfunction. Monitor amikacin levels and serum creatinine concentration on days 3 and 7 and weekly thereafter (safe and effective therapeutic peak concentration of 15–25 mg/mL). Brainstem audiometry to assess hearing if treated for 7 or more days. May be inactivated by ticarcillin or piperacillin if mixed in same infusion. May interfere with neuromuscular junction transmission. ***Do not administer to infants of mothers with myasthenia gravis.***

III.   Amphotericin B

A. Dosage regimen: 0.25 mg/kg infused over 6 hr. Increase gradually to 1.0 mg/kg/24 hr.

After involved sites sterilized, may change to every other day administration for remainder of course.

B. Route

IV only

Concentration for infusion 0.1 mg/mL with 5% dextrose; infuse over 4–6 hr once a day.

C. Comments/cautions

Do not use in-line membrane filter unless mean pore diameter is 1.0 micron or greater. Monitor serum potassium, magnesium and renal, liver, and hematopoietic function. Decrease daily dose or prolong interval if toxicity develops. If infant develops fever, tremors, or other symptoms with infusion, may require pretreatment with acetaminophen or diphenhydramine.

IV.   Amphotericin B (Liposomal)

A. Dosage regimen

3–5 mg/kg/24h, given as a once daily infusion

B. Route

IV over 2 hr as a 1–2 mg/mL infusion.

C. Comments/cautions

Monitor renal, hepatic, electrolyte, and hematologic status closely. Do not use in-line membrane filter unless mean pore diameter is 1.0 micron or greater. Monitor serum potassium, magnesium and renal, liver, and hematopoietic function. Decrease daily dose or prolong interval if toxicity develops. If infant develops fever, tremors, or other symptoms with infusion, may require pretreatment with acetaminophen or diphenhydramine.

V. Ampicillin Sodium

A. Dosage regimen
   1. If ≤ 2000 g and PNA ≤ 7 d: 100 mg/kg/d divided every 12 hr
   2. If > 2000 g and ≤ 7 d: 150 mg/kg/d divided every 8 hr. Group B strep meningitis 300 mg/kg/d divided every 8 hr
   3. If ≤ 2000 g and > 7 d: 150 mg/kg/d divided every 8 hr. Group B strep meningitis 200 mg/kg/d divided every 8 hr
   4. If > 2000 g and > 7 d: 200 mg/kg/d divided every 6 hr

B. Route
   IV as 15- to 30-min infusion or IM

VI. Aztreonam Arginine

A. Dosage regimen
   1. If ≤ 2000 g and ≤ 7 d: 60 mg/kg/d divided every 12 hr
   2. If > 2000 g and < 7 d: 90 mg/kg/d divided every 8 hr
   3. If < 1200 g and > 7 d: 60 mg/kg/d divided every 12 hr
   4. If > 1200–2000 g and > 7 d: 90 mg/kg/d divided every 8 hr
   5. If > 2000 g and > 7 d: 120 mg/kg/d divided every 6 hr

B. Route
   IV or IM

C. Comments/cautions
   Consult with attending physician before use. Excellent gram-negative coverage, but essentially no activity against gram-positive organisms. Good CSF penetration with inflamed meninges, moderate penetration without. Much decreased potential for ototoxicity, nephrotoxicity, or interference with neuromuscular transmission compared to aminoglycosides. Monitor glucose and indirect bilirubin carefully, since treatable abnormalities have been associated with the arginine salt. Better activity in abscesses and necrotic tissue than aminoglycosides. Much less problem with emergence of resistant organisms than with third-generation cephalosporins. Suitable for penicillin allergic infants.

VII. Cefotaxime Sodium

A. Dosage regimen
   1. Newborn infants 0–4 wks and < 1200 g: 100 mg/kg/d divided every 12 hr
   2. If > 1200–2000 g and < 7 d: 100 mg/kg/d divided every 12 hr
   3. If > 2000 g and < 7 d: 150 mg/kg/d divided every 12 hr
   4. If ≥ 1200 g and > 7 d: 150 mg/kg/d divided every 8 hr
   5. If > 2000 g and > 7 d: 150–200 mg/kg/d divided every 6–8 hr

B. Route

IV over 15–30 min; IM

C. Comments/cautions

Effective against many coliforms and penetrates CSF well, hence useful for gram-negative CNS infections. Widespread use in a confined population (e.g., NICU) may facilitate rapid emergence of resistant organisms. No significant interference with bilirubin-albumin binding. Preferred agent for gram-negative coverage among infants with underlying renal or auditory dysfunction and those who are born to mothers with myasthenia gravis. Better activity in abscesses and necrotic tissue than aminoglycosides.

VIII. Cefazolin Sodium

A. Dosage regimen

1. If ≤ 7 d: 40 mg/kg/d divided every 12 hr
2. If > 2000 g and < 7 d: 40 mg/kg/d divided every 12 hr
3. If > 2000 g and > 7 d: 60 mg/kg/d divided every 8 hr

B. Route

IV as 15- to 30-min infusion; IM reported to be less painful than other first-generation cephalosporins (e.g., cephalothin)

C. Comments/cautions

Poor CNS penetration; not effective for gram-negative infection

IX. Ceftazidime Sodium

A. Dosage regimen

1. If ≤ 1200 g: 100 mg/kg/d divided every 12 hr
2. If 1200–2000 g and ≤ 7 d: 100 mg/kg/d divided every 12 hr
3. If > 2000 g and < 7 d: 100–150 mg/kg/d divided every 12 hr
4. If ≥ 1200 g and > 7 d: 150 mg/kg divided every 8 hr

B. Route

IM or IV

C. Comments/cautions

As for cefotaxime, except interference with bilirubin-albumin binding less well studied. Only real advantage compared to cefotaxime is increased activity against *Pseudomonas aeruginosa*.

X. Ceftriaxone Sodium

A. Dosage regimen

Meningitis dose: 75–100 mg/kg/d divided every 12 hr

B. Route

IV or IM; IV over 5–15 min

C. Comments/cautions

Reported effective against many gram-negative organisms. Penetrates CSF well. Use with caution in renal dysfunction; follow for nephrotoxicity. In vitro data suggest significant interference with bilirubin-albumin binding and attendant theoretical increased risk of bilirubin neurotoxicity.

XI. Clindamycin

A. Dosage regimen

1. If ≤ 2000 g and ≤ 7 d: 10 mg/kg/d divided every 12 hr
2. If ≤ 2000 g and > 7 d: 15 mg/kg/d divided every 8 hr
3. If > 2000 g and ≤ 7 d: 15 mg/kg/d divided every 8 hr
4. If > 2000 g and > 7 d: 20–30 mg/kg/d divided every 6 hr

B. Route

IV/IM

C. Comments/cautions

Effective against many coagulase-positive staphylococci as well as some anaerobes, including *Bacteroides fragilis*. Limited neonatal experience. Pseudomembranous enterocolitis appears to be very rare in newborns. Association with development of intestinal strictures when used for treatment of medical NEC has been reported, but unclear if association is causal.

XII. Erythromycin

A. Dosage regimen

1. If IV, 25–40 mg/kg/d as lactobionate divided every 6 hr
2. If PO, ≤ 7 d, 20 mg/kg/d divided every 12 hr
3. If PO, > 7 d < 1200 g, 20 mg/kg/d divided every 12 hr
4. If PO, > 7 d ≥ 1200 g, 30–40 mg/kg/d divided every 6–8 hr
5. Treatment of chlamydia conjunctivitis/pneumonia: oral as erylsuccinate 50 mg/kg/d divided every 6 hr for 14 d

B. Route

PO as ethylsuccinate; IV as lactobionate

C. Comments/cautions

May cause gastric irritation or feeding intolerance. Rare case reports of infants receiving high doses and prolonged course resulting in pyloric stenosis. May interfere with theophylline and caffeine metabolism, producing toxic levels and adverse effects. Intravenous formulation associated with high incidence of phlebitis and rare occurrence of cardiotoxicity.

XIII. Fluconazole

   A. Dosage regimen

     1. 5–6 mg/kg/dose every 24 hr

     2. ≤ 29 weeks GA: 0–14 d, dose every 72 hr; > 14 d, dose every 48 hr

     3. 30–36 weeks GA: 0–14 d, dose every 48 hr; > 14 d, dose every 24 hr

     4. Requires dosage adjustment in renal failure. Reduce dose by 50% if serum creatinine is 0.8–1.1 mg/dL and urine output < 0.5 mL/kg/h. For serum creatinine > 1.1 mg/dL and urine output < 0.5 mL/kg/h give 25% of recommended dose at intervals appropriate for age.

   B. Route

     IV infusion over 45–60 min; PO

   C. Comments/cautions

     Must consult with attending physician before use. Good activity against *Candida albicans* and many other *Candida* species, although clinically important resistance necessitating change to amphotericin has been reported; excellent CNS penetration. Good absorption and bioavailability via PO route. Limited, but increasing, experience in newborns. Much less toxicity than amphotericin B or flucytosine, although careful monitoring of electrolytes and renal, hepatic, and hematopoietic function is still indicated. Monitor at baseline periodically during the course of treatment.

XIV. Flucytosine (5-Fluorocytosine)

   A. Dosage regimen

     75–100 mg/kg/d divided every 6 hr

   B. Route

     PO

   C. Comments/cautions

     Should not be used as *sole* antifungal agent in newborns. Monitor liver, renal and hematopoietic function. Decrease daily dose if hepatotoxicity or bone marrow suppression develops. CNS penetration excellent. Serum levels with PO route are 85% of those with IV route although IV product no longer available. Monitor serum levels to minimize toxicity (nontoxic range < 60 mg/mL). Significant interindividual pharmacokinetic variability.

XV. Gentamicin Sulfate

   A. Dosage regimen

     1. ≤ 1200 g and 0–4 weeks old, 2.5 mg/kg/dose every 18–24 hr

2. ≤ 7 d:
   1200–2000 g: 2.5 mg/kg/dose every 12 hr
   > 2000 g: 2.5 mg/kg/dose every 8 hr
3. > 7 d:
   1200–2000 g: 2.5 mg/kg/dose every 12 hr
   > 2000 g: 2.5 mg/kg/dose every 8 hr
4. Once daily dosing for term infants with normal renal function:
   5–6 mg/kg/ 24 hr
5. If significant renal dysfunction, may load with 2.5 mg/kg and
   then dose according to serum levels.
6. Initial dose for term newborns on ECMO: 2.5 mg/kg/dose
   every 18–24 hr. Follow levels.

B. Route
   IM; IV as 30-min infusion

C. Comments/cautions
   Follow serum levels closely. Peak level should be < 9 μg/mL,
   trough < 2 μg/mL. May need to decrease dose or prolong interval
   if renal dysfunction present. Check levels and serum creatinine on
   days 3 and 7 and weekly thereafter. Infants treated with aminoglycosides for ≥ 7 d should have brainstem audiometry. Extensive
   experience indicates virtually no clinically important ototoxicity or
   nephrotoxicity when recommended dosages are given and therapeutic concentrations are monitored for 7–10 d; increased potential for toxicity with more prolonged administration. May be inactivated by ticarcillin or piperacillin if combined in an IV infusion
   with one of these drugs. May interfere with neuromuscular transmission at toxic levels or at therapeutic levels in infants born to
   mothers with myasthenia gravis. ***Do not administer to infants of
   mothers with myasthenia gravis.***

XVII. Metronidazole

A. Dosage regimen
   1. < 1200 g, 0–4 wks: 7.5 mg/kg/dose every 48 hr
   2. 1200–2000 g, < 7 d: 7.5 mg/kg/24 hr; > 7 d: 7.5 mg/kg/dose
      every 12 hr
   3. > 2000 g, < 7 d: 7.5 mg/kg/dose every 12 hr; > 7 d: 15
      mg/kg/dose every 12 hr

B. Route
   IV or PO

C. Comments/cautions
   Effective against many anaerobic organisms, but ineffective
   against aerobic microbes. Penetrates central nervous system,

abscess, and other sequestered sites well. Primary excretion is renal.

XVIII. Nafcillin Disodium

A. Dosage regimen
1. If < 1200 g: 50 mg/kg/d divided every 12 hr
2. If 1200–2000 g and ≤ 7 d: 50 mg/kg/d divided every 12 hr
3. If 1200–2000 g and > 7 d: 75 mg/kg/d divided every 8 hr
4. If > 2000 g and ≤ 7 d: 75 mg/kg/d divided every 8 hr
5. If > 2000 g and > 7 d: 100 mg/kg/d divided every 6 hr

B. Route
IV as 15- to 30-min infusion; IM

C. Comments/cautions
Major route of excretion is biliary; therefore use with caution if cholestasis is present.

XIX. Penicillin G

A. Dosage regimen
1. For group B streptococcal infection: 250,000 U/kg/d divided every 6–12 hr; some authorities recommend 300–400,000 U/kg/d divided every 6–12 hr for GBS meningitis.
2. For infection by other susceptible organisms:
   a. If < 1200 g: 50,000 U/kg/d divided every 12 hr
   b. If 1200–2000 g and ≤ 7 d: 50,000 U/kg/d divided every 12 hr
   c. If 1200–2000 g and > 7 d: 75,000 U/kg/d divided every 8 hr
   d. If > 2000 g and ≤ 7 d: 75,000 U/kg/d divided every 8 hr
   e. If > 2000 g and > 7 d: 100,000 U/kg/d divided every 6 hr
   f. Double these doses if meningitis is present.

B. Route
1. IV as 15- to 30-min infusion of crystalline aqueous formulation
2. IM as procaine or crystalline aqueous formulation

C. Comments/cautions
IM benzathine formulation not recommended for most infections in newborn infants.

XX. Piperacillin Sodium

A. Dosage regimen
1. ≤ 7 d, ≤ 36 weeks' GA: 150 mg/kg/24 hr divided every 12 hr
2. ≤ 7 d, > 36 weeks' GA: 150 mg/kg/24 hr divided every 8 hr

3. > 7 d, ≤ 36 weeks' GA: 200 mg/kg/24 hr divided every 8 hr
4. > 7 d, > 36 weeks' GA: 200 mg/kg/24 hr divided every 6 hr

B. Route
IV as 20- to 30-min infusion; IM

C. Comments/cautions
Used for infections caused by *Pseudomonas aeruginosa*. Enters CSF well if meninges inflamed. May inactivate aminoglycosides if the two are mixed. Excreted by both renal and biliary routes. May cause hypernatremia or exacerbate hypokalemia.

XXI. Ribavirin

A. Dosage regimen
20 mg/mL in liquid reservoir of SPAG (small particle aerosol generator); aerosol administered 16–24h/d for 3–7 d

B. Route
Oxygen hood or tent; endotracheal

C. Comments/cautions
Monitor hepatic, hematopoietic, and renal function. Precipitates easily in respiratory tubing; careful surveillance necessary to assure airway patency. Efficacy against respiratory syncytial virus is controversial.

XXII. Rifampin

A. Dose regimen
10–20 mg/kg every day in divided doses every 12–24 hr

B. Route
PO; IV over 60 min

C. May be useful in treatment of infections caused by coagulase-negative staphylococci that fail to respond to vancomycin alone. Monitor ALT and bilirubin; use with caution in patients with preexisting hepatopathy. May cause secretions, urine, and stool to turn red-orange. Because of hepatic enzyme induction, may reduce serum concentrations/activity of glucocorticoids, digoxin, analgesics, barbiturates, benzodiazepines, theophylline, anticonvulsants, and others.

XXIII. Sulfamethoxazole-Trimethoprim

A. Dosage regimen (based on trimethoprim)
6–12 mg/kg/24 hr in divided doses every 12 hr. (*Note:* agent is a fixed combination with 5:1 ratio of SMX:TMP)

B. Route

IV

C. Comments/cautions

Consider drug levels on day 3 to assure therapeutic range. Therapeutic levels are generally:

SMX: 150 mg/mL

TMP: 3.0 mg/mL

with adjustments based on susceptibility of organism. In vitro tests suggest little or no interference with bilirubin-albumin binding at usual therapeutic concentrations. Nevertheless, use with caution in infants with indirect hyperbilirubinemia. Penetrates CNS well. *Must consult with attending physician before use.* Follow hematopoietic function.

XXIV. Ticarcillin Sodium

A. Dosage regimen

1. If ≤ 2000 g and ≤ 7 d: 150 mg/kg/d divided every 12 hr
2. If 1200–2000 g and > 7 d: 225 mg/kg/d divided every 8 hr
3. If > 2000 g and ≤ 7 d: 225 mg/kg/d divided every 8 hr
4. If > 2000 g and > 7 d: 300 mg/kg/d divided every 6–8 hr
5. If ≤ 1200 g and > 7 d: 150 mg/kg/24 hr divided every 12 hr

B. Route

IV over 30–120 min; IM

C. Cautions/comments

Useful for infections caused by *Pseudomonas aeruginosa.* Enters CSF well if meninges inflamed. May inactivate aminoglycosides if the two are mixed. Excreted predominantly by renal route. May cause hypernatremia or exacerbate hypokalemia (has three times the sodium content of piperacillin).

XXV. Tobramycin Sulfate

A. Dosage regimen

1. If ≤ 1200 g and 0–4 weeks old: 2.5 mg/kg/dose every 18–24 hr
2. If 1200–2000 g, ≤ 7 d: 2.5 mg/kg/dose every 12 hr
3. If > 2000 g, ≤ 7 d: 2.5 mg/kg/dose every 8 hr
4. If 1200–2000 g, > 7 d: 2.5 mg/kg/dose every 8–12 hr
5. If > 2000 g, > 7 d: 2.5 mg/kg/dose every 8 hr

B. Route

IV as 30-min infusion; IM

C. Comments/cautions

Same as gentamicin and amikacin. Therapeutic peak < 9 μg/mL, trough < 2 μg/mL. Ticarcillin or piperacillin in same infusion may inactivate tobramycin. ***Do not administer to infants of mothers with myasthenia gravis.***

XXVI. Vancomycin Hydrochloride
   A. Dosage regimen
1. If < 27 weeks postconceptional age, 15 mg/kg every 36 hr
2. If 27–30 weeks postconceptional age, 15 mg/kg every 24 hr
3. If 31–34 weeks postconceptional age, 15 mg/kg every 18 hr
4. If 34–40 weeks postconceptional age, 15 mg/kg every 12 hr
5. For meningitis in term infant, may give 15 mg/kg as often as every 8 hr
6. If renal dysfunction, load with 20 mg/kg and then follow serum concentration to determine dosing intervals

   B. Route
IV over 60 min

   C. Comments/cautions
May produce nephrotoxicity or ototoxicity. Monitor trough serum levels and creatinine on days 3 and 7 and weekly thereafter. Very effective agent for coagulase-negative staphylococci and methicillin-resistant coagulase-positive staphylococci. Peak serum levels > 60 μg/mL have been associated with nephrotoxicity and ototoxicity. Due to low incidence of toxicity with currently recommended doses, peak serum levels are measured only if toxicity is suspected. Maintain peak < 30 μg/mL and trough < 10 μg/mL. To minimize selection of resistant organisms for which no alternative agent exists, use for > 3 d should be restricted to circumstances where a gram-positive organism has been recovered from a normally sterile site and is resistant or highly likely to be resistant to β-lactam agents (penicillins and cephalosporins).

Chapter 17

Effects of Maternal Drug Administration on the Fetus and Newborn

Varsha Bhatt-Mehta, Pharm.D., and Steven M. Donn, M.D.

TABLE 24
Fetal and Neonatal Effects of Maternal Drug Administration

Drug	Fetal and Neonatal Effects
Acebutolol	Reduced birthweight, hypotension, bradycardia, hypoglycemia. Observe newborn closely for 3–4 days.
Acetazolamide	Hyperbilirubinemia, hypocalcemia, hypomagnesemia, metabolic acidosis.
Acetohexamide	Prolonged symptomatic hypoglycemia. Should be discontinued at least 48 hours before delivery.
Albuterol	Possibly teratogenic (cleft palate, limb defects). Causes transient hyperglycemia followed by increase in serum insulin, tachycardia, and hypoglycemia.
Alprazolam	Withdrawal (within 2 days of delivery). Possible association with anomalies (*see* Diazepam).
Amikacin	*See* Gentamicin
Aminophylline	*See* Theophylline
Amiodarone	Contains iodine; risk of goiter and congenital hypothyroidism. May be useful for fetal tachycardia.
Amitriptyline	Possible malformations (limb deformities, incomplete ossification), developmental delay, CNS effects, urinary retention, withdrawal syndrome.
Amphetamines	Abruptio placentae, prematurity, IUGR, hypertension, poor feeding, drowsiness, irritability, withdrawal syndrome (congenital heart defects, abnormal sleep, poor feeding, tremor, hypertonia), cerebral injuries (secondary to vasoconstriction).
Aspirin	Premature closure of ductus arteriosus (last trimester), IUGR, congenital salicylate intoxication, depressed albumin-binding capacity, hemorrhage (antiplatelet effect, depressed factor XII), IVH in VLBWs. Chronic, high doses may be teratogenic.
Atenolol	IUGR, persistent bradycardia/hypotension, transient tachypnea, hypoglycemia.

(*Table continues on following page*)

TABLE 24
Fetal and Neonatal Effects of Maternal
Drug Administration (*Continued*)

Drug	Fetal and Neonatal Effects
Azathioprine	Several case reports of malformations (limb, neural tube defect), pancytopenia, immunosuppression. Risk of infections and neoplasia. IUGR.
Bismuth subsalicylate	*See* Aspirin. (Note: sodium salicylate does not alter platelet function.)
Brompheniramine	Possible increased risk of retinopathy in premature infants.
Butalbital	Severe neonatal withdrawal.
Captopril	Renal failure (anuria), oligohydramnios, pulmonary hypoplasia, IUGR, prematurity, skull hypoplasia, severe hypotension, death.
Carbamazepine	Congenital malformations (spina bifida, craniofacial defects, fingernail hypoplasia, developmental delay).
Ceftriaxone	Reversible biliary pseudolithiasis in newborns; no reports of in utero exposure.
Chloramphenicol	"Gray baby syndrome" (abdominal distention, pallid cyanosis, vasomotor collapse, death).
Chlordiazepoxide	Withdrawal (up to 26 days after delivery), prolonged neonatal depression.
Chlorothiazide	Thrombocytopenia, hypoglycemia, hyponatremia, hypokalemia, hemolytic anemia.
Chlorpromazine	Maternal hypotension with resultant fetal hypoxia, extrapyramidal signs (prolonged), hyper-/hyporeflexia, prolonged jaundice.
Chlorpropamide	Prolonged severe hypoglycemia (4–10 days). If used during pregnancy, should be discontinued at least 48 hours before delivery. Insulin preferred for blood glucose management during pregnancy. Possible association with facial, ear, skeletal anomalies.
Ciprofloxacin	Possible cartilage damage, arthropathy, fatal interaction with theophylline.
Clomipramine	Withdrawal (colic, cyanosis, tachypnea, irritability), seizures, hypotonia.
Clonazepam	Hypotonia, apnea, lethargy, hypothermia.
Cocaine	Abruptio placentae, PROM, congenital anomalies (CNS, GU, cardiac, limb, craniofacial), IUGR, cerebrovascular accidents, bowel atresia, NEC, irritability, tremulousness, muscular rigidity, vomiting, diarrhea, seizures, SIDS, neurobehavioral abnormalities.

(*Table continues on following page*)

TABLE 24
Fetal and Neonatal Effects of Maternal
Drug Administration (*Continued*)

Drug	Fetal and Neonatal Effects
Codeine	Respiratory depression, withdrawal.
Cortisone	Cleft palate, risk of adrenal suppression.
Coumadin	Fetal warfarin syndrome: nasal hypoplasia, IUGR, eye defects, extremity hypoplasia, seizures, hearing loss, congenital heart disease (25% if exposed between 6–9 weeks' gestation). CNS defects with later exposure. Hemorrhage (3%). Most (70%) exposed infants are normal. Heparin preferred from 6–12 weeks' gestation and at term.
Desipramine	*See* Clomipramine
Diazepam	Possible risk of craniofacial defects (especially cleft lip/palate), inguinal hernia, cardiac defects, pyloric stenosis. "Floppy infant" syndrome (hypotonia, lethargy, poor suck), withdrawal syndrome (tremor, irritability, hypertonicity, diarrhea, vomiting), hypothermia.
Diphenhydramine	Possible increased risk of ROP in premature infants. Withdrawal in high doses.
Enalapril	*See* Captopril
Ephedrine	Tachycardia, hypertension.
Ergotamines	Fetal death from placental vasoconstriction.
Ethosuximide	Malformations (cleft lip/palate), spontaneous hemorrhage, PDA.
Fenoprofen	*See* Ibuprofen
Fentanyl	Respiratory depression and withdrawal if used for prolonged periods or high doses. Narcan-reversible.
Flurazepam	Lethargy. One case with reported seizure.
Furosemide	Possible association with hypospadias.
Gentamicin	Potentially ototoxic. Interferes with transmission at neuromuscular junction potentiating the effect of anesthetics, $MgSO_4$, and neuromuscular blockers resulting in weakness and respiratory paralysis.
Glyburide	Prolonged severe hypoglycemia (4–10 days). If used during pregnancy, should be discontinued at lest 48 hours before delivery. Insulin preferred for blood glucose management during pregnancy. Possible association with facial (ear) anomalies.
Heparin	Does not cross placenta, possible hypocalcemia.
Heroin	Multiple varied anomalies, SGA, narcotic withdrawal (hyperactivity, respiratory distress, fever, diarrhea, mucus secretion, sweating, convulsions, yawning; appears

(Table continues on following page)

TABLE 24
Fetal and Neonatal Effects of Maternal
Drug Administration (*Continued*)

Drug	Fetal and Neonatal Effects
	usually within 48 hours but up to 6 days), increased perinatal mortality.
Hydralazine	Thrombocytopenia and bleeding. One case of lupus-like syndrome reported.
Hydrochlorothiazide	*See* Chlorothiazide
Hydromorphone	Respiratory depression.
Hydroxyzine	Possible association with oral clefts. Withdrawal syndrome with prolonged exposure.
Ibuprofen	Like other prostaglandin syntheses inhibitors, may cause oligohydramnios, reduced urine output, premature closure of the ductus arteriosus (if administered in third trimester), PPHN, and prolonged labor.
Imipramine	Limb reduction, cardiovascular anomalies, withdrawal (colic, cyanosis, tachypnea, irritability), urinary retention.
Indomethacin	Like other prostaglandin synthetase inhibitors, may cause oligohydramnios, reduced urine output, premature closure of the ductus arteriosus (if administered in third trimester), PPHN, and prolonged labor. GI hemorrhage and intestinal perforation reported.
Iodine, Iodide	Hypothyroidism and goiter when used for long periods (10-day course for maternal thyroid surgery is safe). Tracheal compression from large goiters. Transient hypothyroidism has been demonstrated following topical or vaginal use in the mother before delivery. Present in many OTC medications.
Isoniazid	Possible hemorrhagic disease of the newborn. Unlikely teratogen.
Isotretinoin	Severe anomalies (CNS, craniofacial, conotruncal malformations, neural tube).
Ketoprofen	*See* Ibuprofen
Labetalol	Bradycardia (possibly marked and persistent), hypoglycemia, transient hypotension. Observe closely for 24–48 hours.
Lidocaine	CNS depression, seizures, hypotension, cardiac arrhythmias from high maternal levels or inadvertent fetal injection.
Lisinopril	*See* Captopril
Lithium	Cardiac defects (especially Ebstein's disease) when used in first trimester; toxicity (cyanosis, hypotonia, bradycardia, goiter with hypothyroidism, GI bleeding, diabetes insipidus, seizures) at term. Toxic effects resolve in 1–2 weeks.

(*Table continues on following page*)

TABLE 24
Fetal and Neonatal Effects of Maternal
Drug Administration (*Continued*)

Drug	Fetal and Neonatal Effects
Lorazepam	Respiratory depression, "floppy infant." Other benzodiazepines (diazepam, chlordiazepoxide) have been associated with malformations.
Magnesium sulfate	Respiratory depression, hypotonia, hyporeflexia, decreased GI motility. Toxicity poorly correlated with serum Mg concentration. Impaired fetal bone mineralization and hypocalcemia with prolonged use.
Meclizine	Possible increased malformations.
Meclofenamate	Like other prostaglandin synthetase inhibitors, may cause oligohydramnios, reduced urine output, premature closure of the ductus arteriosus (if administered in third trimester), PPHN, and prolonged labor.
Medroxyprogesterone	Possible increased risk of cardiac malformations.
Menadione (Vit K3)	Hyperbilirubinemia, kernicterus in premature infants.
Meperidine	Respiratory depression (peak if delivery occurs 2–3 hours after maternal dose), withdrawal syndrome.
Methadone	Low birthweight, narcotic withdrawal (60–90% of fetuses exposed, usually within 48 hours of delivery, may be delayed 7–14 days), SIDS, jaundice, thrombocytosis (marked and persistent). Respiratory depression not common.
Methamphetamine	*See* Amphetamine
Methyldopa	Mild systolic hypotension lasting up to 2 days.
Metolozone	*See* Chlorothiazide
Metoprolol	No reports of adverse effects, however, close monitoring for bradycardia, hypotension, and hypoglycemia indicated for 24–48 hours
Metronidazole	Possibly teratogenic.
Midazolam	Respiratory depression, hypoglycemia, jaundice, hypotonia, hypothermia.
Minoxidil	Hypertrichosis, hypotension, possible association with malformations.
Morphine	Respiratory depression, narcotic withdrawal, possible association with inguinal hernia.
Nadolol	Persistent, severe beta blockage (cardiorespiratory depression, hypothermia, hypoglycemia). Close monitoring for at least 48 hours indicated (24-hour half-life).
Nalbuphine	Respiratory depression, narcotic withdrawal.
Naproxen	*See* Ibuprofen

(*Table continues on following page*)

TABLE 24
Fetal and Neonatal Effects of Maternal
Drug Administration (*Continued*)

Drug	Fetal and Neonatal Effects
Neostigmine	Insignificant placental transfer, safe for treatment of maternal myasthenia gravis. Transient muscle weakness occurs in 20% infants of mothers with myasthenia gravis.
Nifedipine	Risk of reduced uterine blood flow with resultant fetal hypoxia.
Nitrofurantoin	May cause hemolytic anemia, particularly with G6PD deficiency.
Nitroglycerin	Fetal decelerations, bradycardia.
Nitroprusside	Transient bradycardia, risk of cyanide toxicity.
Nortriptyline	Possible risk of limb reduction anomalies. Urinary retention.
Oral contraceptives	Generally contain both a progestin and synthetic estrogen. Masculinization of female infants. Increased bilirubin.
Penicillamine	Cutis laxa, inguinal hernia, possibly other malformations.
Pentazocine	Withdrawal (jitters, tremor, irritability, hypertonia, high-pitched cry, diaphoresis, diarrhea, vomiting, opisthotonic posturing) appearing within 48 hours of delivery following chronic maternal ingestion. Severe respiratory depression.
Pentobarbital	Hemorrhagic disease of the newborn, barbiturate withdrawal.
Phencyclidine (PCP)	Irritability, jitters, hypertonicity, poor feeding, abnormal neurobehavior.
Phenobarbital	Possible increased risk of minor congenital defects, hemorrhagic disease of the newborn (vitamin K depletion), barbiturate withdrawal (3–14 days after delivery). May reduce the incidence/severity of IVH in preterm infants when given to mother.
Phenytoin	Fetal hydantoin syndrome (hypoplasia of distal phalanges, small or absent nails, various craniofacial anomalies, congenital heart defects, cleft lip/palate). Possible increased risk of neoplasms, hemorrhagic disease of the newborn (vitamin K depletion).
Piroxicam	*See* Ibuprofen
Prednisone/prednisolone	Very small increased risk of anomalies. Individual case reports of immunosuppression and cataracts. May prevent RDS.
Primaquine	Hemolytic anemia with G6PD deficiency.
Primidone	Anomalies similar to fetal hydantoin syndrome. Tremors, hemorrhagic disease of the newborn.

(*Table continues on following page*)

TABLE 24
Fetal and Neonatal Effects of Maternal
Drug Administration (Continued)

Drug	Fetal and Neonatal Effects
Prochlorperazine	Isolated reports of congenital anomalies, probably safe in low doses.
Promethazine	Impaired platelet aggregation. Possible respiratory depression.
Propoxyphene	Possible congenital anomalies (extremities, craniofacial), neonatal withdrawal (irritability, tremors, fever, high-pitched cry, hypertonicity, diaphoresis, seizures) within hours of delivery, subsiding by 4 days.
Propranolol	IUGR (chronic dosing), bradycardia, hypotension, hypoglycemia, respiratory depression, hyperbilirubinemia. Observe closely for beta blockade for 24–48 hours.
Propylthiouracil	Mild hypothyroidism (resolves in days), goiter (12%) if used near term. Small risk of tracheal compression from goiter. Drug of choice for maternal hyperthyroidism during pregnancy.
Pseudoephedrine	See Phenylephrine
Pyridostigmine	See Neostigmine
Quinapril	See Captopril
Quinidine	Thrombocytopenia. Useful for fetal supraventricular tachycardia.
Quinine	Congenital anomalies (CNS, limb), optic nerve damage, thrombocytopenia, hemolytic anemia in infants with G6PD deficiency.
Ribavirin	Teratogenic.
Rifampin	Hemorrhagic disease of the newborn.
Ritodrine	Tachycardia, arrhythmias, septal hypertrophy (> 2 wk exposure), hyper- or hypoglycemia (more common with IV dosing).
Streptomycin	Ototoxicity.
Sulfonamides	Possible association with congenital defects (especially sulfamethoxazole-trimethoprim). Severe jaundice, hemolytic anemia. Compete for bilirubin-binding sites on albumin. Sulfasalazine, used for ulcerative colitis, has not been shown to cause severe neonatal jaundice.
Sulindac	See Ibuprofen
Terbutaline	Tachycardia, hypoglycemia.
Terfenadine	Possible association with polydactyly.
Tetracycline	Possible risk of minor anomalies, yellow staining of deciduous teeth, inhibition of fibula growth (premature infants).

(Table continues on following page)

TABLE 24
Fetal and Neonatal Effects of Maternal
Drug Administration (*Continued*)

Drug	Fetal and Neonatal Effects
Theophylline	Transient tachycardia, irritability, vomiting with high maternal levels (> 20 µg/mL). Single case of apnea reported.
Tobramycin	*See* Gentamicin
Tolbutamide	Prolonged hypoglycemia not reported, but has been seen with other oral hypoglycemics. Should be discontinued at least 48 hours before delivery.
Tolmetin	*See* Ibuprofen
Tretinoin topical	Unlikely to cause significant malformations because of the limited systemic absorption of this topical medicine.
Trimethadione	Congenital anomalies (craniofacial, cardiac, GU, TEF), IUGR, mental retardation.
Valproic acid	Congenital anomalies in 1–2% of those exposed between 17 and 30 days gestation (neural tube, cardiac, craniofacial, GU, limb), IUGR, hyperbilirubinemia, hepatotoxicity, transient hyperglycinemia, afibrinogenemia.
Verapamil	Useful for fetal SVT. Risk of reduced uterine blood flow with resultant fetal hypoxia.
Vitamin A	Congenital anomalies (CNS, microtia, clefts, limb reduction).
Warfarin	*See* Coumadin

Suggested Reading

Briggs GG, Freeman RK, Yaffe SJ (eds): Drugs in Pregnancy and Lactation, 6th ed. Baltimore, Williams & Wilkins, 2002.

Chapter 18

Drugs in Breastfeeding

Varsha Bhatt-Mehta, Pharm.D.

I. **Issues to Consider in Lactating Women**
    A. Is the drug really necessary?
    B. Use the safest drug when alternatives exist (e.g., acetaminophen rather than aspirin for simple analgesia).
    C. If the drug is potentially harmful to the infant, consider obtaining plasma concentrations (e.g., phenobarbital, phenytoin).
    D. Drug exposure to the nursing infant may be minimized by adjusting maternal administration schedule to just after completion of nursing or just before the infant is to have a lengthy sleep period.

II. **Decisions Should Be Individualized**
    A. Specific illness
    B. Therapeutic modalities (e.g., avoid breastfeeding after ingestion of diagnostic radioactive pharmaceuticals).
    C. Risk-benefit analysis

III. **Difficulties in Interpreting Existing Information**
    A. Inadequate study design
    B. Lack of controlled clinical trials

IV. **Recommendations (Tables 25–27)**
    A. Accompanying tables are to be used as a quick guide.
    B. Consult the original reference for complete information.
    C. Commonly administered drugs are listed alphabetically by generic name.
    D. *Do not assume that drugs not listed are safe.*
    E. Information that follows has been extracted from several well-known references. However, it should be used with caution, and the original references should be consulted if there is a question regarding interpretation of the information that follows.

TABLE 25
Maternal Medication Usually Compatible with Breastfeeding*

Drug Class and Subclass	Reported Sign or Symptom in Infant or Effect on Lactation	Reference
Anesthetics		
General		
Halothane	None	3
Lidocaine	None	3
Magnesium sulfate	None	1, 3
Methyprylon	Drowsiness	3
Secobarbital	None	3
Thiopental	None	3
Local		
Bupivacaine (Marcaine)	Effect of this subclass is unknown,	2
Chloroprocaine (Nesacaine)	but systemic effects are not expected since very small	2
Etodocaine (Duraest)	amounts are excreted in milk.	1
Mepivacaine (Carbocaine)		1
Anticoagulants		
Bishydroxycoumarin	None	1, 3
Warfarin	None	1, 3
Antidepressants		
Amitriptyline	Unknown, but may be of concern	1
Amoxapine	Galactorrhea; unknown, may be of concern	1
Desipramine	Effect on infant unknown, but may be of concern	1
Dothiepin	Effect on infant unknown, but may be of concern	1
Doxepin	Muscle hypotonia, drowsiness, poor sucking and swallowing, vomiting, should be avoided during lactation	1
Fluoxetine	*See* Table 27	
Lithium	*See* Tables 26, 27	
Haloperidol	Decline in mental and psycho-motor development, Effect on infant unknown, but may be of concern	3
Imipramine	Effect on infant unknown, but may be of concern	3
Trazodone	Effect on infant unknown, but may be of concern	3
Antiepileptics		
Carbamazepine	None	1
Ethosuximide	None	1

(*Table continued on following page*)

TABLE 25
Maternal Medication Usually Compatible
with Breastfeeding* (*Continued*)

Drug Class and Subclass	Reported Sign or Symptom in Infant or Effect on Lactation	Reference
Phenobarbital	Sedation: infantile spasms after weaning from milk containing phenobarbital. Methemoglobinemia.	1
Phenytoin	Methemoglobinemia, drowsiness, decreased sucking	1
Primidone	Sedation, feeding problems	1
Valproic acid	None	1
Felbamate	Caution in infant. Effects unknown, but causes aplastic anemia and hepatic failure at therapeutic doses in adults.	1
Bronchodilators and Decongestants		
Pseudoephedrine	None	1
Terbutaline	None	1
Theophylline	Irritability	1
Antihypertensive and Cardiovascular Drugs		
Atenolol	Cyanosis, bradycardia; use with caution	3
Captopril	None	3
Digoxin	None	3
Diltiazem	None	3
Hydralazine	None	3
Labetalol	Cyanosis, bradycardia; use with caution	3
Lidocaine	None	3
Methyldopa	None	3
Metoprolol	Cyanosis, bradycardia; use with caution	3
Procainamide	None	3
Propranolol	None	3
Verapamil	None	3
Anti-infective Drugs (All antibiotics transfer into breast milk in limited amounts)		
Acyclovir	None	3
Amoxicillin	None	3
Aztreonam	None	3
Cefazolin	None	3
Cefotaxime	None	3
Cefotetan	None	1
Cefoxitin	None	3
Ceftazidime	None	3
Ceftriaxone	None	3
Clindamycin	None	3

(Table continued on following page)

TABLE 25
Maternal Medication Usually Compatible
with Breastfeeding* (*Continued*)

Drug Class and Subclass	Reported Sign or Symptom in Infant or Effect on Lactation	Reference
Erythromycin	None	3
Ethambutol	None	3
Isoniazid	None; acetyl metabolite also secreted; Hepatoxicity	3
Nitrofurantoin	Hemolysis in infants with G6PD deficiency	3
Rifampin	None	3
Sulbactam	None	3
Sulfisoxazole	Caution in infants with G6PD deficiency or jaundice	3
Tetracycline	None; negligible absorption by infant	3
Ticarcillin	None	3
Trimethoprim-sulfamethoxazole	None	3
Antithyroid Drugs		
Levothyroxine	None	1
Diuretics		
Chlorothiazide	None	3
Hydrochlorothiazide	None	3
Spironolactone	None	3
Furosemide	None	1
Hormones		
Contraceptive pill with estrogen/progesterone	Rare breast enlargement; decrease in milk production and protein content (some studies only)	3
Estradiol	Withdrawal, vaginal bleeding	3
Medroxyprogesterone	None	3
Prednisone/Prednisolone	None	3
Muscle Relaxants		
Baclofen	None	3
Narcotics, Nonnarcotic Analgesics, Anti-inflammatory Agents		
Acetaminophen	None	3
Butorphanol	None	3
Codeine	None	3
Gold salts	None	3
Ibuprofen	None	3
Indomethacin	Seizure (1 case)	3
Mefenamic acid	None	3
Methadone	None (if mother gets < 20 mg/24 hr)	3

(*Table continued on following page*)

TABLE 25
Maternal Medication Usually Compatible
with Breastfeeding* (*Continued*)

Drug Class and Subclass	Reported Sign or Symptom in Infant or Effect on Lactation	Reference
Morphine	None	3
Propoxyphene	None	3
Salicylates	*See* Table 27	3
Tolmetin	None	3
CNS Stimulants		
Caffeine	Irritability, poor sleep pattern; no effects with usual amounts of caffeine beverages (2–3 cups/day)	3
Miscellaneous		
Atropine	None	3
Cimetidine†	None	3
Cisapride	None	3
Metoclopramide	Caution: although transmitted into milk in very small amounts, potential for CNS adverse effects; dopaminergic blocking agent	1, 3
Antidepressants/Antipsychotics		
Fluoxetine	*See* Table 27	3
Lithium	⅓ to ½ therapeutic blood concentration in infants	3

*Drugs included in this table have the effects listed or no effect. The word *none* implies that no adverse effects were seen in the infant while the mother was taking that drug. Most literature consists of single case reports or case report series.
†Drug concentrates in breast milk.

TABLE 26
Maternal Medication Contraindicated During Breastfeeding

Drug Class and Subclass	Effect	Reference
Miscellaneous		
Bromocriptine	Suppresses lactation; may be hazardous to mother	3
Cyclophosphamide	Possible immune suppression; unknown effect on growth or association with carcinogenesis; neutropenia	3
Cyclosporine	Same as above	3
Doxorubicin*	Same as above	3
Ergotamine	Vomiting, diarrhea, convulsions	3
Lithium	$\frac{1}{3}$ to $\frac{1}{2}$ therapeutic blood concentration in infants	3
Methotrexate	Possible immune suppression; unknown effect on growth or association with carcinogenesis; neutropenia	3
Drugs of Abuse		
Amphetamine	Irritability, poor sleep pattern	3
Cocaine	Cocaine intoxication	3
Heroin	Addiction in infant, tremors, restlessness, vomiting, poor feeding	3
Marijuana	Effect unknown; avoid	3
Nicotine (smoking)	Shock, vomiting, diarrhea, rapid heart rate, restlessness; decreased milk production	3
Phencyclidine (PCP)	Potent hallucinogen	3

*Drug is concentrated in human milk

TABLE 27
Drugs with Significant Effects on Some Nursing Infants (to Be Used with Caution)*

Drug	Effect	Reference
Aspirin	Metabolic acidosis (dose-related) may affect platelet function; rash	3
Fluoxetine	Irritability, diarrhea, vomiting	1
Lithium	$\frac{1}{3}$ to $\frac{1}{2}$ therapeutic blood concentration in infants	1, 3
Phenobarbital	Sedation; infantile spasms after weaning from milk containing phenobarbital. Methemoglobinemia	3

*Measure blood concentration in the infant if possible.

References

1. Briggs GG, Freeman RK, Yaffe SJ (eds): Drugs in Pregnancy and Lactation, 6th ed. Baltimore, Williams & Wilkins, 2002.
2. Committee on Drugs, American Academy of Pediatrics: The transfer of drugs and other chemicals into human milk. Pediatrics 108:776–789, 2001.
3. Felbanate monograph. In McEvoy GK (ed): American Hospital Formulary Service. Bethesda, MD, American Society of Health System Pharmacists, 1995.

Fluids and Electrolytes

Robert E. Schumacher, M.D., and Jennifer L. Grow, M.D.

I. **Neonatal Fluid Physiology**
   A. Percent total body water exceeds that of adult
   B. Expanded extracellular space which contracts during first week of life
      1. Increasing glomerular filtration rate
         a. Over first few days of life
         b. Until glomerulogenesis complete (34 weeks)
      2. Physiologic diuresis occurs with loss of about 10% of total body weight
      3. Some SGA/dysmature infants may not have expanded extracellular space
   C. Fluid losses
      1. Measurable (urine, feces, sweat)
      2. Insensible
         a. Respiratory
            i. Water vapor density of inspired-expired air $\times$ ventilatory rate $\div$ diffusion surface area
            ii. Increases with low humidity of inspired air and/or increased minute ventilation
         b. Transepidermal water loss (TEWL)
            i. Water vapor density of skin $-$ air $\div$ resistance of air and skin to diffusion
            ii. Affected by:
               (a) Skin keratin thickness
               (b) Surface:mass ratio
               (c) Postnatal age
               (d) Activity
               (e) Body temperature
               (f) Ambient humidity
               (g) Ambient temperature
               (h) Phototherapy ($\uparrow$ 20–50%)
               (i) Radiant warmer ($\uparrow$ 50–150%)
   D. Other disturbances in fluid balance
      1. Third spacing (sepsis, NEC, burns)
      2. Diarrhea

3. Diabetes insipidus—rare
4. SIADH
5. Renal failure
6. Osmotic diuresis

E. Basal fluid requirements (mL/kg/d)
1. Vary tremendously
2. Estimate fluid requirement and revise frequently based on clinical and laboratory studies (Table 28)

TABLE 28
Estimated Initial Fluid Requirements (mL/kg/d)

Day	< 1000 g	< 1250 g	> 1250 g	Term
1	120–200	100	75	60–75
2	120–225	100–120	75–100	75–85
3	120–180	≥ 120	≥ 100	≥ 85

3. May range from 40 (term) to > 200 (VLBW infant under radiant warmer)

F. Monitoring fluid status
1. Weight (daily or more frequently)
2. Urine output (normal 0.5–3.0 mL/kg/hr)
3. Urine specific gravity
4. Skin turgor
5. Fontanel tension
6. Central venous pressure
7. Serum electrolytes

II. Electrolytes

A. Sodium (*see also* pages 151 and 157)
1. Maintenance: 2–4 mEq/kg/d for infants > 30 weeks' gestation, 3–5 mEq/kg/d for infants < 30 weeks' gestation. ELBWs (especially with diuretic use) may require > 10 mEq/kg/d.
2. Generally not required in first 24 hours
3. In VLBW infant and infant born to mother who received large amounts of intrapartum fluids, check baseline electrolytes at birth.
4. Excessive fluid intake (and glomerular filtration rate) can lead to significant sodium loss in urine.
5. Bicarbonate is a *sodium* salt: 1 mEq $NaHCO_3$ = 1 mEq Na. Avoid iatrogenic hypernatremia.

B. Potassium (*see* page 135)
1. Generally not required before 24 hours of age

2. Maintenance requirement: 2 mEq/kg/d as KCl
3. Decreased need with renal compromise or extensive tissue breakdown
4. Increased need with diuretics, some drugs (e.g., amphotericin B)
5. Premature kidney may not tolerate large potassium load.

C. Calcium (*see* pages 130–132)
   1. The most abundant mineral in the body
   2. Can be given IV or PO
   3. Calcium accretion occurs in the third trimester. Preterm and SGA infants are at risk for osteopenia.
   4. In utero bone accretion rates average 150 mg/kg/d for Ca and 75 mg/kg/d for P. This cannot be met via parenteral route.
   5. Maintenance of serum calcium requires 50–75 mg elemental Ca/kg/d.

D. Magnesium (*see* pages 133–134)
   1. The second most abundant intracellular electrolyte
   2. Maintenance requirement: 7–10 mg/kg/d
   3. Serum values often high in infants born to mothers treated with magnesium sulfate

Suggested Reading

Doyle LW, Sinclair JC: Insensible water loss in newborn infants. Clin Perinatol 9:453–482, 1982.

Tsang RC, Nichols BL: Nutrition during Infancy. Philadelphia, Hanley & Belfus, 1988.

Chapter 20

Hyperglycemia

Jennifer L. Grow, M.D., and Robert E. Schumacher, M.D.

I. Definition

Blood glucose > 125 mg/dL or plasma glucose > 150 mg/dL. Occurs in < 5% of term newborns, > 50% of "micropremies."

II. Etiologic Factors

A. Immaturity—very small preterm infants are relatively glucose intolerant, secondary to decreased peripheral sensitivity to insulin and hepatic unresponsiveness to glucose.

B. Stress—surgery, RDS, sepsis/infection, shock, intracranial hemorrhage

C. Drugs—steroid therapy, excessive glucose

III. Prevention

A. Avoid excessive glucose loads. Calculate the glucose infusion rate (GIR, mg/kg/min) the baby is receiving. Do not increase the IV rate without reassessing the impact of the increase in glucose infusion.

B. Monitor closely in high-risk situations.

IV. Treatment

A. Decrease GIR by 2 mg/kg/min every 4–6 hr until glucose values normalize. Decrease more rapidly if glucose > 200 mg/dL. Do not give less than basal glucose requirement 4–8 mg/kg/min. Avoid hypotonic fluids.

B. Insulin—give if glucose remains > 250 mg/dL despite the above measures. Use regular insulin.

1. Intravenous insulin: infuse starting at 0.01 U/kg/hr
2. Follow K^+ carefully whenever giving insulin.

Suggested Reading

Farraq HM, Cowett RM: Glucose homeostasis in the micropremie. Clin Perinatol 27:1–22, 2000.

Chapter 21

Hypoglycemia

Jennifer L. Grow, M.D., and Robert E. Schumacher, M.D.

I. Definition

A. In most newborns, low blood glucose concentrations are not reflective of any problem but rather representative of a transition to an extrauterine metabolic state. Although recurrent or prolonged low glucose values may cause long-term sequelae, for any one infant the exact level and duration of "hypoglycemia" needed to do so remains uncertain.

B. Neonatal brains have the capacity to oxidize ketone bodies and lactate.

C. For practical/working purposes infants can be classified as:
1. Having/not having signs of hypoglycemia
2. Having glucose screen values of
   a. < 20 mg/dL
   b. > 20 mg/dL and < 40 mg/dL
   c. ≥ 40 mg/dL

II. Signs and Symptoms

A. Tremors
B. Apnea
C. Cyanosis
D. Diaphoresis
E. Lethargy/irritability
F. Hypotonia
G. Tachypnea/grunting
H. Hypothermia
I. Poor feeding (after feeding well)
J. Tachycardia
K. Seizures

III. Risk Classification

A. Healthy term infants. Healthy term infants born following uncomplicated pregnancy and delivery need not be screened. Follow for development of clinical signs.

B. Infants at risk because of clinical signs (see above) should prompt screening.

C. Infants at risk by history/condition
  1. Maternal factors
     a. Diabetes
     b. Large amounts IV glucose
     c. Oral hypoglycemic agents (propranolol, ritodrine, terbutaline)
  2. Neonatal factors
     a. IUGR/SGA
     b. Prematurity
     c. Twin
     d. Perinatal distress, hypoxia/ischemia
     e. Polycythemia
     f. Hypothermia
     g. Infection
     h. Clinical signs/history compatible with hyperinsulinemic state
     i. Other endocrine disorders/suspicion

IV. Guidelines for Screening and Prevention

A. Screening of infants consists of a series of capillary blood glucose determinations.
  1. Infants at historical risk
     a. Capillary blood glucose at approximately 30 minutes, 2 hours, and 4 hours of age
     b. Correlate before and after first feed and before second feed.
  2. At any time infant exhibits signs/symptoms
     a. Serial capillary blood glucose determinations: when signs/symptoms are first observed, then repeat at approximately 30 minutes and at 2 hours, to correlate with appropriate interventions based on symptoms
     b. Assess for additional and/or related problems.

V. Management

A. For at-risk infants with signs (other than infants of insulin-dependent diabetic mothers)
  1. If capillary blood glucose is:
     a. > 20 mg/dL, < 40 mg/dL, feed if able and repeat capillary blood glucose in 30 minutes, and before refeeding, in approximately 2 hours.
     b. > 20, < 40 mg/dL and unstable for PO feed, notify attending physician, consider OG/NG feed vs. intravenous glucose.
     c. < 40 mg/dL repeat; initiate IV therapy.

2. If capillary blood glucose < 20 mg/dL and asymptomatic:
   a. Stat serum glucose
   b. Feed PO if able, or per NG or OG tube.
   c. Repeat capillary blood glucose 30 minutes before feeding and 1 hour after feeding; repeat before feeding or PRN.
   d. If glucose < 40 mg/dL at repeat, anticipate IV therapy
3. If < 20 mg/dL and symptomatic:
   a. Stat serum glucose
   b. Initiate IV therapy
B. Parenteral treatment doses
1. Intravenous
   a. Asymptomatic: intravenous infusion 10% dextrose at 6–8 mg/kg/min (3–5 mL/kg/hr).
   b. Symptomatic: 200 mg/kg/IV push stat (2 mL/kg $D_{10}W$). Follow with 8 mg/kg/min (4.8 mL/kg/hr $D_{10}W$) and recheck glucose in 10–20 minutes.
2. In refractory cases: IM/SC as directed by physician
   a. Glucagon may be effective acutely in full-term infants (AGA or LGA only). Dose is 100 μg/kg (maximum dose is 300 μg) subcutaneously or IM.
   b. Susphrine 0.005 mL/kg IM or SC every 8 hr. Also works best in term AGA or LGA infants.
   c. Infants not responding to above should have plasma insulin, cortisol, and growth hormone concentrations measured and be started on hydrocortisone. Total daily dose: 5 mg/kg (IM) divided into two doses.
   d. If still hypoglycemic, diazoxide may be used in a total daily dose of 10–25 mg/kg/d divided TID PO.

Suggested Reading

Cornblath M, Hawdon JM, Williams AF, et al: Controversies regarding definition of neonatal hypoglycemia: Suggested operational thresholds. Pediatrics 105:1141–1145, 2000.

Halamek LP, Stevenson DK: Neonatal hypoglycemia. Part II. Pathophysiology and therapy. Clin Pediatr 37:11–16, 1998.

Vannucci RC, Vannucci SJ: Hypoglycemic brain injury. Semin Neonatol 6:147–155, 2001.

Chapter 22

Hypocalcemia

Jennifer L. Grow, M.D., and Robert E. Schumacher, M.D.

I. Definition

A. Ionized Ca^{2+} (iCa) is a better measure then total Ca^{2+}. "Low" values are similar in premature and term infants. Consider values < 1.1 mmol as low.

B. Normative total serum calcium values can only represent estimates of ionized values. Of clinical necessity, the definition of "low" values is conservative in nature and are action values, not "danger" values. Normative values vary with gestational age. For term infants, low is < 8 mg/dL; for preterm, < 7 mg/dL.

C. A functional measure of calcium is to look at its effect on the electrocardiogram, the QoTc interval. QoTc > 0.20 in term infants, > 0.19 in preterm infants.

D. $QoTc = \dfrac{Q - oT}{\sqrt{RR}}$ $oT =$ origin of T wave (in sec)
$\sqrt{RR} =$ interval between R waves (in sec)

E. In addition, it may be helpful to classify as having/not having signs of hypocalcemia.

II. Signs

A. Irritability

B. Tremors

C. Twitching

D. Bradycardia/hypotension

E. Convulsions

III. Associated Conditions

A. Infant of diabetic mother

B. Asphyxia

C. Prematurity

D. DiGeorge syndrome

E. Bicarbonate therapy

F. Exchange transfusion

G. Tocolytic agents

H. Congenital hypoparathyroidism

    I. Maternal hyperparathyroidism

    J. Malabsorption syndrome

IV. Treatment

    A. No signs; early onset, on oral feeding

       1. Consider the need to treat. Continue to monitor. The usual history of this state includes resolution without treatment.

       2. Elemental calcium (75 mg/kg/d as 10% calcium gluconate). May give this dose followed by ½ this dose for 24 hours and then ¼ for an additional 24 hours.

       3. Avoid hypertonic calcium solutions (e.g., Neocalglucon), which are hyperosmolar.

    B. No or "mild" signs; not on oral feeding

       1. Consider the need to treat. Continue to monitor. The usual history of this state includes resolution without treatment.

       2. May be treated or prevented with a continuous infusion containing 50–75 mg (1.25–1.88 mmol) elemental calcium/kg/d during the first 2–3 days of life. *Note:* Calcium is *very* sclerosing if it infuses subcutaneously. If there is any question of patency of IV, *stop* infusion and use a new vein. With a continuous infusion, however, care must be taken to not infuse the calcium at a high rate (e.g., flushing of an umbilical vein catheter, which is near the heart, may be particularly dangerous).

    C. Signs compatible with hypocalcemia and ill

       1. A single dose of 100 mg/kg of calcium gluconate decreases signs and corrects the blood values. (1 mL of 10% calcium gluconate = 100 mg calcium gluconate = 9.2 mg of elemental Ca^{2+}.) *Dilute at least* 1:2 (more if possible). Effect can be short-lived.

       2. If biochemical abnormalities and/or signs are to be avoided, follow bolus with continuous infusion

    D. Tetany

    Immediate treatment consists of 1–2 mL/kg of 10% calcium gluconate with IV fluid via intravenous route (preferred), no faster than 1 mL per minute. Monitor heart rate. Stop infusion at first sign of falling heart rate or when signs abate. Too rapid infusion may induce severe bradycardia or asystole. Continue therapy as mentioned for asymptomatic infant.

V. Comments

    A. Never mix calcium gluconate with IV fluid containing $NaHCO_3$. It will precipitate as calcium carbonate.

B. If hypocalcemia persists despite adequate treatment, further work-up, as well as dietary manipulations, may be necessary.

C. Hypocalcemia will not be corrected by calcium administration if baby is *hypomagnesemic;* thus, assess magnesium level and treat that problem if present.

D. Late hypocalcemia, onset at 5–10 days. Results from high phosphate load or inability of the kidney to excrete phosphate adequately, or inadequate dietary intake.

E. Once treatment is initiated, the QoTc interval is not a reliable way to follow calcium homeostasis.

Suggested Reading

Brown DR, Salsburey DJ: Short-term biochemical effects of parenteral calcium treatment of early-onset neonatal hypocalcemia. J Pediatr 100:777–781, 1982.

Brown DR, Steranka BH, Taylor FH: Treatment of early-onset neonatal hypocalcemia: Effects on serum calcium and ionized calcium. Am J Dis Child 135:24–28, 1981.

Porcelli PJ Jr, Oh W: Effects of single dose calcium gluconate infusion in hypocalcemic preterm infants. Am J Perinatol 12:18–21, 1995.

Salsburey DJ, Brown DR: Effect of parenteral calcium treatment on blood pressure and heart rate in neonatal hypocalcemia. Pediatrics 69:605–609, 1982.

Sauder SE: Endocrinological emergencies. In Donn SM, Faix RG (eds): Neonatal Emergencies. Mt. Kisco, NY, Futura Publishing, 1991, pp 477–500.

Scott SM, Ladenson JH, Aguanna JJ, et al: Effect of calcium therapy in the sick premature infant with early neonatal hypocalcemia. J Pediatr 104:747–751, 1984.

Chapter 23

Hypermagnesemia

Jennifer L. Grow, M.D., and Robert E. Schumacher, M.D.

I. Definition
Serum Mg^{2+} > 2.8 mg/dL

II. Signs and Symptoms
A. Neuromuscular depression/flaccidity
B. Hypotension
C. CNS depression
D. Respiratory depression
E. Tachycardia or bradycardia
F. Ileus

III. Treatment for Symptomatic Hypermagnesemia
A. Supportive
B. Adequate hydration (excretion is renal)
C. Correct acidosis if present
D. Furosemide after hydration
E. Exchange transfusion if *severe* depression

IV. Comments
A. Typically results from maternal $MgSO_4$ administration (preterm labor, preeclampsia)
B. May be intermittent with high doses or inappropriate ratios of Ca, P, and Mg in TPN, especially when maximized to prevent osteopenia of prematurity.
C. Potentiation of hypermagnesemic weakness by gentamicin has been suggested.

Chapter 24

Hypomagnesemia

Jennifer L. Grow, M.D., and Robert E. Schumacher, M.D.

I. Definition
Serum Mg^{2+} < 1.7 mg/dL

II. Signs and Symptoms
  A. Neuromuscular hyperexcitability
  B. Muscle twitching
  C. Seizures
  D. Depression of ST segments and inverted T in precordial leads of ECG

III. Treatment
0.05–0.1 mL of 50% magnesium sulfate (2.5–5 mg elemental magnesium)/kg, IM, or IV. May be repeated every 8–12 hr if necessary (rare).

IV. Maintenance Dose
0.25 mL/kg of 50% $MgSO_4$ PO/d (dilute to 10% concentration)

V. Comments, Etiologies
  A. Etiology: decreased Mg^{2+} supply
    1. Malabsorption
      a. Primary (rare)
      b. Short bowel syndrome
    2. Decreased placental transfer
      a. IUGR
      b. Maternal hypomagnesemia (IDM)
  B. Etiology: increased Mg^{2+} loss
    1. Exchange transfusion with acid citrate blood
    2. Renal dysfunction or diuretics
    3. Inappropriate Ca, P, Mg concentrations or ratios in TPN
  C. Etiology: disordered Mg^{2+} homeostasis
    1. Neonatal hypoparathyroidism
    2. Infant of diabetic mother
    3. Birth asphyxia (controversial)
    4. Hyperphosphatemia

Chapter 25

Hyperkalemia

Jennifer L. Grow, M.D., and Robert E. Schumacher, M.D.

I. Definition

Serum potassium > 7.0 mEq/L* or electrocardiographic evidence at lower levels (tall peaked T waves, S-T depression, QRS widening, prolonged P-R interval). *Exact definition is controversial as population normative values are gestational age-dependent and "action levels" vary according to the clinical situation.

II. Etiologies

A. Increased intake

B. Impaired excretion

    1. Renal failure

    2. Extreme prematurity with immature distal tubular function

    3. Adrenal insufficiency

C. Increased movement into extracellular space

    1. Acidosis

    2. Tissue catabolism

    3. Cell destruction

III. Diagnosis

A. Serum should be obtained from "clean" arterial or venous specimen. Capillary sticks or blood drawn through indwelling catheters usually have excessive hemolysis, falsely elevating the result.

B. ECG (Lead II usually is best)

IV. Treatment

A. Stop all potassium-containing intake

B. Alkalinization

    1. $NaHCO_3$ 1.5–2.0 mEq/kg over 10–15 min

    2. Transient effect 30–60 min later

    3. Temporizing therapy only

C. Calcium gluconate (10%)

    1. 0.5–1.0 mL/kg over 2–5 min

    2. Monitor ECG effects (changes ECG findings but not serum K^+)

D. Glucose/insulin

    1. 0.5–1.0 g/kg glucose

    2. 0.1 units/kg insulin
    3. Give over 15–30 min
    4. Effect in 1 hour, transient
    5. Monitor serum glucose closely

E. Sodium chloride (normal saline)
    1. 10 mL/kg over 10–15 min
    2. Expands extracellular fluids
    3. Increases renal excretion if kidneys normal
    4. More effective in hyponatremia

F. Furosemide

G. Nebulized beta-agonists (albuterol)
    1. 1–2 puffs standardized MDI
    2. Caution: may alter pulmonary mechanics
    3. Fast onset, but do not use as sole therapy.

H. Kayexalate
    1. Ion exchange enema
    2. 0.5–1.0 g/kg PR (or PO)
    3. Effects are delayed. Other acute treatments should be started concomitantly.

I. Peritoneal dialysis or hemodialysis for refractory cases (*see* pages 367 and 368).

Chapter 26

Parenteral Nutrition

Theresa Han-Markey, M.S., R.D., and Robert E. Schumacher, M.D.

I. Indication

Indication for parenteral nutrition is an inability of the neonatal patient to tolerate a minimum of 60 kcal/kg/d via enteral feedings.

II. Administration

Parenteral nutrition may be administered through either peripheral or central venous access.

A. Parenteral nutrition solutions administered via central venous access should be limited to a maximum dextrose concentration of 35% and a maximum amino acid concentration of 6%. Central TPN should contain 0.5–1.0 unit of heparin/mL.

    1. Central TPN solutions may be administered through an umbilical venous catheter (UVC), percutaneous central venous catheter (PCVC), or surgically placed central venous catheter (CVC), once proper line placement is confirmed.

    2. If unable to confirm placement of the catheter tip, parenteral nutrition should be limited to peripheral formulations.

B. Parenteral nutrition solutions administered via peripheral access should be limited to a maximum dextrose concentration of 12.5%.

    1. Umbilical artery catheters (UACs) may be used for parenteral nutrition administration with care if other sites are unavailable.

    2. Infusion through the UAC is against blood flow and, therefore, parenteral nutrition solutions should be limited to peripheral formulations to minimize the risk of thrombosis.

III. Content

Total parenteral nutrition includes dextrose, amino acids, and lipid emulsion, as well as vitamins, minerals, and electrolytes.

A. The majority of calories in parenteral nutrition are generally provided by dextrose.

    1. For full-term infants, the estimated hepatic glycogen mobilization rate is 4–6 mg/kg/min; therefore, most newborns should be able to tolerate a comparable glucose load.

    2. Infants < 1000 g body weight may be unable to tolerate this glucose load during the first few days of life.

    a. Calculations for the glucose load are as follows: percent dextrose $\times$ 0.01 $\times$ total volume = grams dextrose infused.

$$\text{glucose load (mg/kg/min)} = \frac{(\text{g dextrose})(1000 \text{ mg/g})}{(\text{kg body wt})(1440 \text{ min/d})}$$

    b. Increases in dextrose concentration of 1.5–2 mg/kg/min per day to a maximum of 11–14 mg/kg/min may be tolerated by most newborns.

3. Tolerance of glucose administration is indicated by glucose screening values of 60–150 mg/dL with negative to trace glucose in urine.

    a. Serum glucose provides a more accurate measurement of glucose tolerance.

    b. Because of immature renal function, urine glucose of up to 2+ with a normal serum glucose level does not necessarily indicate glucose intolerance.

    c. Sudden intolerance to a previously tolerated glucose load may be an early indication of sepsis or stress, or IVH in the premature infant.

    d. For those patients demonstrating glucose intolerance, dextrose concentration should be returned to the concentration most recently tolerated.

    e. Insulin administration should be considered when the patient demonstrates extreme glucose intolerance.

        i. The response of newborns to insulin therapy is unpredictable, and therefore requires careful monitoring.

        ii. An insulin pump should be used for insulin administration for more consistent dosage.

4. Calories from dextrose are calculated as follows: (0.01)(% dextrose)(mL infused) = g dextrose. g dextrose $\times$ 3.4 kcal/g = kcal from dextrose.

5. Avoid interruption of dextrose administration for more than 30 minutes as this may result in reactive hypoglycemia.

B. Protein is supplied in the form of crystalline amino acids.

1. Amino acids (AA) are ordered on the first day of TPN.

    a. AA can be administered beginning at 1.0 g/kg/d and advanced by 0.5–1 g/kg/d to maximum of 3.5 g/kg/d.

    b. AA infusions greater than 3.0 g/kg/d can result in increased BUN, the clinical consequences of which are speculative.

    c. To avoid the use of AA as an energy source, the total nonprotein calories must be sufficient to spare AA for protein synthesis (Table 29).

TABLE 29
Nonprotein-to-Protein Ratios

Nonprotein cal/kg	g/protein/kg
25	1.0
35	1.5
50	2.0
70+	2.5

2. Infants < 1000 g have limited energy and can receive TPN as early as day 1 of life.
3. For patients with renal insufficiency and increased serum BUN, limit AA to 1.5 g/kg/d until there is a downward trend in BUN.
4. Calories from protein = g/kg AA × body weight (kg) × 4.

C. Lipids provide a concentrated calorie source and may provide up to 60% of total calories.
1. Fat is provided as a 20% safflower/soybean oil emulsion. The 10% solution contains excessive phospholipids and is not recommended.
2. Lipids can be administered on day 1 of TPN beginning at 0.5–1.0 g/kg/d and advanced 0.5–1 g/kg/d to a maximum of 3 g/kg/d.
   Note: Calculations for grams of lipid are: mL lipid × % lipid × 0.01 = grams of lipid.
   a. Lipid administration should be at ≤ 0.25 mg/kg/hr to minimize complications associated with lipid administration.
   b. Lipid tolerance improves with a longer duration of infusion. Infusion should run at least 12 hr/day, preferably up to 24 hr/day.
   c. A minimum of 0.5–1.0 g/kg/d intravenous lipid (2–4% of total calories) is required to meet daily essential fatty acid requirements.
3. It is impossible to provide adequate calories for growth without intravenous lipids.
4. Lipid intolerance may be indicated by a serum triglyceride level ≥ 200 mg/dL. Elevated triglyceride levels may be associated with normal lipid metabolism. A more accurate test, which is not currently standardized, is serum-free fatty acid levels. Currently, intralipids are decreased for triglyceride levels > 200 mg/dL.
   a. A sudden increase in serum triglycerides not associated with an increase in lipid dose may be an indication of sepsis or stress.

      b. VLBW or septic infants may not tolerate maximum dosage of lipids.

    5. Calories from lipids can be calculated as:
      kcal from 20% = mL lipid $\times$ 2.0 kcal/mL.

    6. As IV lipid administration may affect bilirubin binding, bacterial clearance, pulmonary arterial resistance, oxygen diffusion ratio, pulmonary fat accumulation, and thrombocytopenia, the maximum dose of lipids may be contraindicated for infants with these problems (*see* VII *below*).

    7. The need for carnitine is controversial and currently neonatal TPN is not supplemented with it.

D. Suggested amounts of electrolytes to be added to TPN are as follows:

Sodium	2–5 mEq/kg/d
Potassium	2–4 mEq/kg/d
Magnesium	0.3–1 mEq/kg/d
Calcium	1–3 mEq/kg/d
Phosphorus	0.5–2.0 mM/kg/d

    1. Phosphorus can be provided as a salt of potassium or sodium (1 mM K_3PO_4 provides 1.47 mEq K^+; 1 mM Na_3PO_4 provides 1.33 mEq Na^+).

    2. To avoid precipitation of Ca and P in solution, pharmacists must calculate the precipitation factor.

    3. The amount of Ca and P in the TPN solution should be maximized within the precipitation guidelines to minimize the effects of osteopenia of prematurity. A Ca/P mg ratio of 2:1 maximizes retention. Only a maximum of 60% of calcium requirements can be met parenterally. Alternate day calcium and phosphorous infusions are ineffective. The efficacy of additional vitamin D supplements has not been proven.

    4. The ratio of Ca:P that may promote the greatest retention of both Ca and P is > 1.1:1 to 2:1 (mEq/mM) for most infants; however, a ratio of 1.7:1 is probably best for VLBW infants.

    5. Intravenous nutrition cannot provide sufficient minerals for bone accretion. Significantly more minerals are present in enteral formulas, and feeds should be initiated as soon as reasonable.

E. Current daily vitamin recommendations can be met by the following daily doses of Infuvite Pediatric Solution:
    < 1750 g infant: 3.3 mL
    $\geq$ 1750 g infant: 5 mL

F. Current daily trace element recommendations can be met by 0.2 mL of Pediatric Trace Element Solution for all birthweights.

G. Intravenous iron is potentially quite dangerous; therefore, its use is restricted to the rare circumstance of an infant remaining NPO > 2 months without receiving blood transfusions. Once feeding enterally, 2 mg/kg/d of elemental iron should meet maintenance needs. Treatment of anemia and/or use of erythropoietin will increase iron requirement to 5–6 mg/kg/d.

H. To avoid thromboses and facilitate intravenous lipid utilization, heparin is routinely added to central TPN solution. In smaller infants at high infusion rates excessive heparin can be inadvertently administered. To avoid these complications, the following is suggested:

1. $\geq$ 1500 g infant: 1.0 unit/mL heparin is added to the TPN
2. $<$ 1500 g infant: 0.5 unit/mL heparin is added to the TPN, if the volume of solution is $>$ 150 mL; if TPN volume $<$ 150 mL, 1 unit/mL is added

IV. Recommendations for Ordering TPN

A. Calculate the total TPN fluid to be administered to the infant [total daily fluid − (arterial line + other IV)]

B. Calculate amount of lipids to be administered to patient (*see* III., C.) and subtract this volume from total TPN fluid.

C. Calculate dextrose concentration (*see* III, A).

D. Calculate protein to be delivered (*see* III, B).

E. Calculate electrolyte needs (*see* III, D).

V. Caloric Requirements

Although caloric requirements vary with clinical status, total parenteral calorie requirements have been estimated at approximately 80–105 kcal/kg/d for the premature infant.

A. Caloric intake should be adjusted to the amount of calories necessary to promote appropriate weight gain.

B. Total caloric intake must be carefully monitored during the transition from parenteral nutrition to enteral nutrition.

1. The volume of enteral feedings necessary to provide adequate calories should be calculated.
2. Parenteral nutrition should be continued until the patient tolerates 75% of the estimated enteral caloric needs.
3. Calories from lipids should not exceed 60% of total.
4. Amino acids from combined, enteral, and parenteral nutrition should not exceed 3 g/kg/d.

VI. Recommended Parameters to Be Monitored While the Patient Is Receiving Parenteral Nutrition

A. Weight

B. Electrolytes, daily for at least the first week; thereafter, every 2–3 days depending on the patient's status.

C. Baseline serum magnesium concentration

D. CBC, BUN, creatinine, Ca, P, Mg, alkaline phosphatase, and total and direct bilirubin, weekly.

E. Triglycerides, when at maximum IV lipid administration, and weekly thereafter.

VII. Complications

Three basic types of complications associated with the use of TPN include mechanical, infectious, and metabolic.

A. Mechanical complications may include those associated with insertion or use of the catheter, such as pneumothorax, hematoma, or vessel lacerations; catheter malposition or dislodgment; pulmonary embolism; skin slough; phlebitis; thrombosis; or catheter occlusion.

    1. Complications arising from administration of TPN through a UAC in newborns may be associated with vasospasm, thrombosis, embolization, hypertension, hemorrhage, and necrotizing enterocolitis.

    2. Occlusion of 2.7-Fr Broviac catheters may be treated as follows:

       a. Calculate the intraluminal volume of the catheter: volume = length (cm) $\times$ 0.002 mL/cm (volume/length).

       b. Reconstitute urokinase (5000 U/mL).

       c. Instill calculated amount of agent into each occluded lumen and let sit for 30 minutes. Aspirate contents into a syringe. Repeat if necessary.

B. Infection is considered the major complication of centrally infused parenteral nutrition.

    1. Placement of catheters under strict aseptic conditions, and meticulous care of the catheter site with standardized dressing changes will reduce the incidence of septic complications.

    2. Avoidance of the use of the TPN catheter for blood drawing and administration of medications or blood products whenever possible will minimize the risk of contamination.

C. Only the more common metabolic complications of TPN administration are listed below:

    1. For information regarding hyperglycemia/hypoglycemia, see Chapters 20 and 21.

    2. Possible lipid-related disorders include alterations in glucose homeostasis, bilirubin binding, oxygenation, immune function, and coagulation function.

    a. Incidents of hyperglycemia during lipid infusion, which continued for up to 1–9 hours after discontinuing the infusion, have been reported in infants.

    b. Free fatty acids may compete with bilirubin for binding sites on serum albumin.

3. Clinical signs of essential fatty acid deficiency (EFAD) may occur with as little as 1 week of fat-free parenteral nutrition.

    a. Clinical signs of EFAD include scaly dermatitis, sparse hair growth, increased susceptibility to infection, thrombocytopenia, and poor growth.

    b. As little as 1–3% of total calories as linoleic acid prevents EFAD.

    c. Controversy exists regarding whether intravenous lipids increase alveolar-arterial oxygen gradients. Phospholipids maybe the injurious component.

    d. There is some controversy concerning the effect lipids may have on the immune function of the infant.

      i. Most current in vivo studies do not indicate compromise of immune function with lipid infusion.

      ii. However, the effect of lipid infusion on the immune system may depend on the type of lipid used.

    e. Although some investigators have reported thrombocytopenia in infants after lipid infusion, others have reported improvement of platelet counts with lipid infusion and correction of fatty acid deficiency.

4. For information related to mineral deficiencies, see Chapters 22 and 24.

5. For information related to osteopenia of prematurity, see Chapter 29.

6. TPN-related cholestasis can be defined as a direct bilirubin of greater than 2 mg/dL in a patient who has been on TPN for 2 weeks or more. Amino acids appear to be the important agent.

    a. All other possible causes of cholestasis should be ruled out.

    b. Because TPN-related cholestasis may progress to end-stage liver disease, the goal is to discontinue TPN as soon as possible.

    c. If the patient is unable to tolerate full enteral feeds, other suggested treatments include initiating hypocaloric enteral feeds; arranging TPN solution so that amino acid administration is given on a cyclic schedule (as opposed to continuously); protecting the TPN solution from photo-oxidation; and decreasing the amino acids in solution to 1.5–2 g/kg/d.

    d. Minimize use of drugs contributing to GI dysmotility (e.g., morphine).

    e. Low-dose phenobarbital may help treat direct hyperbilirubinemia.

Suggested Reading

American Society for Parenteral and Enteral Nutrition (ASPEN) Board of Directors: Standards for Hospitalized Pediatric Patients. Nutr Clin Pract 11:217–228, 1996.

ASPEN. Board of Directors and the Clinical Guidelines Task Force: Guidelines for the Use of Parenteral and Enteral Nutrition in Adult and Pediatric Patients. J Parenter Enteral Nutr 26:1SA–138SA, 2002.

Baker RD Jr, Baker SS, Davis AM (eds): Pediatric Parenteral Nutrition. New York, Chapman & Hall, 1997.

Baugh N, Recupero MA, Kerner JA: Nutritional requirements for pediatric patients. In Merritt RJ (ed): The ASPEN Nutrition Support Practice Manual. Silver Spring, MD, American Society for Parenteral and Enteral Nutrition, 1998.

Cairns PA, Stalker DJ: Carnitine supplementation of parenterally fed neonates. Cochrane Database Syst Rev 1:CD001016, 2002.

Greene HL, Hambridge KM, Schanler R, Tsang RC: Guidelines for the use of vitamins, trace elements, calcium, magnesium and phosphorus in infants and children receiving total parenteral nutrition: Report of the Subcommittee on Pediatric Parenteral Nutrient Requirements from the Committee on Clinical Practice Issues of the American Society for Clinical Nutrition. Am J Clin Nutr 48:1324–1342, 1988.

Groh-Wargo S, Thompson M, Cox JH (eds): Nutritional Care for High-Risk Newborns. Chicago, Precept Press, 2000.

Haumont D, Deckelbaum RJ, Richelle M, et al: Plasma lipid and plasma lipoprotein concentrations in low birth weight infants given parenteral nutrition with twenty or ten percent lipid emulsion. J Pediatr 115:787–793, 1989.

Hay WW Jr, Lucas A, Heird WC, et al: Workshop summary: Nutrition of the extremely low birth weight infant. Pediatrics 104:1360–1368, 1999.

Heron P, Bourchier D: Insulin infusions in infants of birthweight less than 1250 g and with glucose intolerance. Aust Pediatr J 24:362–365, 1988.

Kalhan S, Bier D, Yaffe S, et al: Protein/amino acid metabolism and nutrition in very low birth weight infants. J Perinatol 21:320–323, 2001.

Kanarek KS, Santeiro ML, Malone JI: Continuous infusion of insulin in hyperglycemic low-birth weight infants receiving parenteral nutrition with and without lipids. J Parenter Enteral Nutr 15:417–420, 1991.

Kennedy KA, Tyson JE, Chamnanvanakij S: Rapid versus slow rate of advancement of feedings for promoting growth and preventing necrotizing enterocolitis in parenterally fed low-birth-weight infants. Cochrane Database Syst Rev 2:CD001241, 2000.

Khalidi N, Btaiche I, Kovacevich D: The University of Michigan Parenteral and Enteral Nutrition Manual, 8th ed. Ann Arbor, MI, University of Michigan Health System, 2002.

Kleinman RE (ed): Pediatric Nutrition Handbook, 4th ed. Elk Grove Village, IL, American Academy of Pediatrics, Committee on Nutrition, 1998.

Ostertag SG, Jovanovic L, Lewis B, Auld PAM: Insulin pump therapy in the very low birth weight infant. Pediatrics 78:625–630, 1986.

Pelegano JF, Rowe JC, Carey DE, et al: Simultaneous infusion of calcium and phosphorus in parenteral nutrition for premature infants: Use of physiologic calcium/phosphorus ratio. J Pediatr 114:115–119, 1989.

Safe Practices of Parenteral Nutrition Formulations. National Advisory Group and Practice Guidelines for Parenteral Nutrition. J Parenter Enteral Nutr 22:49–66, 1998.

Samour PQ, Helm KK, Lang C (eds): Handbook of Pediatric Nutrition, 2nd ed. Gaithersburg, MD, Aspen Publishers, 1999.

Stahl GE, Spear ML, Hamosh M: Intravenous administration of lipid emulsions to premature infants. Clin Perinatol 13:133–162, 1986.

Taylor R, Baker A: Enteral nutrition in critical illness: Part One. Paediatr Nurs 11:16, 1999.

Taylor R, Baker A: Enteral nutrition in critical illness: Part Two. Paediatr Nurs 11:26–31, 1999.

Teitelbaum DH, Tracy T: Parenteral nutrition-associated cholestasis. Semin Pediatr Surg 10:72–80, 2001.

Thureen PJ, Hay WW Jr: Intravenous nutrition and postnatal growth of the micropremie. Clin Perinatol 27:197–219, 2000.

Chapter 27

Enteral Nutrition

Theresa Han-Markey, M.S., R.D., and Robert E. Schumacher, M.D.

I. Goals

A. Energy (E) stored = E intake − E expended − E excreted.

B. An energy intake of 105–135 kcal/kg/d is recommended for growth in most preterm infants. Higher intakes may improve growth in cases with increased energy expenditure, such as BPD or IUGR.

C. Exogenous protein will also be necessary if endogenous protein stores are to be preserved.

D. Specific recommendations for fluid and electrolyte management are included on pages 123–125.

E. Although the optimal rate of growth and retention of nutrients for preterm infants is still not known, present standards are based on in utero growth rates.

F. The quality of postnatal growth may vary from the quality of fetal growth because of the difference in source of nutrients.

II. Enteral Feedings

A. Indications for use

1. Early enteral feedings (*trophic feedings*) may promote the secretion and the induction of intestinal hormones that enhance growth and maturation of villi and stimulate intestinal motility.

2. Enteral feedings may increase intestinal motility and excretion of bilirubin, thereby reducing physiologic jaundice of prematurity.

3. Enteral feedings may protect against TPN-induced cholestasis.

4. Enteral feedings provide more calcium and phosphorous than TPN and appear to reduce the incidence of osteopenia of prematurity.

5. Enteral feedings decrease the risk of catheter-related sepsis.

B. Routes of enteral feeding and feeding techniques

1. Tube feedings are indicated for infants with immature suck/swallow (≤ 34 weeks' gestation), those neurologically impaired, and those recovering from respiratory distress.

   a. Orally placed tubes are preferred because nasal tubes increase upper airway resistance.

      i. An orogastric tube is used if gastric function is normal.

      ii. Infrequently, an orojejunal tube may be trialed with infants who have significant GE reflux, excessive gastric residuals, or in some infants receiving CPAP.

   b. Continuous tube feedings are an uninterrupted cycle of feeding given by infusion pump.

      i. Advantages

         (a) Continuous feedings may be useful for the VLBW infant in transition from TPN.

         (b) Continuous feedings may be preferred for ELBW infants or infants who are intolerant of intermittent feedings.

         (c) Continuous feedings may be used following gastrointestinal surgery.

         (d) Continuous feedings may allow the ELBW infant to achieve full enteral feedings sooner.

      ii. Disadvantages

         (a) Continuous feedings are more susceptible to bacterial contamination.

         (b) Continuous infusion at low rates (< 5 mL/hr) may result in decreased delivery of minerals from infant formula or loss of fat from human milk secondary to separation.

         (c) Continuous feedings do not allow cycling of enteric hormones.

   c. Intermittent tube feedings are given at timed intervals (usually every 2–3 hr) by gravity drip, syringe, or infusion pump.

      i. Intermittent feedings more closely approximate normal "cyclic" physiology of feeding.

      ii. Intermittent feedings may not be tolerated by the ELBW baby because of immaturity of the GI system.

      iii. Intermittent feedings should be given to an infant placed in a prone or right lateral decubitus position to facilitate gastric emptying.

   d. Trials of continuous versus intermittent feedings have been reviewed.

      i. Infants fed continuously reach full feeds faster.

      ii. Neither method has been shown to reliably confer any benefits vs. the other method.

2. Nipple feeding may be initiated in infants over 34 weeks' gestation who demonstrate the ability to suck and swallow, and who are stable.

    a. Oral feeding guidelines
       i. Initiate one nipple feed per shift with a maximum of 10 minutes per feeding and a minimum of 3 feedings before advancing.
      ii. Advance as tolerated, monitoring for adequate weight gain and evidence of satiety.
    b. Breastfeeding (*see* Chapter 28)
       i. Appropriate lactation counseling should be provided soon after birth for mothers whose infants are unable to initially breastfeed.
      ii. Indicators of success are maintenance of the infant's pattern of weight gain and evidence of satiety.
     iii. Social feeding or skin-to-skin contact (as in kangaroo care) preceding true attempts at breastfeeding may help maintain maternal milk supply and promote success.
     iv. Breastfeeding should be encouraged as soon as oral feedings are initiated. There is no need to learn to bottle feed before breastfeeding.
      v. Breastfeeding mothers should be given as much privacy and encouragement as possible. The practice of weighing an infant before and after breastfeeding is discouraged, unless there is strong evidence of inadequate intake.

C. Initiation of enteral feedings
  1. Early hypocaloric enteral feeds may promote development of the bowel, enzyme induction in the brush border, release of gut hormones and prohormones, and facilitate earlier tolerance of full feeds. Trophic feeds of 0.5–1.0 mL/hr (without advancement) may be sufficient and should be considered in all stable infants, including the ELBW infant.
  2. Larger infants (> 1000 g) may receive a test feeding of 1–3 mL formula or human milk at 2–4 hours of age. Some stable smaller infants tolerate bolus feedings. The volume of the "unfed" stomach is approximately 3 mL/kg.
  3. Caution should be exercised in the following circumstances:
    a. Extreme immaturity of neurologic and gastrointestinal systems will predispose infants to delayed gastric emptying and hypomotility of the gut.
    b. Significant hypotension, hypothermia, or generalized instability may be reasons to defer enteral feedings.
    c. Asphyxia may predispose the newborn to ileus, NEC, malabsorption, and increased risk of aspiration.

    d. Pancuronium and morphine significantly reduce the rate of gastric emptying and cause hypomotility of the gut.

    e. Respiratory distress or tachypnea may predispose to aspiration.

    f. The presence of a UAC may indicate that the infant is still not stable enough to consider initiating enteral feedings.

D. Progression of enteral feedings

1. The progression to full feeding (approximately 105–135 kcal/kg) in the low birthweight infant should be gradual (6–10 d), based on gestational age and birthweight.

2. Increases of 10–20 mL/kg/d are usually tolerated.

3. Do not change strength and volume of feeding at the same time.

4. There should be continuous evaluation of feeding tolerance.

    a. Significant emesis, abdominal distention, absence of bowel sounds, visible bowel loops, significant gastric residuals, and guaiac positive stools are signs of intolerance and may indicate the need to decrease or stop the feedings.

       i. Delayed gastric emptying may be associated with GE reflux, RDS, CHD, opiates, or beta-adrenergic drugs, and hyperosmolar formulas.

       ii. Gastric emptying may be promoted by continuous tube feedings, small frequent feedings, or metoclopramide administration.

    b. Acceptable quantities of aspirates range from 2 to 4 mL/kg (but can be higher).

       i. Pay attention to trends.

       ii. If aspirates seem excessive but continued feeds are planned, subtract the excessive amount from the volume of the next feed.

       iii. Aspirates may be re-fed to help maintain electrolyte balance.

III. Choices for Enteral Feeding

A. Human milk

1. Human milk from an infant's own mother offers macrophages, immunoglobulins, complement, and lactoferrin to provide immunity; prostaglandins and intestinal growth factor to stimulate gastrointestinal development; easily digested fat; a desirable protein composition; nucleotides; and unique long-chain fatty acids.

2. Human milk is variable in nutrient composition. Mature human milk has less protein and fat than early postpartum milk. Caloric content averages 20 kcal/oz, but maybe as few as 12 kcal/oz.

3. Human milk must be supplemented to meet the energy, protein, vitamin, and mineral requirements for optimal growth of the VLBW infant. Supplementation of human milk with protein, sodium, calcium, phosphorus, magnesium, and vitamin D should be considered when the preterm infant is tolerating a volume that will promote growth.

4. Vitamin supplementation is suggested for full-term infants consuming only human milk; iron supplementation should be considered at discharge.

B. Formula (Tables 30–33)

1. Premature formulas have been developed to provide nutrients in the amounts appropriate to support growth for preterm infants approaching intrauterine rates.

2. Standard infant formulas intended for full-term infants or elemental formulas (such as Pregestimil) are inadequate in protein, minerals, and vitamins and must be supplemented if consumed by the preterm infant.

3. Soy formulas are not recommended for standard use in premature infants because of the questionable availability of minerals.

IV. Meeting Nutrient Needs Enterally

A. Calories

1. A calorie range of 105–135 kcal/kg/d will allow most infants to achieve satisfactory growth rates.

2. Energy requirements may be increased above 135 kcal/kg/d for growth-restricted infants, or infants with chronic illness, major surgery, or infection.

B. Protein

1. The estimated enteral protein requirement for the premature infant is 3.5–4 g/kg/d based on fetal accretion rates.

2. The estimated enteral protein requirement for the full-term infant is 2.2 g/kg/d.

3. Human milk is appropriate for full-term infants but may have an inadequate amount of protein to satisfy calculated requirements for VLBW infants and should be supplemented with a human milk fortifier. The protein content decreases as human milk matures.

4. The protein requirements and utilization depend on the carbohydrate and fat composition of the diet.

5. Human milk and formula contain taurine.

6. Nucleotides are in human milk and some formulas.

TABLE 30
Formulas for Term Infants

Per 100 kcal	Unit	Human Milk	Enfamil (Mead Johnson)	Enfamil Lipil* (Mead Johnson)	Similac (Ross)	Similac PM 60/40 (Ross)
Protein	g	1.46	2.1	2.1	2.07	2.22
Carbohydrate	g	10.00	10.9	10.9	10.80	10.20
Fat	g	5.42	5.3	5.3	5.40	5.59
Linoleic	g	0.54	0.860	0.860	1.00	1.30
Vitamin A	IU	310.00	300.00	300.00	300.00	300.00
Vitamin D	IU	3.05	60.00	60.00	60.00	60.00
Vitamin E	IU	0.32	2.00	2.00	1.50	2.50
Vitamin K	μg	0.29	8.00	8.00	8.00	8.00
Ascorbate	mg	5.56	12.00	12.00	9.00	9.00
Thiamin	μg	29.17	80.00	80.00	100.00	100.00
Riboflavin	μg	48.61	140.00	140.00	150.00	150.00
Pyridoxine	μg	28.50	60.00	60.00	60.00	60.00
Niacin	μg	208.00	1000.00	1000.00	1050.00	1050.00
Pantothenate	μg	250.00	500.00	500.00	450.00	450.00
Biotin	μg	0.56	3.00	3.00	4.40	4.0
Folic acid	μg	6.94	16.0	16.0	15.00	15.00
Vitamin B_{12}	μg	0.07	0.30	0.30	0.25	0.25
Sodium	mg	25.00	27.00	27.00	30.00	24.00
Potassium	mg	73.00	108.00	108.00	107.00	86.00
Magnesium	mg	4.86	8.00	8.00	6.00	6.00
Iron	mg	0.04	1.80	1.80	1.8	0.22
Zinc	μg	0.17	1.00	1.00	0.75	0.75
Copper	μg	35.00	75.00	75.00	90.00	90.00

(Table continues on following page)

TABLE 30
Formulas for Term Infants (Continued)

Per 100 kcal	Unit	Human Milk	Enfamil (Mead Johnson)	Enfamil Lipil* (Mead Johnson)	Similac (Ross)	Similac PM 60/40 (Ross)
Selenium	μg	—	2.80	2.80	2.20	—
Chromium	μg	—	—	—	—	—
Manganese	μg	0.08	15.00	15.00	5.00	5.00
Molybdenum	μg	—	—	—	—	—
Iodine	μg	15.28	10.0	10.0	6.0	6.00
Taurine	mg	5.56	yes	yes	yes	yes
Carnitine	mg	yes	no	no	yes	yes
Inositol	mg	yes	6.00	6.00	4.70	24.00
Choline	mg	12.50	12.0	12.0	16.00	12.00

*Available with or without iron and 20 or 24 kcal/oz. Contains arachidonic acid, docosahexaenoic acid.

TABLE 31
Nutrient Profiles of Formulas for Premature Infants (20 and 24 kcal/oz)

Per 100 kcal	Unit	Similac Special Care (Ross)	Enfamil Premature LIPIL (Mead Johnson)	Enfamil Human Milk Fortifier Mixed (Mead Johnson)	Enfamil Enfacare (Mead Johnson)	Similac Natural Care (Ross)	Similac Human Milk Fortifier + Preterm Human Milk 1 pkt:25 mL	Similac NeoSure (Ross)
Protein	g	2.71	3.00	2.90	2.80	2.71	2.97	2.60
Carbohydrate	g	10.60	11.10	12.50	10.70	10.60	10.40	10.30
Lactose	g	5.30	4.60	9.10	—	5.30	—	5.15
Oligomers	g	5.30	6.50	2.60	—	—	—	—
Fat	g	5.43	5.10	4.40	5.30	5.43	5.24	5.50
Linoleic	g	0.70	0.81	—	0.95	0.70	—	0.75
Linolenic	mg	—	90.00	—	—	—	—	—
Vitamin A	iu	1250.00	1250.00	1250.00	450.00	1250.00	1245.00	460.00
Vitamin D	iu	150.00	240.00	270.00	80.00	150.00	150.00	70.00
Vitamin E	iu	4.00	6.30	6.20	4.00	4.00	5.30	3.60
Vitamin K	µg	12.00	8.00	8.00	8.00	12.00	11.00	11.00
Ascorbate	mg	37.00	20.00	20.00	16.00	37.00	44.00	15.00
Thiamin	µg	250.00	200.00	200.00	200.00	250.00	313.00	220.00
Riboflavin	µg	620.00	300.00	300.00	200.00	620.00	574.00	150.00
Pyridoxine	µg	250.00	150.00	150.00	100.00	250.00	278.00	100.00
Niacin	mg	5.00	4.00	4.00	2.00	5.00	4.58	1.95
Pantothenate	mg	1.90	1.20	1.20	850.00	1.90	2.07	0.80
Biotin	µg	37.00	4.00	4.10	6.00	37.00	32.60	9.00
Folate	µg	37.00	40.00	35.00	26.00	37.00	32.00	25.00

(Table continues on following page)

TABLE 31

Nutrient Profiles of Formulas for Premature Infants (20 and 24 kcal/oz) (Continued)

Per 100 kcal	Unit	Similac Special Care (Ross)	Enfamil Premature LIPIL (Mead Johnson)	Enfamil Human Milk Fortifier Mixed (Mead Johnson)	Enfamil Enfacare (Mead Johnson)	Similac Natural Care (Ross)	Similac Human Milk Fortifier + Preterm Human Milk 1 pkt:25 mL	Similac NeoSure (Ross)
Vitamin B_{12}	µg	0.55	0.25	0.25	0.30	0.55	0.85	0.40
Sodium	mg	43.00	39.00	44.00	35.00	43.00	49.00	33.00
Potassium	mg	129.00	103.00	82.00	105.00	129.00	148.00	142.00
Chloride	mg	81.00	85.00	95.00	78.00	81.00	115.00	75.00
Calcium	mg	180.00	165.00	144.00	120.00	210.00	175.00	105.00
Phosphorus	mg	90.00	83.00	74.00	66.00	116.00	98.00	62.00
Magnesium	mg	12.00	9.00	5.40	8.00	12.00	12.40	9.00
Iron	mg	0.37	1.80	0.11	1.80	0.37	0.60	1.80
Zinc	µg	1500.00	1500.00	1350.00	1250.00	1500.00	1650.00	1200.00
Copper	µg	250.00	120.00	125.00	120.00	250.00	289.00	120.00
Selenium	µg	1.80	2.8	—	2.30	1.80	6.20	2.30
Chromium	µg	—	0.0	—	—	—	—	—
Manganese	µg	12.00	6.3	6.30	15.00	12.00	10.00	—
Molybdenum	µg	—	0.0	—	—	—	—	—
Iodine	µg	20.00	25.00	22.00	15.00	6.00	6.20	—
Taurine	mg	6.70	6.0	55.00	Yes	6.70	—	yes
Carnitine	mg	5.90	2.4	—	Yes	—	—	yes
Inositol	mg	5.50	44.00	—	15.00	5.50	23.00	—
Choline	mg	10.00	20.00	12.50	30.00	10.00	14.00	—

TABLE 32
Special and Soy-Based Formulas 20 kcal/oz (67 kcal/dL)

	Enfamil 20+ Premature (Mead Johnson)	Enfamil 24+ Premature (Mead Johnson)	Similac Special Care 20 (Ross)	Similac Special Care 24 (Ross)
Indications for use	Premature infants	Growing premature infants	Premature infants	Growing premature infants
kcal/mL	0.67	0.81	0.67	0.81
Protein g/dL source	2.00 whey & nonfat milk	2.41 whey & nonfat milk	1.83 whey & nonfat milk	2.19 whey & nonfat milk
Fat g/dL source	3.40 MCT, soy oils	4.10 MCT, soy oils	3.70 MCT, soy & coconut oils	4.38 MCT, soy & coconut oils
Carbohydrate g/dL source	7.40 corn syrup solids, lactose	9.00 corn syrup solids, lactose	7.16 corn syrup solids, lactose	8.5 corn syrup solids, lactose
Water Osm/kg	240.00	300.00	235.00	280.00
Sodium Eq/L	11.30	13.70	12.60	15.10
Potassium Eq/L	17.60	21.30	22.30	26.6
Calcium g/L	1110.00	1340.00	1216.00	1452.00
Phosphorus g/L	560.00	680.00	676.00	806.00

C. Fat
   1. Fat in formulas and human milk provides approximately 40–50% of calories and greater than 3% as linoleic acid.
   2. Fat in human milk is well absorbed because of distribution of fatty acids in the triglyceride molecule and the presence of bile salt-activated lipase and human milk lipase. The fat content in human milk decreases as it matures.
   3. Fat absorption from human milk may be decreased by calcium supplementation.
   4. Special formulas for premature infants contain a mixture of medium-chain triglycerides (MCT can be absorbed without chylomicron formulation) and mostly unsaturated long-chain triglycerides.
   5. Human milk and all formulas contain carnitine.
   6. Omega-3, omega-6 long-chain polyunsaturated fatty acids may be essential nutrients for premature infants. Docosahexaenoic acid and arachidonic acid are present in variable amounts in human milk and in lesser amounts in unsupplemented formulas.

TABLE 33
Guidelines for Initiating Enteral Feedings in Preterm Infants

Birthweight	1000 g	1250 g	1500 g	2000 g	> 2000 g
Volume first feeding schedule of feeding	0.5 mL continuous (tube)	3 mL q3h, OR 1.0 mL continuous (tube)	4 mL q3h	5 mL q34h	0 mL q3h
Type of first feeding	Human milk or formula	Human milk or formula	Human milk or formula	Human milk or formula	Human milk or formula
Volume/rate of milk increase	10–20 mL/kg/d	10–20 mL/kg/d	20 mL/kg/d	20 mL/kg/d: may increase faster if tolerating feedings well	5 mL every other feed; may increase faster if tolerating feedings well

Formulas supplemented with the same may have effects on the developmental processes of premature infants.

D. Carbohydrates

1. The premature infant has low intestinal lactase activity, which may limit the ability to digest lactose.
2. Standard infant formulas are intended for use with full-term infants and contain lactose as the carbohydrate source.
3. Premature infant formulas contain 50–60% glucose polymers (which are easily digested by glycosidase enzymes) and 40–50% lactose.
4. Human milk contains principally lactose, with trace amounts of glucose, oligosaccharides, and glycoproteins. The lactose content of human milk increases as it matures.

E. Selected minerals

1. Sodium
   a. Renal sodium conservation mechanisms are not well developed in the low birthweight infant.
   b. Some VLBW infants may require 4–8 mEq/kg/d of sodium to prevent hyponatremia.
   c. Premature formulas provide 2 mEq Na/100 kcal.
   d. Human milk provides 1.1–1.3 mEq Na/100 kcal.
2. The potassium requirement of low birthweight infants is similar to that of full-term, e.g., 2–3 mEq/kg/d. Careful adjustment is necessary with renal impairment, hemolysis, or the use of drugs such as furosemide or amphotericin B.
3. Calcium, phosphorus, and magnesium
   a. The advisable intakes of calcium (140–160 mg/l00 kcal) and phosphorus (95–108 mg/100 kcal) for the preterm infant are based on anticipated fetal accretion rates in the last trimester.
   b. Human milk and standard infant formulas do not provide enough calcium and phosphorus to enable the preterm infant to meet normal fetal accretion rates and should be supplemented until the infant reaches 3–3.5 kg.
   c. Only the specialized premature formulas (e.g., Enfamil Premature and Similac Special Care) approach the advisable intakes for calcium and phosphorus.
   d. The duration of supplementation required is controversial. The smallest infants will need supplements for longer periods. The use of premature follow-up formulas may be beneficial.
   e. While soy formulas provide for adequate bone mineralization

in term infants, they may not meet mineral needs of preterm infants.

   f. If calcium and phosphorus are supplemented to the level intended to meet fetal accretion rates, additional magnesium supplementation (up to 20 mg/kg/d) may be needed. Serum magnesium values do not necessarily reflect overall magnesium balance.

  4. Iron

    a. Premature infants have low iron stores at birth.

    b. Iron supplementation (2–3 mg/kg/d) of elemental iron in the form of ferrous sulfate, may begin by age 2–4 weeks of life or whenever full enteral feedings are tolerated. Full formula feeds provide this amount of iron.

    c. Premature infants fed human milk and receiving iron, should also be supplemented with 4–5 IU vitamin E per day, available in fortifier or 1 mL of MVI.

    d. Physiologic anemia of prematurity is not prevented by iron therapy.

    e. Large supplements of iron ($\geq$ 6 mg/kg/d) may be required with use of erythropoietin.

F. Selected vitamins

  1. Vitamin A

    a. Vitamin A is recommended at 450 μg/kg/d or 1500 IU/kg/d.

    b. Supplementation with the above doses results in normal serum values.

    c. Supplementation with much larger repeated doses of vitamin A is associated with benefit in terms of reducing oxygen requirements at 36 weeks' postmenstrual age. The relative benefit in relation to the number needed to treat with multiple IM injections is debatable.

  2. Vitamin D

    a. Vitamin D is recommended at 400 IU/d. Exposure to sunshine provides insignificant amounts of vitamin D.

    b. Premature infants consuming human milk can receive vitamin D daily via human milk fortifier (HMF) or liquid multivitamin supplements.

    c. Full-term infants consuming human milk should receive 400 IU of vitamin D daily via 1.0 mL liquid multiple vitamin supplement (although not currently recommended by the American Academy of Pediatrics [AAP]).

    d. Healthy full-term or preterm infants consuming formula will not require vitamin supplementation.

3. Vitamin E
   a. The majority of infants < 1500 g at birth are deficient in vitamin E.
   b. The AAP suggests supplementation of 5–25 IU vitamin E per day for preterm infants because of concerns related to adequacy of vitamin E absorption.
   c. The majority of premature infants consuming a full volume (105 kcal/d) of any of the current formulas designed for low birthweight infants will generally achieve satisfactory plasma vitamin E concentrations by 2 weeks of age.
   d. Preterm infants receiving less than full amounts of enteral feeds should receive multivitamins in their TPN solution.
   e. Current formulas developed for the premature infant provide an adequate vitamin E-to-PUFA ratio, even if the infant is being supplemented with iron at 2 mg/kg/d.
   f. Preterm infants fed exclusively human milk and supplemented with iron may also require a supplement of 5 IU vitamin E per day, available in human milk fortifiers or 1 mL of MVI.
   g. Signs of vitamin E deficiency include hemolytic anemia, edema, and thrombocytosis.
   h. Full-term infants have adequate vitamin E stores at birth.
4. Folic acid
   a. Premature infants have approximately 2 weeks' folate stores at birth.
   b. An intake of 15 mg/kg/d of folic acid should be sufficient, and will be adequately provided either by human milk or current premature infant formulas fed at full volume (105 kcal/kg/d). Breastfeeding mothers should continue to take prenatal vitamins daily.
   c. Anticonvulsants such as Dilantin and phenobarbital may interfere with folate metabolism. Folate status should be carefully monitored and supplementation considered if necessary.
   d. Folate is unstable in liquid form and is not contained in multivitamins.

V. Considerations for the Growing Preterm Infant

A. Preterm infants can meet vitamin requirements by consuming at least 150 mL of human milk fortified with 4 pkts/100 mL of HMF or at least 150 mL of Premature Enfamil with Iron. A larger volume of Similac Special Care or human milk supplemented with Similac Natural Care is required to provide similar vitamins,

    although the exact vitamin requirements remain unproven. Ross
Laboratories' data show adequate mineral and fat retention in premature infants feeding Similac SC.

B. Infants not feeding the above volumes, especially those who are
ELBW, should receive daily MVI in TPN or receive MVI supplements. A multivitamin supplement of 1.0 mL/d should also be provided for premature infants consuming formula intended for full-
term infants.

C. Poly-Vi-Sol with iron contains (1 mL):

Vitamin A	1500 IU
Vitamin C	35 mg
Vitamin D	400 IU
Vitamin E	5 IU
Thiamin	0.5 mg
Riboflavin	0.6 mg
Niacin	8 mg
Vitamin B_6	0.4 mg
Iron	10 mg

Note that there is no folate. Breastfeeding mothers should continue
to take prenatal vitamins.

D. Liquid multivitamin preparations are hypertonic and should be
given in divided doses.

VI. Mineral Supplementation

A. Human milk should be fortified to provide additional minerals, especially calcium and phosphorus.

B. Iron (2–3 mg/kg/d):
1. Fer-In-Sol (0.3 mL) provides 7.5 mg elemental iron.
2. All preterm and standard term formulas *with iron* provide 1.88
mg elemental iron/100 kcal.
3. Standard formulas *with iron* should be used for full-term infants.

C. Formulas intended for full-term infants provide inadequate minerals for the growing premature infant.

D. Calorie supplementation
1. Formula concentration
   a. Less water may be added to formula resulting in a higher
     caloric density.
   b. Concentrated formulas provide a more balanced nutrient in-
     take than carbohydrate or fat supplements.
   c. Concentrated formulas increase renal solute load. Urine os-
     molarity should be monitored.
2. Fortification of human milk

    a. Enfamil and Similac human milk fortifiers contain corn syrup solids, whey protein, casein, and selected vitamins and minerals.

        i. Add only after the infant has achieved an intake of 100 mL human milk per day.

        ii. Begin with 2 pkt per 100 mL human milk and increase to 4 pkt per 100 mL as tolerated.

        iii. Four pkt per 100 mL human milk will increase calorie density to approximately 24 kcal/oz.

        iv. Adding a powdered fortifier still allows for full volume of breast milk.

        v. Fortifier contains soluble calcium, a controversial area.

    b. Similac Natural Care contains the same nutrients as Similac Special Care Formula but with added calcium and phosphorus.

        i. The supplement is designed to be mixed in equal portions with human milk when fed to preterm infants. It may be helpful when breast milk supply is limited.

        ii. Similac Natural Care may be added to human milk after enteral feeding is well established.

        iii. When fed in equal volume with human milk, caloric density will be increased to 22 kcal/oz with additional protein, vitamins, and minerals provided.

3. Added carbohydrates

    a. Powdered glucose polymers are easily digested and absorbed and will contribute less to the osmolality of formulas than mono- or disaccharides.

    b. Increasing caloric density by 20% with carbohydrate will decrease the relative proportions of protein from 2.2 g/100 kcal to 1.85 g/100 kcal.

    c. Powdered glucose polymers provide 3.8 cal/g powder or 2 cal/mL of liquid.

    d. If used in large amounts, carbohydrate supplements may increase CO_2 production and may produce diarrhea.

4. Added fat

    a. Emulsified MCTs require minimal digestion, are absorbed into the portal system and provide 7.7 cal/mL.

    b. Microlipid is an emulsified safflower oil product containing 75% of its fatty acids as linoleic, and provides 4.5 cal/mL.

    c. Fat calories should not exceed 60% of total calories.

    d. Adding fat will decrease the relative proportions of protein and carbohydrate in a formula.

E. Discharge considerations

  1. Switching from premature to "follow-up" or full-term infant formulas

   a. The first 6 months of life appear to be the optimal time for VLBW infants to recover from accumulated bone mineral deficits.

   b. For the VLBW infant feeding a nutrient-enriched postdischarge formula (PDF) such as Enfacare or NeoSure is desirable.

   c. Some studies suggest a benefit for PDF used as long as 9 months. Most studies show benefit for at least 4 months.

  2. Human milk fortification

   a. Mineral supplementation to 6 months postnatal age may be considered if human milk is the major source of nutrition for the VLBW infant at risk for hypocalcemia.

   b. Although not yet proven to increase bone density, mineral fortification of human milk may be accomplished by offering 1–2 supplemental bottles of premature infant formula or a nutrient enriched postdischarge formula daily.

   c. Fluoride supplements should not begin before 6 months of age to minimize the risk of fluorosis.

  3. Vitamins/minerals for discharge

   a. Preterm infant
     i. Breast milk—Poly-Vi-Sol with iron (1 mL)
     ii. Iron fortified standard or premature formula—none

   b. Term infant
     i. Breast milk—Poly-Vi-Sol with iron (1 mL) (the AAP does not currently advise MVI if adequate iron fortified cereal is established.)
     ii. Standard or soy iron fortified formula—none

  4. Women, Infants, and Children (WIC) program eligibility

   a. Low-income mothers may qualify for the WIC program, which provides free infant formula or food vouchers for breastfeeding mothers.

   b. Contact a continuing care or public health nurse for evaluation.

Suggested Reading

American Academy of Pediatrics Committee on Nutrition: Nutritional needs of low-birth-weight infants. Pediatrics 75:976–986, 1985.

Cowett RM (ed): Nutrition and Metabolism of the Micropremie. Clinics in Perinatology, vol. 27, no. 1. Philadelphia, W.B. Saunders, 2000.

Dunn L, Hulman S, Weiner J, Kliegman R: Beneficial effects of early hypocaloric enteral feeding on neonatal gastrointestinal function: Preliminary report of a randomized trial. J Pediatr 112:622–629, 1988.

Hay WW Jr (ed): Neonatal Nutrition and Metabolism. St. Louis, Mosby, 1991.

Kennedy KA, Tyson JE, Chamnanvanikij S: Early versus delayed initiation of progressive enteral feedings for parenterally fed low birth weight or preterm infants (Cochrane Review). In The Cochrane Library. Oxford, Update Software, 2002, Issue 2.

Nutrition Committee, Canadian Paediatric Society (CPS): Nutrient needs and feeding of premature infants. Can Med Assoc J 152:1765–1785, 1995.

Premji S, Chessell L: Continuous nasogastric milk feeding versus intermittent bolus milk feeding for premature infants less than 1500 grams (Cochrane Review). In The Cochrane Library. Oxford, Update Software, 2002, Issue 2.

Tsang RC, Lucas A, Uauy R, Zlotkin S (eds): Nutritional Needs of the Preterm Infant. Baltimore, Williams & Wilkins, 1993.

Chapter 28

Breastfeeding and Premature or Sick Infants

Jennifer L. Grow, M.D., and Robert E. Schumacher, M.D.

I. **Introduction**
   A. The American Academy of Pediatrics has recommended that human milk is the preferred feeding for all infants, including premature and sick newborns, with rare exceptions.
   B. Health care providers should provide parents with complete, current information on the benefits and methods of breastfeeding to ensure that the feeding decision is fully informed.
   C. When direct breastfeeding is not possible, expressed human milk, fortified when necessary for the premature infant, should be provided.
   D. Experts in the area of nutrition strongly encourage the use of human milk, specifically preterm milk, as the optimal food for preterm infants.
   E. Mothers of infants in intensive care nurseries should be encouraged to breastfeed and need to be given instruction on how to use a breast pump to establish and maintain a milk supply as soon as possible after delivery.
   F. Breast milk collected may be frozen and stored until enteral feeds begin. Mothers should be instructed to contact their nurse and/or their baby's nurse to obtain instruction and supplies for the breast pump. Lactation consultants are helpful in assisting mothers with pumping and to provide support and guidance with the transition to breastfeeding.

II. **Reasons for Use of Breast Pump**
   A. Premature/ill infant
   B. To increase milk supply
   C. Mother working or away from the home
   D. Relief of engorgement
   E. Mother on medication contraindicated in breastfeeding

III. **Types of Breast Pumps**
   A. Hand pumps—usually not sufficient or adequate to establish or maintain milk supply when mother and baby are separated
   B. Electric

    1. Hospital-grade (Ameda-Egnell or Medela)
      a. Recommended for long-term pumping
      b. Available in most hospitals
      c. Can be rented for home use
      d. Individual kit needed for each mother to be used with electric pump
      e. Dual pump kit preferable
    2. Battery operated
      a. Various brands available
      b. *Not* effective for establishing or maintaining milk supply

IV. Avoiding Contamination

A. Wash hands prior to pumping.
B. Wash kit after each use with hot soapy water and rinse well.
C. Sterilize kit once every 24 hours by one of the following methods:
    1. Sterilizer in NICU
    2. Boiling in water 20 minutes
    3. Using top rack of dishwasher
D. Wash breast with plain water (no soap) in shower each day.

V. Storing Breast Milk

A. Plastic, sterile container—collect in small amounts (up to 60 mL). Containers can be obtained from mother's or baby's nurse or in pump rooms.
B. Keep amount from each pumping session separate. Refrigerate if breast milk is to be used within 48 hours, or freeze.
C. Label—record baby's name, registration number, date, time collected, date frozen, date thawed on container.
D. Refrigerator/freezing
    1. Freeze fresh, not previously frozen, milk
    2. Refrigerator—keeps up to 48 hours
    3. Previously frozen, thawed milk: thaw in refrigerator, use within 24 hours
    4. Freezer compartment inside refrigerator—keeps 2 weeks
    5. Freezers with separate outside door—keeps 4–6 months
E. Bring chilled milk to hospital from home in a cooler, then freeze if baby is not feeding.

VI. Pumping Guidelines/Considerations

A. Recommended pumping intervals
    1. Usual timing—every 2–3 hours during the day
    2. One 5-hour stretch during the night

    3. Begin as soon as possible after delivery (even if baby is not being fed).

B. Encouraging milk ejection reflex. Some mothers find hand massage of nipple, areola, and breast or warm compresses prior to pumping may encourage milk ejection reflex.

C. Ambiance of room
    1. Private, quiet, warm
    2. Comfortable chair
    3. Picture of baby, diaper, baby blanket

D. Double pumping is encouraged. If mother is unable to do this, she should pump first breast until milk stops dripping, then switch sides. Alternate back and forth until breasts feel soft. Massaging breast during pumping may help.

E. Suggestions for improving milk supply
    1. Reassurance/support
    2. Decrease the interval between pumping sessions (pump more frequently).
    3. Ensure adequate fluid intake. Drink when thirsty.
    4. Encourage rest periods.
    5. When infant is stable enough, holding, particularly skin-to-skin care
    6. Support from other breastfeeding mothers
    7. Pump at the hospital after visiting the baby or being at the baby's bedside.
    8. Obtain help with other family responsibilities to allow time and energy to both visit the baby and find time for pumping.

VII. Transition to Breastfeeding

A. No universally agreed upon criteria for initiation of breastfeeding by preterm infants exist.

B. Gradual transition of the infant to breastfeeding may be optimal.

C. Kangaroo care often allows infant opportunity for "practice" feeding.

D. Non-nutritive breastfeeding can be offered by allowing the mother to offer the infant an opportunity to suckle on the breast *after* pumping.

E. Nutritive sucking can be offered as the infant matures.

F. Mothers may pump before putting the infant to breast to reduce the effect of the milk ejection reflex, which allows the preterm infant to be introduced to small droplets of milk.

G. As the infant demonstrates more ability to coordinate suck, swallow, and breathing, the mother may cease pumping before feedings.

H. When the infant becomes more adept at feeding at the breast, test weights may be obtained to determine the amount of supplementation needed. The scale used needs to be electronic and accurate to within 2 g (1 g = 1 mL).

I. Lactation consultants can assist the mother, infant, and staff with techniques to provide the most support for both mother and infant to insure optimal milk transfer.

J. Most infants will make the transition to full breastfeeding close to their original due date.

K. Mothers need to continue to supplement either at the breast or after breastfeeding until the infant is able to transfer enough milk to maintain an adequate growth pattern.

L. The mother will need to continue to pump after the feedings to empty the breasts and maintain her milk supply.

M. Referrals may be made for follow-up support of the breastfeeding premature infant/mother dyad.

Suggested Reading

American Academy of Pediatrics Work Group on Breastfeeding: Breastfeeding and the use of human milk. Pediatrics 100:1035–1039, 1997.

Auerbach K, Riordan J: Breastfeeding and Human Lactation, 2nd ed. Sudbury, MA, Jones & Bartlett, 1999.

Briggs GG, Freeman RK, Yaffe SJ: Drugs in Pregnancy and Lactation, 5th ed. Baltimore, Williams & Wilkins, 1998.

Hale T: Medications and Mothers' Milk, 10th ed. Amarillo, TX, Pharmasoft Publishing, 2002.

Lang S: Breastfeeding Special Care Babies. London, W.B. Saunders, 1997.

Chapter 29

Osteopenia of Prematurity

Jennifer L. Grow, M.D., and Robert E. Schumacher, M.D.

I. Problem

Fetal accretion of calcium and phosphorus peaks after 34 weeks' gestation. Preterm infants and infants from pregnancies complicated by placental insufficiency are at risk of developing osteopenia of prematurity. Vitamin D absorption and metabolism appears adequate even in ELBW infants. In general, calcium and phosphorus absorption is also adequate even in ELBW infants. The primary problem is inadequate mineral intake. Exact vitamin requirements for ELBW infants are controversial.

II. Etiology

A. Multifactorial—inadequate mineral intake is the major etiologic factor
  1. Standard formulas or unfortified human breast milk contain insufficient Ca and P for the premature infant, leading to bone demineralization.
  2. It is very difficult to provide adequate Ca and P intake by total parenteral nutrition.
  3. Furosemide therapy promotes calcium excretion.
  4. It is impossible to provide adequate Ca and P absorption in the presence of high aluminum concentrations, as occurs with TPN amino acids. The amount and ratios of Ca, P, Mg, and amino acids in TPN may affect mineral retention and urinary excretion.
  5. Bone demineralization is enhanced with physical immobility.

B. Abnormalities of vitamin D absorption, metabolism
  1. Most premature infants can absorb and hydroxylate vitamin D_3 to form 1–25OHD, such that 400 IU/day of vitamin D_3 is sufficient.
  2. In the presence of liver disease (such as severe cholestasis), vitamin D malabsorption may occur.
  3. Renal disease may impair conversion of 25-OHD to 1–25OHD.
  4. Anticonvulsant therapy has been associated with increased vitamin D metabolism, low 25-OHD levels, and rickets.

C. Miscellaneous

1. Because of placental insufficiency, IUGR infants may have decreased stores of Ca and P.
2. Unwarranted use of 1–25OHD may lead to bone resorption.
3. Prolonged TPN use may be directly toxic to bone (vitamin D, aluminum?).
4. Severe osteopenia is rare with current formulas. Those at high risk are critically ill preterm infants who remain NPO on TPN > 1 month, concomitantly requiring furosemide and fluid restriction.
5. Renal calcium excretion varies depending on TPN content and ratios of Ca, P, Mg, and amino acids.

III. Physical and Laboratory Findings in Neonatal Bone Disease

A. Radiographs show demineralization relatively late (osteopenia), fractures are variable.

B. Craniotabes or rachitic rosary may be seen (rare), but are late findings.

C. Laboratory findings may include normal serum Ca and low serum phosphorus (less than 4.0 mg/dL), normal or low serum 25-OHD, and normal or high 1–25OHD. Serum alkaline phosphatase is often elevated, but is not a measure of osteopenia.

D. Consider measuring serum Ca, P, Mg, parathyroid hormone, calcitonin, 25-OHD, 1–25OHD, renal P excretion, and serum aluminum levels when etiology is unknown *and* if any of the values will cause one to act.

IV. Treatment

A. Adequate provision of dietary mineral is of paramount importance. Premature infant formulas should therefore be used (see above). Consider supplementing breast milk for those infants receiving breast milk and showing signs of osteopenia, with Ca and P (available in standard breast milk supplements/fortifiers). For reference, the average in utero accretion rate of Ca is 150 mg/kg/d; P is 75 mg/kg/d.

B. Enteral feeds provide significantly more minerals than parenteral.

C. Furosemide, spironolactone, and theophylline are calciuric. Diuril may be calcium-sparing. Limit furosemide use, changing to thiazide when possible.

D. Vitamin D, 400 IU every day should be sufficient. Standard premature formulas contain vitamin D. Breast milk fortifiers mixed with milk will have variable amounts; intake should be monitored.

E. One trial of a program of physical activity/therapy showed evidence of increased bone mineralization.

F. In cases of severe cholestasis, consider the use of 25-OHD supplements (4 mg/kg/d).

G. Consider continued Ca and P supplementation after discharge in extremely preterm infants. Nutrition enriched follow-up formulas (such as Neocare or Enfacare) may be helpful.

Suggested Reading

Rigo J, De Curtis M, Pieltain C, et al: Bone mineral metabolism in the micropremie. Clin Perinatol 27:147–170, 2000.

Ryan S: Nutritional aspects of metabolic bone disease in the newborn. Arch Dis Child 74:F145–F148, 1996.

Chapter 30

Asphyxia Neonatorum

John D.E. Barks, M.D., and Steven M. Donn, M.D.

I. Definition

The inability to provide adequate oxygen to, or remove carbon dioxide or hydrogen ions from the fetus or newborn (alternatively, failure of the organ of respiration)

II. Pathophysiology

During prolonged partial asphyxia there is a redistribution of available cardiac output to more vital organs (brain, heart, adrenals) at the expense of less vital organs (e.g., lungs, gut, kidneys, skin). This may lead to hypoxic-ischemic injury and forms the pathophysiologic basis for systemic complications.

III. Etiologies

A. Fetal (e.g., severe anemia)
B. Placental (e.g., abruptio placentae)
C. Maternal (e.g., toxemia)
D. Neonatal (e.g., infection)

IV. Systemic Complications

A. Biochemical changes
　1. Respiratory, metabolic, or mixed acidosis
　2. Disordered carbohydrate metabolism (hypo/hyperglycemia)
　3. Hypocalcemia, hyponatremia
　4. Hyperkalemia, aminoaciduria
　5. Increased glycerol, free fatty acids
　6. Hyperammonemia
　7. Hyperuricemia
B. Cardiovascular system
　1. Transient myocardial insufficiency
　2. Transient tricuspid insufficiency
　3. Dysrhythmias
　4. Persistent pulmonary hypertension
C. Hematologic system—disseminated intravascular coagulopathy; transient "left shift"; nucleated RBCs
D. Pulmonary system

    1. Shock lung
    2. Pulmonary hemorrhage
E. Gastrointestinal system
    1. Necrotizing enterocolitis
    2. Feeding disturbances
F. Genitourinary system
    1. Renal failure
      a. Tubular necrosis
      b. Medullary necrosis
      c. Cortical necrosis
      d. Papillary necrosis
    2. Asphyxiated bladder syndrome
G. Endocrine system
    1. Adrenal hemorrhage
    2. Syndrome of inappropriate antidiuretic hormone secretion (SIADH)
    3. Transient hyperglycemia (pancreatic insufficiency)
    4. Transient hypoparathyroidism (hypocalcemia)
H. Integument—subcutaneous fat necrosis
I. Central nervous system
    1. Structural brain injury
      a. Cerebral edema
      b. Ischemic lesions
      c. Hemorrhagic lesions
    2. Clinical features of hypoxic-ischemic encephalopathy
      a. Decreased level of consciousness
      b. Hypotonia
      c. Depressed reflex status
      d. Seizures (30–69%)
    3. Clinicopathologic correlates
      a. Selective neuronal necrosis
      b. Status marmoratus
      c. Parasagittal cerebral injury
      d. Periventricular leukomalacia (preterm infants)
      e. Focal and multifocal ischemic necrosis
        (1) Porencephaly
        (2) Hydranencephaly
        (3) Multicystic encephalomalacia

V.   Management
A. The key to successful management is **anticipation** of postasphyxial sequelae and initiation of treatment *before* significant complications transpire.

TABLE 34
Sarnat Staging Criteria

	Stage 1	Stage 2	Stage 3
Level of consciousness	Hyperalert	Lethargic or obtunded	Stuporous
Neuromuscular control			
Muscle tone	None	Mild hypotonia	Flaccid
Posture	Mild distal flexion	Strong distal flexion	Intermittent decerebration
Stretch reflexes	Overactive	Overactive	Decreased or absent
Segmental myoclonus	Present	Present	Absent
Complex reflexes			
Suck	Weak	Weak or absent	Absent
Moro	Strong; low threshold	Weak; incomplete high threshold	Absent
Oculovestibular	Normal	Overactive	Weak or absent
Tonic neck	Slight	Strong	Absent
Autonomic function	Generalized sympathetic	Generalized parasympathetic	Both systems depressed
Pupils	Mydriasis	Miosis	Variable; often unequal; poor light reflex
Heart rate	Tachycardia	Bradycardia	Variable
Bronchial and salivary secretions	Sparse	Profuse	Variable
Gastrointestinal motility	Normal or decreased	Increased diarrhea	Variable
Seizures	None	Common; focal or multifocal	Uncommon (exceeding decerebration)
Electroencephalogram findings	Normal (awake)	*Early:* low-voltage continuous delta and theta *Later:* periodic pattern (awake) Seizures: focal 1–1½ Hz spike and wave	*Early:* periodic pattern with isopotential phases *Later:* totally isopotential
Duration	< 24 hours	2–14 days	Hours to weeks

From Sarnat HB, Sarnat MS: Neonatal encephalopathy following fetal distress. Arch Neurol 33:696–705, 1976, with permission.

      1. Maintain blood pressure.
      2. Maintain normal blood glucose.
      3. Treat seizures.

B. Infants may be at higher risk for neurodevelopmental sequelae if:
      1. Apgar score $\leq$ 3 at $\geq$ 20 minutes.
      2. Seizures are difficult to control.
      3. EEG shows burst suppression pattern.
      4. Severe, protracted oliguria or renal failure is seen.
      5. The infant has an abnormal neurologic examination at $\geq$ 5 days postnatal age (term infants).

C. Sarnat staging criteria are prognostically useful (Table 34).
      1. Infants who are only in stage 1 are usually normal on follow-up.
      2. Infants in stage 3 are almost always abnormal.
      3. The longer an infant is in stage 2, the more guarded the prognosis (especially > 5 days).

D. Other tests, planning, considerations
      1. Brain imaging—CT or MRI
      2. BAERs
      3. VERs
      4. Evaluation by someone skilled in neurobehavioral assessment of the newborn
      5. Longitudinal follow-up

E. Sequelae
      1. Most infants with a history of asphyxia will be normal.
      2. Cerebral palsy or motor abnormalities with or without mental retardation may be seen.
      3. Speech and language delays are common sequelae.

F. Experimental therapies
      1. Hypothermia, both generalized and selective (head)
      2. Prophylactic high-dose phenobarbital
      3. Anti-inflammatory agents
      4. Magnesium sulfate

Suggested Reading

Donn SM, Sinha SK, Chiswick ML (eds): Birth Asphyxia and the Brain: Basic Science and Clinical Implications. Armonk, NY, Futura Publishing, 2002.

Fenichel GM: Hypoxic-ischemic encephalopathy in the newborn. Arch Neurol 40:261–266, 1983.

Johnston MV, Donn SM: Hypoxic-ischemic encephalopathy. In Nelson NM (ed): Current Therapy in Neonatal-Perinatal Medicine—2. Philadelphia, B.C. Decker, 1990, pp 276–279.

Sarnat HB, Sarnat MS: Neonatal encephalopathy following fetal distress: A clinical and electroencephalographic study. Arch Neurol 33:696–705, 1976.

Volpe JJ: Neurology of the Newborn, 4th ed. Philadelphia, W.B. Saunders, 2001.

Chapter 31

Intracranial Hemorrhage

John D.E. Barks, M.D., and Steven M. Donn, M.D.

I. **Subdural Hemorrhage (SDH)**

A. Severe, symptomatic cases are rarely seen, especially in preterm infants. Most often seen in term infant, often (but not always) with an instrumented (vacuum or forceps) or traumatic birth history. Lesser severity of injury (i.e., asymptomatic) may be more common than previously appreciated.

B. Most often birth-related
1. Large baby, with small maternal pelvis
2. Precipitous or very prolonged active labor
3. Forceps or vacuum-assisted delivery

C. Diagnosis
1. CT brain scan is the gold standard.
2. MRI scan may be useful in evaluating status of adjacent brain tissue.
3. LP is not necessary, but if done, it may show increased RBCs and protein in the CSF.
4. Cranial sonography does not visualize posterior fossa or cerebral convexities well.

D. Classification
1. Falx/tentorium laceration-associated
2. Occipital osteodiastasis with posterior fossa subdural hematoma
3. Convexity subdural hemorrhage

E. Management
1. Most symptomatic cases can be managed supportively, including:
   a. Correction of any coagulation defects, either congenital or acquired (e.g., FFP, platelets, vitamin K)
   b. Protect airway and provide respiratory support in case of stridor, apnea, or hypoventilation.
   c. Anticonvulsant therapy of seizures
   d. Frequent neurologic examination
   e. Sonographic monitoring for posthemorrhagic ventriculomegaly
2. Prompt neurosurgical evacuation may be indicated if the patient shows signs of neurologic deterioration, particularly of

brainstem compression, but is fraught with difficulty given fragility of neonatal brain and frequent adherence of clot to CNS tissue.

F. Prognosis

1. Very poor for major lacerations of the tentorium or falx. Virtually all are fatal.
2. There is a 90% chance of good outcome in survivors of less severe posterior fossa hemorrhages, whether or not surgical drainage is provided. There is a lack of randomized trials comparing surgical vs. nonsurgical approaches.
3. Majority of infants with convexity SDH do well.
4. Posthemorrhagic hydrocephalus can occur, particularly after posterior fossa SDH.

II. Subarachnoid Hemorrhage (SAH)

A. Relatively common, especially in term infants

B. Sometimes associated with trauma or hypoxic events

C. May present as benign, undetected by exam (e.g., incidental finding on LP or CT for other indication)

1. More severe bleeds present with seizures or apnea.
2. Catastrophic deterioration with major bleed is rare.

D. Diagnosis

1. CT brain scan is the gold standard. Cranial sonography is generally unhelpful.
2. LP is not necessary but, if done, usually (but not always) shows increased RBCs and protein.

E. Prognosis is usually good.

1. Up to 50% of patients with seizures develop normally.
2. The principal concerning sequela is hydrocephalus, which can have a delayed onset.

III. Intracerebellar Hemorrhage

A. Very rare, usually associated with a traumatic delivery or hypoxia

1. More commonly seen in premature newborns
2. Seen in up to 15–25% of autopsy cases < 1500 g, but is uncommon in normal newborns or living premature infants (by CT)

B. Four types of hemorrhages described

1. Primary intracerebellar hemorrhage
2. Venous infarction
3. Extension of IVH or subarachnoid hemorrhage
4. Traumatic laceration

C. Clinically presents with signs of brainstem compression or increased ventricular size secondary to decreased CSF absorption.
   1. Apnea, irregular respirations, and bradycardia are common with large bleeds.
   2. Full fontanel may be observed.
D. Diagnosis follows a high index of suspicion. CT or MRI is necessary to obtain full cerebellar views.
E. Management
   1. Supportive (*see* I, E, above)
   2. If the patient develops hydrocephalus, serial LPs or reservoir/VP shunt may be necessary to relieve pressure.
F. Prognosis
   1. Very poor in premature newborns
   2. Much better in term newborns

IV. Periventricular-Intraventricular Hemorrhage

A. IVH is the most common and serious form of neonatal intracranial hemorrhage.
   1. In the premature newborn, the germinal matrix adjacent to the lateral ventricles is highly vascular and susceptible to bleeding. Most IVH originates in this area.
   2. Later in gestation (> 34 wks) this vascular network involutes and the infant is not as susceptible to hemorrhage, decreasing the risk of IVH with advancing gestational age.
   3. In term infants, IVH may originate from the choroid plexus.
B. Risk factors
   1. Prematurity
   2. Factors causing abrupt changes in cerebral blood flow
      a. Rapid changes in PaO_2 or $PaCO_2$
      b. Rapid changes in aortic pressure from rapid volume infusions or rapid addition of pressors
   3. Factors potentially interfering with normal cerebral blood flow
      a. Asphyxia disrupting cerebral autoregulation
      b. Hypocarbia
      c. Systemic hypotension
      d. Large PDA and left-to-right shunt
      e. Elevated venous pressure from pneumothorax or increased intrathoracic pressure
   4. Traumatic birth injury
   5. Rapid infusions of hypertonic solutions
      a. Bicarbonate
      b. Hypertonic dextrose

C. Clinical presentation

    1. Catastrophic—occurs with acute, large bleeds

        a. Rapid evolution (minutes to hours) of severe symptoms, often progressing rapidly to death

        b. Neurologic signs include stupor, coma, generalized seizures, decerebrate posturing, pupillary fixation, absence of nystagmus with vestibular stimulation, hypoventilation, apnea, and flaccid quadriparesis.

        c. Associated findings may include bulging fontanel, split sutures, drop in hematocrit, bradycardia, hypotension, temperature instability, metabolic acidosis, glucose intolerance, and SIADH.

        d. The above signs can appear very similar to sepsis. Keep IVH in mind in this differential diagnosis.

    2. Saltatory syndrome—more subtle in presentation, evolving over many hours. Rarely fatal.

        a. Common signs are changes in level of alertness, alteration in spontaneous and elicited movements, hypotonia, subtle changes in eye position/movement, and respiratory abnormalities.

        b. Unexplained fall in hematocrit

    3. Silent hemorrhage—most common

        a. There are no signs at the time of the IVH, but the patient may become symptomatic later if hydrocephalus develops.

        b. Signs of hydrocephalus:

           i. Accelerated head growth

          ii. Bulging fontanel with split sutures

         iii. Apnea or inability to wean from the ventilator

         iv. Lethargy, poor feeding

D. Diagnosis

    1. Cranial ultrasonography is the study of choice. Brain CT and MRI may be helpful for follow-up or prognosis, but are not necessary for diagnosis and evaluation of the acute hemorrhage.

    2. If an LP is done, the CSF may show increased red blood cell count, increased protein (usually marked), and decreased glucose (hypoglycorrhachia).

E. Screening

    1. Obtain cranial sonogram within first 72 hours, then again between 7–10 days of age. Majority of IVH occurs within 4 days of birth.

    2. Obtain a study any time IVH is clinically suspected.

    3. Very low birthweight infants (< 1000 g) or infants suspected

of having hypoxic-ischemic lesions or septic episodes (risk factors for periventricular leukomalacia) should receive additional later follow-up, such as monthly and prior to discharge.

F. Grades of IVH (Papile classification)
1. Grade I = germinal matrix only (subependymal, not within ventricle)
2. Grade II = IVH without ventricular distention
3. Grade III = IVH severe enough to cause ventricular distension
4. Grade IV = ventricular and parenchymal involvement. Sometimes referred to as intraparenchymal echodensity (IPE). This may actually represent a hemorrhagic venous infarction.

G. Recommended management
1. Phenobarbital prophylaxis for infants < 1800 g that are intubated and ventilated; 20 mg/kg IV loading dose, then 5 mg/kg/d for additional 4 days IV/IM/PO. Indomethacin has also been shown to reduce incidence of IVH but without improvement in neurodevelopmental outcome.
2. Supportive care—red cell transfusion if associated with acute fall in Hbg/Hct.
3. Anticonvulsant(s) for seizures
4. For grade I hemorrhage, obtain serial ultrasounds to rule out extension of the hemorrhage (20% extend).
5. For grade II hemorrhage, serial ultrasounds
   a. If ventricles remain stable, treat as for grade I.
   b. If ventricles enlarge, treat as for grade III.
6. For grades III and IV
   a. Serial ultrasound scans to assess ventricular size
   b. If progressive ventricular dilation occurs, consider serial lumbar punctures. Volume of CSF removed should be that which flows freely. The frequency of LPs is determined by clinical condition, response to therapy, and ease of procedure.
7. Diuretics (used to decrease rate of CSF formation)
   a. Furosemide or acetazolamide are used.
   b. They may cause metabolic acidosis, so use with caution in infants with chronic lung disease.
8. Stop LPs when ventricles are stable in size over 1 week and CSF cell counts and chemistries normal. Repeat ultrasound scan 1 week later. If ventricles enlarge, resume LPs.
9. Infants refractory to serial LPs (e.g., do not tolerate procedure, inadequate CSF volumes obtained) should be considered for ventricular reservoir or ventriculo-peritoneal shunt placement.

H. Complications

1. Acute
   a. Multiplicity of "centrally mediated" physiologic aberrations including apnea, arrhythmias, vasomotor instability
   b. SIADH
   c. Seizures
2. Long-term
   a. Psychomotor disabilities
   b. Intellectual impairment
   c. Porencephaly
   d. Speech and language delays
3. Hydrocephalus
   a. Communicating is the most common form and may occur in up to 20% of cases of IVH. May respond to diuretics and/or serial LPs.
   b. Noncommunicating is rare and seen in only 5–10% of posthemorrhagic hydrocephalus. It can occur if the aqueduct or foramina are obstructed, and it requires neurosurgical intervention.
   c. The above conditions may be distinguished by radionuclide lumbar cisternography, if necessary.

Suggested Reading

Bowerman RA, Donn SM, Silver TM, et al: Natural history of neonatal periventricular/intraventricular hemorrhage and its complications: Sonographic observations. Am J Roentgenol 143:1041–1052, 1984.

Bozynski ME, Nelson MN, Rosati-Skeetich C, et al: Two year longitudinal follow-up of the premature infant weighing ≤ 1200 g at birth: Sequelae of intracranial hemorrhage. J Dev Behav Pediatr 5:346–352, 1984.

Donn SM, Roloff DW, Keyes JW Jr: Lumbar cisternography in evaluation of hydrocephalus in the preterm infant. Pediatrics 72:670–676, 1983.

Goldstein GW, Donn SM: Periventricular and intraventricular hemorrhages. In Sarnat HB (ed): Topics in Neonatal Neurology. New York, Grune & Stratton, 1984, pp 83–108.

Volpe JJ: Neurology of the Newborn, 4th ed. Philadelphia, W.B. Saunders, 2001.

Chapter 32

Seizures

John D.E. Barks, M.D., and Steven M. Donn, M.D.

I. Introduction

A. Neonatal seizures can be caused by a wide variety of underlying conditions. Repetitive seizures are associated with increased mortality and morbidity.

1. Seizure activity differs clinically from that of older children and adults. Recognition may be difficult clinically, and EEG documentation is sometimes required.

2. Neonatal tremulousness or jitteriness can be confused with neonatal seizures, and can be distinguished by the damping effect of extremity flexion, swaddling, or a pacifier.

3. Seizures in a paralyzed infant on a ventilator may only present as cyclic oscillation in heart rate and/or blood pressure. EEG documentation may be the only means of diagnosis of seizures.

B. Timing and etiologies—50% percent of neonatal seizures begin on the first day of life, 75% have their onset within the first 3 days of life.

1. Bacterial meningitis can present at any time.

2. Nonbacterial meningitis/encephalitis seizures from entities such as HSV or coxsackie B usually begin in the first 7–10 days of life.

3. Hypoxic-ischemic encephalopathy—seizures usually start 6–12 hours after insult and tend to be difficult to control.

4. Intracranial hemorrhage (subdural/subarachnoid)
   a. Usually in term infants with a history of traumatic delivery
   b. Onset of most seizures is in the first 24–48 hours of life.

5. IVH (seen primarily in preterm infants)—seizures are usually seen in first week of life.

6. Metabolic disorders
   a. Hyponatremia
   b. Hypernatremia
   c. Hypomagnesemia
   d. Hypocalcemia
   e. Hypoglycemia
   f. Kernicterus (hyperbilirubinemia)
   g. Pyridoxine deficiency/dependency

      h. Aminoacidopathies and other inborn errors of metabolism (hyperammonemia)

      i. Hyperthermia

      j. Drug toxicity (e.g., theophylline)

   7. Developmental defects/genetic syndromes

   8. Benign familial epilepsy

   9. Drug withdrawal—prominent in opiate-exposed and sedative-hypnotic–exposed newborns

  10. Idiopathic neonatal seizures

II. Types of Seizures

A. Subtle—the most frequent in both term and preterm infants. Tonic eye deviation, blinking, eyelid fluttering, orofacial movements, rowing, swimming, pedaling motions of extremities, and apnea may be observed.

B. Multifocal clonic—clonic jerking of extremities, either simultaneous or sequential; if sequential, order is random.

C. Focal clonic—in one extremity, less commonly seen and often associated with focal CNS injury or metabolic abnormalities

D. Tonic—generalized hypertonus of all limbs

   1. May be accompanied by subtle signs

   2. More common in preterm infants

   3. Often associated with intracranial hemorrhage

E. Myoclonic—single or multiple jerks of extremities, very uncommon in the newborn period and associated with profound CNS abnormalities

III. Diagnostic Evaluation

A. It is important to begin with the most probable cause and most likely etiology given the circumstances. History should include questions concerning perinatal asphyxia, delivery trauma, sepsis risks, family seizure history, and maternal substance abuse. Evaluate rapidly for treatable causes (e.g., hypoglycemia, hypocalcemia)

B. Data collection

   1. Laboratory data

      a. Complete blood count and blood culture

      b. Serum electrolytes, Ca, Mg, glucose

      c. Lumbar puncture—send for WBC, RBC, protein, glucose, bacterial and viral cultures, HSV PCR

      d. Nasopharyngeal and rectal swab for HSV

      e. Urine and/or meconium toxicology screen

2. EEG — ideally during a clinical episode, but in practice may be interictal
3. Brain imaging study
    a. Ultrasound if premature and concerned about possible IVH
    b. CT or MRI scans may be indicated
4. Video EEG
    a. May be useful in determining whether atypical paroxysmal phenomena correspond to electrographic seizures
    b. May be useful in monitoring patients whose seizures are difficult to control

IV. General Management

A. Seizures should be considered a medical emergency and treated aggressively. During seizures there is an imbalance in brain perfusion, depletion of CNS glucose and ATP, and increased intracranial pressure; all may jeopardize central nervous system homeostasis.
1. Support ventilation and oxygenation as necessary.
2. Perform appropriate studies *before* treating.
3. Treat underlying cause or suspected diagnosis (e.g., glucose for hypoglycemia, calcium for hypocalcemia).
4. IV antibiotics at meningitis doses until cultures prove this is not meningitis or sepsis

B. Pharmacologic management
1. Phenobarbital
    a. Loading dose in the term infant = 30 mg/kg. If infant is breathing spontaneously, give very slowly or as divided dose, 10 mg/kg × 3, 20 min apart. Infants receiving assisted ventilation may receive 30 mg/kg by *slow* IV push (over 15–30 min). Obtain therapeutic range of 20–50 μg/mL.
    b. Maintenance = 3–5 mg/kg/d. It is important to monitor serum concentration.
    c. Phenobarbital monotherapy may require very high concentrations (80–100 μg/mL) in some instances. This should be discussed with a pediatric neurologist.
2. Diphenylhydantoin (phenytoin, administered as parenteral fosphenytoin; ordered at University of Michigan as phenytoin equivalent) — use if phenobarbital alone is ineffective.
    a. Give in incremental doses of 5–10 mg/kg by slow IV infusion up to a maximum of 20 mg/kg.
    b. Maintenance dose 5 mg/kg/d IV (not absorbed well from the GI tract in infants). Therapeutic range = 10–20 μg/mL.
3. Diazepam (Valium) — loading dose of 0.05–0.10 mg/kg should

be given over 2 minutes. May be repeated several times for persistent seizures, e.g., in status epilepticus, if phenobarbital and phenytoin (Dilantin) have been ineffective.

4. Pyridoxine—50 mg IV, preferably with EEG running, as a diagnostic-therapeutic trial.
5. Pentobarbital—rare use may be indicated in infant in status epilepticus refractory to all therapy.
   a. Dose is 4 mg/kg × 1–2 doses
   b. Infant *must* be receiving assisted ventilation with arterial line and continuous blood pressure monitoring *before* dose is given.

Suggested Reading

Johnston MV: Neurologic emergencies. In Donn SM, Faix RG (eds): Neonatal Emergencies. Mt. Kisco, NY, Futura Publishing, 1991, pp 585–596.

Mizrahi EM, Kellaway P: Characterization and classification of neonatal seizures. Neurology 34:1837–1844, 1987.

Painter MJ, Scher MS, Stein AD, et al: Phenobarbital compared with phenytoin for the treatment of neonatal seizures. N Engl J Med 341:485–489, 1999.

Volpe JJ: Neonatal seizures: Current concepts and revised classification. Pediatrics 84:422–428, 1989.

Volpe JJ: Neurology of the Newborn, 4th ed. Philadelphia, W.B. Saunders, 2001, pp 178–214.

Chapter 33

Transient Neonatal Myasthenia Gravis

John D.E. Barks, M.D.

I. Introduction

Affected infants born to mothers with myasthenia gravis may develop transient generalized weakness during the newborn period.

A. Incidence: 10–15% of infants of MG mother. The birth of a previously affected infant increases the risk in subsequent children (approximately 75%).

B. The severity or duration of maternal disease does not correlate with the degree of weakness in the infant; *asymptomatic mothers may have severely affected infants.*

II. Pathophysiology

Maternal antibody against the neuromuscular junction passively crosses the placenta and interferes with function in the newborn infant. Some symptomatic infants may also synthesize antibody *de novo.*

III. Clinical Presentation

Signs usually begin within hours of birth, but may be delayed. The mean duration of signs is 18 days with a range of 5 days to 2 months. Complete recovery usually occurs within 4–6 weeks.

A. Difficulty in feeding; infant may have a good initial sucking response which rapidly fatigues.

B. Generalized hypotonia

C. Weak cry

D. Lack of facial expression

E. Limited extraocular movements and ptosis

F. Apnea/hypoventilation

G. *Acute cardiorespiratory failure may be the presenting sign.*

IV. Diagnosis

A. High plasma concentrations of antiacetyl cholinesterase receptor antibody

B. Characteristic EMG: repetitive nerve stimulation produces decremental neuromuscular fatigue.

C. Anticholinesterase challenge produces rapid improvement.

1. Neostigmine methylsulfate 0.04 mg/kg IM (maximal effect in approximately 30 min)
2. Pretreatment with atropine should be considered to minimize muscarinic effects, e.g., diarrhea, and profuse tracheal secretions.
3. One should not attempt an anticholinesterase challenge unless facilities and personnel for intubation, ventilation, and CPR are immediately available.

D. Diagnosis is best made with simultaneous EMG and anticholinesterase challenge.

V. Management

A. Careful monitoring, prompt diagnosis, and early initiation of therapy is most important.
   1. All infants born to mothers with MG should receive cardiorespiratory monitoring for at least 7 days.
   2. Nutritional support in the affected infant is best achieved with frequent, small volume feedings via an oro- or nasogastric tube.
   3. Secretions should be suctioned frequently.
   4. Early institution of respiratory support should be provided as needed.

B. Approximately 80% of symptomatic infants may require anticholinesterase therapy.
   1. Neostigmine is preferred at doses of 0.04 mg/kg IM or subcutaneously given approximately 30 minutes prior to feedings.
   2. The dose should be titrated to minimize signs and progressively reduced as signs resolve.
   3. Oral neostigmine may be administered when the suck-swallow mechanism becomes competent. Ten times the parenteral dose is used.
   4. Exchange transfusion has reportedly been successful in treating a few severely affected infants requiring prolonged ventilatory support. Its use, along with plasmaphoresis, remains controversial.

C. *The use of aminoglycoside antibiotics should be avoided* because they may have an adverse affect on neuromuscular function. A third generation cephalosporin or other agent should be used for gram-negative coverage.

VI. Prognosis

A. Most infants will recover spontaneously within a few weeks as maternal passive antibodies are catabolized. Death is rare in the modern NICU era. Older reports of 10% mortality of symptomatic infants were related to delayed diagnosis or treatment.

B. Arthrogryposis may occur in infants born to mothers with MG (as a result of reduced intrauterine movements). This condition may require long-term physical therapy.

C. Assess whether severity of maternal disease may require special plans for home care at discharge.

Suggested Reading

Dunn JM: Neonatal myasthenia. Am J Obstet Gynecol 125:265–266, 1976.

Fenichel GM: Myasthenia gravis. Pediatr Ann 18:432–438, 1989.

Volpe JJ: Neurology of the Newborn, 4th ed. Philadelphia, W.B. Saunders, 2001, pp 658–660.

Chapter 34

Neonatal Abstinence Syndrome

Charles R. Neal, Jr., M.D., Ph.D.

I. Commonly Abused Drugs and Pregnancy

A. Cocaine—milder symptoms than narcotics

B. Narcotics (opiates)—onset of withdrawal depends on which drug and when last used.
   1. Heroin
   2. Methadone
   3. Pentazocine (Talwin), may be used with antihistamines ("T's and Blues")

C. Alcohol—can cause severe withdrawal when its use is mixed with depressants by the pregnant woman

D. Other depressants
   1. Barbiturates
   2. Bromide
   3. Chlordiazepoxide (Librium)
   4. Chloral hydrate
   5. Ethchlorvynol (Placidyl)
   6. Glutethimide (Doriden)
   7. Meprobamate (Miltown)

E. Cannabinoids

F. Phencyclidine (PCP)

G. Tobacco and nicotine

II. Screening

A. Fetal drug exposure occurs in up to 15% of pregnancies. The majority of women use multiple drugs. Polysubstance abuse increases risks of fetal/neonatal complications and may lead to neonatal withdrawal symptoms.
   1. Question the mother directly about use of illicit drugs, alcohol, prescription medications, and over-the-counter medications taken during pregnancy.
   2. Women using drugs during pregnancy also have an increased incidence of sexually transmitted diseases. The mother should be questioned about this and the baby should be screened appropriately.

B. When to do toxicology screening

1. With an admission of use or documented past positive toxicology screens
2. Physical or behavioral signs of maternal drug abuse
3. Mother who received no or inadequate prenatal care
4. Placental abruption or precipitous delivery without a known cause
5. Infant who has unexplained signs that may be consistent with withdrawal

III. Signs of Neonatal Abstinence Syndrome

W = **W**akefulness

I = **I**rritability

T = **T**remulousness, **t**emperature instability, **t**achypnea

H = **H**yperactivity, **h**igh-pitched persistent cry, **h**yperacusis, **h**yper-reflexia, **h**ypertonia

D = **D**iarrhea, **d**iaphoresis, **d**isorganized or voracious suck

R = **R**ub marks, **r**hinorrhea, **r**espiratory distress

A = **A**pnea, **a**utonomic dysfunction

W = **W**eight loss or failure to thrive

A = **A**lkalosis

L = **L**acrimation

Also: hiccups, yawning, stuffy nose, sneezing, photophobia, twitching, myoclonic jerks, opisthotonus, or seizures.

For nonopiate drugs, onset of withdrawal is usually soon after birth, peaking at 3–4 days and usually resolved by the end of the first week of life. With heroin, onset is usually after the first 24 hours and peaks by 7 days of life. Methadone withdrawal may not appear until 3–7 days of life and may peak at 10 days. With opiates, subacute signs may persist for 4–6 months.

IV. Other Neonatal Effects

A. Dysmorphology

B. IUGR

C. Asphyxia—meconium aspiration syndrome

D. Polycythemia

E. Prematurity

F. Respiratory distress

G. Hypoglycemia

H. Hypocalcemia

I. Infection
1. Hepatitis B
2. HIV

3. CMV

4. Syphilis, other STDs

J. Increased incidence of SIDS in children of drug-abusing mother

K. Reduced incidence of RDS, feeding problems, hyperbilirubinemia

V.   Obstetric Concerns

A. Spontaneous abortion

B. Ectopic pregnancy

C. Premature labor

D. Preeclampsia

E. Abruption

F. Placental insufficiency

G. Malpresentation

H. Sexually transmitted diseases

I. Poor/absent prenatal care

J. Intrauterine fetal death

K. Withdrawal (maternal)

VI.   Management

A. If the infant needs resuscitation at birth, *do not use Narcan,* because it may provoke acute withdrawal and seizures in infants exposed to opiates *in utero.*

B. Observe the infant in the hospital until adequate time for onset of withdrawal syndrome has passed. The infant should be discharged only after withdrawal has regressed and the primary caregiver (parent or foster parent) is able to care for the child.

C. Have the nursing staff utilize withdrawal scoring (Finnegan system) during each shift.

D. Administer HBIG within 24 hours of birth and hepatitis vaccine within 72 hours of birth if the mother's hepatitis B status is positive or unknown.

E. Refer for Social Service evaluation in cases where the toxicology screen is positive. Child protective services may need to be notified.

F. If drug screen is positive and HIV status is unknown, recommend HIV antibody testing of mother or cord blood with appropriate pre- and post-test counseling.

G. Treatment is primarily supportive. 30–50% of all opiate-exposed infants do not require pharmacologic therapy. Cocaine, marijuana, nicotine, and alcohol-exposed infants almost never need pharmacologic intervention.

1. Swaddling, pacifier

2. Frequent feeding—may need 150–250 cal/kg/d
3. Quiet, dimly lit room with minimal handling and stimulation

VII. Pharmacologic Management

A. Drugs are not necessary unless the infant has seizures or severe withdrawal signs
1. Inability to sleep or feed
2. > 10% weight loss in spite of good caloric intake
3. Severe diarrhea
4. Electrolyte imbalance
5. The goal of therapy is to enable the infant to sleep, feed, and grow without excessive sedation.

B. Tincture of opium—the most specific and the drug of choice
1. Dilute to strength of paregoric = 0.4% opium, 0.04% morphine.
2. Use 0.2–0.5 mL PO every 3–4 hr, increase by 0.05 mL each dose until signs are controlled.
3. Taper drug slowly after 4–6 days of stability until baby is weaned from drug. (***Caution***—respiratory depressant.)
4. ***Do not*** use paregoric; this compound contains camphor, a CNS stimulant.

C. Phenobarbital—*safest* to use if unfamiliar with use of tincture of opium.
1. May load first with 20 mg/kg then 3–5 mg/kg/d
2. Switch to oral when stable.
3. Taper by decreasing daily dosage every 1–2 days.
4. Drug of choice for seizures

D. Methadone
1. Range, 0.1–0.4 mg/kg
2. Start with 0.1 mg/kg every 12 hr and wean by 10% every 2–3 days once patient's withdrawal is stable.
3. No real side effects
4. Methadone has a prolonged half-life and its use and weaning may extend withdrawal hospitalization longer than tincture of opium or phenobarbital.

E. Diazepam (Valium)—may give 1–2 mg every 8 hr, but should be used with caution
1. Limited neonatal ability to metabolize; elimination may require 1 month for maturation.
2. Parenteral diazepam contains sodium benzoate (may displace bilirubin from albumin).
3. Late seizures observed in some infants
4. Depresses sucking reflex

VIII. Disposition of Infants

A. Arrange early follow-up visits with the baby's primary care physician.

B. It is important to educate the parents (or foster parents) about the infant's behavior, which can be irritating and difficult to handle. If the parents are not adequately prepared, this could lead to physical abuse.

C. Recommend drug counseling and rehabilitation to the mother/parents. It is important to include the father in this, because co-users are common in this scenario.

D. Infants with apnea as a sign of withdrawal should be considered for pulmonary evaluation and multichannel study if indicated.

E. Any suspicion of child abuse or neglect must, by law, be reported to the Child Protective Services.

Suggested Reading

Bell G, Lau K: Perinatal and neonatal issues of substance abuse. Pediatr Clin North Am 42:261–281, 1995.

Chasnoff I: Newborn infants with drug withdrawal symptoms. Pediatr Rev 9:273–277, 1988.

Committee on Drugs, American Academy of Pediatrics: Neonatal drug withdrawal. Pediatrics 72:895–903, 1983.

Finnegan LP: Neonatal abstinence scoring system: Assessment and pharmacotherapy. In Rubaltelli FF, Granati B (eds): Neonatal Therapy: An Update. Amsterdam, Excerpta Medica, 1986.

Hadeed A, Siegel S: Maternal cocaine use during pregnancy: Effect on the newborn infant. Pediatrics 84:205–210, 1989.

Palmer TP: Neonatal withdrawal syndrome. In Donn SM, Faix RG (eds): Neonatal Emergencies. Mt. Kisco, NY, Futura Publishing, 1991, pp 611–623.

Chapter 35

Morphine Withdrawal

Charles R. Neal, Jr., M.D., Ph.D.

I. Introduction

Morphine sulfate is often used in sick newborns for sedation, alone and in combination with pancuronium. Possible immediate side effects are hypotension, respiratory depression oversedation, and ileus. Morphine dependence can occur.

II. Signs of Withdrawal

A. Disturbed patterns of sleeping and waking
B. High-pitched cry
C. Hypertonicity
D. Irritability
E. Jitteriness
F. Sweating
G. Tachypnea
H. Tremors
I. Vomiting, diarrhea

III. Withdrawal Management

A. If the infant has received morphine for less than 7 days, the morphine can usually be discontinued and the infant observed for signs of withdrawal.

B. If the infant has been on morphine for longer than 7 days drug dependence may be present.

   1. To avoid withdrawal symptoms, it is recommended that the morphine be tapered slowly rather than suddenly being discontinued.

   2. A tapering schedule is preferred to a PRN dosing schedule.

     a. Usually, decreasing the total daily dose by 10% per day and maintaining the usual dosing schedule (every 4 hr) is well tolerated.

     b. Remember to decrease the dose each day by 10% of the original dose so that the tapering is not prolonged.

   3. If, as the drug dose is lowered, and signs appear, the dose can be increased to a previous dose that prevented signs.

   4. Persistent signs may need treatment. Phenobarbital or lorazepam may be necessary to enable complete withdrawal of morphine.

Section VI.   INFECTIOUS DISEASES

Chapter 36

Neonatal Sepsis and Meningitis

Jennifer L. Grow, M.D., and Steven M. Donn, M.D.

I.   Importance

A. Frequency: 1–5/1000 newborns in the U.S. are afflicted; 40–50/1000 of those < 2500 g, with further increases in incidence as birthweight decreases; as smaller and sicker infants survive and require longer NICU hospitalizations with invasive and immuno-compromising therapies, further increments are possible.

B. Mortality/morbidity: 10–20% of all neonatal deaths are associated with infection; of all infants with sepsis, 10–20% die overall (higher mortality at lower birthweights and gestational ages); survivors may sustain important neurodevelopmental sequelae.

C. Changing spectrum of responsible pathogens; group B streptococcus and coliforms still dominant, but new organisms are becoming important:

1. Community—untypable *Haemophilus influenzae,* possibly resurgent group A streptococcus

2. NICU—untypable *Haemophilus influenzae,* nosocomial infection attributed to coagulase-negative staphlyococci, *Candida, Malassezia,* others

D. Possibility of effective intervention

E. Limitations of intervention—effective therapy may arrest or prevent further injury but will not necessarily reverse damage that has already occurred, or immediately terminate pathophysiologic processes that are already under way.

II.   Mechanisms of Injury

A. Toxic structural components of microorganisms (e.g., endotoxin) activate complement cascade which triggers release of multiple cytokines with resultant leukostasis, release of vasoactive substances, altered tissue perfusion, and derangement of many physiologic processes.

B. Metabolic products of microorganisms (e.g., leukocidin, exotoxins, enzymes, leukotriene/prostaglandins, regulators, endorphin modulators, others) may directly injure or kill host cells.

C. Initiation and amplification of host inflammatory response are meant to eradicate invading organism, but may do substantial injury to "innocent bystander" normal host tissues.

    D. Rechanneling of host cellular metabolism to provide metabolic needs of invader rather than host

    E. Pressure from suppurative accumulations in a confined space injures adjacent tissues (e.g., pus in septic joint may occlude blood supply to underlying bone/cartilage with death of growth plate) or interferes with function of neighboring structures (e.g., purulent pericarditis, empyema).

    F. Others

III. Clinical Manifestations

May be extremely variable and nonspecific, including:

    A. Lethargy

    B. Poor feeding

    C. Jaundice

    D. Apnea

    E. Cyanosis

    F. Irritability

    G. Abdominal distention

    H. Hypotension/oliguria

    I. Petechiae/purpura

    J. Unstable temperature

    K. Diarrhea

    L. Seizures

    M. Tense fontanel

    N. Metabolic acidosis

    O. Respiratory distress

    P. Hyperglycemia

    Q. Hypoglycemia

IV. Associated Possible Risk Factors

    A. Early onset infection (< 5 days of age)

       1. Prolonged (definition varies, but typically 18–24 hrs) rupture of membranes in preterm infant

       2. Premature rupture of membranes (rupture before onset of labor)

       3. Foul-smelling amniotic fluid or baby

       4. Maternal fever or other signs suggestive of infection

       5. Preterm infants in whom there is no evident non-infectious explanation for preterm delivery

    B. Late onset infection (≥ 5 days age)

       1. Anatomic defects (e.g., obstructive uropathy, gastroschisis, myelodysplasia)

       2. Prolonged instrumentation of mucoepithelial surfaces

3. Repetitive or prolonged course(s) of broad spectrum antibiotic therapy
4. Indwelling vascular catheters
5. Long-term glucocorticoid therapy

V. Diagnosis

Sepsis work-up should include consideration of the following:

A. Careful physical examination

B. Blood culture (whenever possible this should be drawn from a peripheral site after sterile preparation of skin); at least 1.0 mL of blood is preferred. Aerobic processing preferable for most neonatal settings, although anaerobic cultures should be considered if intra-abdominal process is suspected. Additional cultures of blood drawn through indwelling vascular catheters may be useful for catheter-associated infection. If infant is already receiving antibiotic therapy, use resin bottles, antimicrobial removal device, or other maneuvers to optimize recovery of organisms.

C. Lumbar puncture—Gram stain and culture. Significant ongoing controversy as to whether it should be routinely included or not. Our own practice is to forego it in the setting of the asymptomatic infant who is being evaluated for early-onset infection on the basis of historical factors only. May be deferred in infants who are unstable. In some series of proven neonatal meningitis, however, CSF yielded the only positive culture in 10–15% of cases (especially in late-onset infection). Some authors have noted this to be especially likely in settings in which infant was exposed to intrapartum maternal antibiotic therapy. Cell counts, protein, glucose may be initially normal in same CSF specimen from which organism is recovered. CSF inflammation without organism recovery may indicate CNS infection in a site not communicating directly with CSF (Table 35).

D. Suprapubic bladder aspiration—Gram stain and culture. May not be helpful in first 3 days of life since isolated UTI is very uncommon in that setting; most helpful in infants ≥ 4 days old. Specimen obtained by bladder catheter may be reasonable alternative, although contamination is more likely (*see* page 202).

E. Urine obtained by catheter or suprapubic aspirate for antigen testing for group B strep, *if* mother is treated with antibiotics prior to delivery or if infant is treated prior to obtaining cultures. Testing in absence of pretreatment may be frequently misleading, given high incidence of false-positive results. (Utility of testing for such antigens as *Streptococcus pneumoniae*, *Haemophilus influenzae*

TABLE 35
Normal Cerebrospinal Fluid Values in High-Risk Newborns

	Term*	Preterm*	VLBW[†]
WBC count (cells/mm^3)			
Mean	8.2	9.0	5.0
Range	0–32	0–29	0–44
Mean % PMN	61.3	57.2	7.0
Range % PMN	NR	NR	(0–66)
Protein (mg/dL)			
Mean	90	115	142
Range	(20–170)	(65–150)	(45–370)
Glucose (mg/dL)			
Mean	52	50	60
Range	(34–119)	(24–63)	(29–217)

PMN = polymorphonuclear cells; NR = not reported.
*Data from Sarff LD, Platt LH, McCracken GH Jr: Cerebrospinal fluid evaluation in
neonates: Comparison of high-risk infants with and without meningitis. J Pediatr
88:473–477, 1976.
[†]Data from Rodriguez AF, Kaplan SL, Mason EO Jr: Cerebrospinal fluid values in the very
low birth weight infant. J Pediatr 116:971–974, 1990.

type B, or others appears to be very limited, as does antigen testing of CSF.)

F. Sterile aspirate of sites suggestive of focal infection— Gram stain
and culture.

G. If no response to 24–48 hours of broad-spectrum antimicrobial
therapy, or if other historic, physical, or epidemiologic factors are
suggestive, viral cultures of urine, throat, rectal swab/stool, conjunctiva, CSF, or other local sites may also be desirable. Consider
also cultures for fungi, mycoplasma.

H. Tracheal aspirate—Gram stain and culture; may be useful if obtained within 8 hours of birth in infant with significant respiratory
signs. Later specimens are more likely to reflect colonization than
infection.

I. Consider syphilis—maternal and infant VDRL, FTA; CSF analysis darkfield microscopy of placenta, lesions; long bone radiography. Clinical signs may overlap those of sepsis.

J. Surface cultures (e.g., umbilicus, ear canal, gastric aspirate) are unlikely to be helpful are frequently misleading, and are expensive.

K. Other tests have been reported to be variably helpful in consider-
ing an early diagnosis in a baby whose clinical appearance is
equivocal. Beware that both false-positives and false-negative results are frequent. Many noninfectious processes are also associated with abnormal studies.

1. CBC and differential. Multiple reference ranges have been published, but most widely used are probably those of Manroe et al. (1979). Norms change with postnatal age in hours. It is controversial whether same ranges should be applied to preterm or low birthweight infants.
2. Micro-ESR. Fill capillary tube to top, wipe excess from top rim. Tape in vertical position. Measure column of serum above cells at one hour.
   0–5 mm: probably normal
   6–8 mm: suspicious
   > 8 mm: strongly suspicious
3. Other acute phase reactants include C-reactive protein, orosomucoid, platelet count, and various cytokines.

VI. Goals of Therapy
A. Kill invading pathogens and prevent further invasion and destruction (lysis of organisms may facilitate release of toxic components and transiently worsen clinical status in some circumstances).
B. Modify or ablate adverse effects of organism-elaborated toxins and mediators (the ability to accomplish A is better than B, so far).

VII. Treatment
A. Sepsis or meningitis—begin with broad-spectrum parenteral antibiotic coverage. Choice of agents will be based on likely organisms for particular institution and clinical circumstances. Recent experience of our institution suggests ampicillin and gentamicin for patients < 5 days old, and vancomycin and gentamicin for patients ≥ 5 days old and continuously hospitalized since birth. If admitted from the community at ≥ 5 days old, ampicillin and cefotaxime are used. Initial drugs of choice may change periodically because of changing dominant pathogens or resistance patterns. For meningitis, alterations in choice of antibiotics, dosage, and duration may be necessary. Therapy must be intravenous if meningitis is suspected, or if peripheral perfusion is impaired. Later modification of antibiotic therapy is guided by results of cultures and susceptibility testing. Attempt to use as narrow spectrum agents as possible for final therapy to minimize selection of resistant organisms.
   1. Common organisms for early-onset sepsis (NICU and community): group B streptococcus, *Escherichia coli*, untypable *Haemophilus influenzae*, enterococcus, *Listeria monocytogenes*
   2. Common organisms for community-acquired late-onset sepsis:

group B streptococcus, *Haemophilus influenzae* type B, *Streptococcus pneumoniae*

3. Common organisms for NICU-acquired late-onset sepsis: coagulase-negative and coagulase-positive staphylococci, *Candida* species, enterococcus, *E. coli, Klebsiella* species, other gram-negatives

B. Strongly consider removal or replacement of indwelling catheters, appliances

C. Incision and drainage of abscesses

D. Meningitis—anticipate complications
1. SIADH—follow serum and urine sodium and osmolality and restrict fluids, if indicated.
2. Ventricular obstruction—serial neurologic exam, cranial sonography
3. Seizures—maintain normal glucose, calcium, electrolytes
4. Brain abscess—CT scan, cranial sonography
5. Ventriculitis
6. Cranial nerve dysfunction

E. If initial cultures were positive, repeat cultures of infected sites should be obtained 24–48 hours after initiation of therapy to assess therapeutic efficacy. If cultures remain positive, consider:
1. Improper antibiotic
2. Inadequate dose
3. Drug not being received (e.g., IV tubing inadvertently changed before dose completely infused)
4. Abscess or other sequestered focus (e.g., osteomyelitis, endocarditis)
5. Infected vascular catheter or other appliance

F. Duration
1. Sepsis: 7–14 days after sterilization of infected body fluid
2. Meningitis: 14–28 days after sterilization of infected body fluid

G. Adjunct therapy to support organ perfusion, oxygenation, and ventilation may be required. The use of fresh frozen plasma, exchange transfusions, granulocyte transfusions, IV immune globulin, granulocyte/monocyte-colony stimulating factor, and others to facilitate immune clearance and/or ablation of adverse pathophysiologic processes remains controversial.

H. Monitor antibiotic levels to assure therapeutic, but nontoxic range. MIC/MBC testing of selected isolates may facilitate decisions.

I. Serial assessment of organs for which host antimicrobial toxicity might be anticipated

J. Follow-up cranial sonography should be considered for all preterm infants with confirmed sepsis to assess for associated periventricular leukomalacia.

K. Careful neurodevelopmental follow-up, including audiology; physical therapy may also be useful.

VIII. Cessation of Therapy in Culture-Negative Suspected Sepsis

A. Low index of suspicion—if clinically well and cultures (antigen tests where appropriate) are negative, antibiotics may be stopped after 48 hours

B. High index of suspicion—exercise clinical judgment. If mother was pretreated (prior to delivery) or if treatment of baby was begun prior to cultures, may wish to consider longer course even if infant is well.

Suggested Reading

American Academy of Pediatrics Committee on Infectious Diseases: 1994 Red Book: Report of the Committee on Infectious Disease, 23rd ed. Elk Grove Village, IL, AAP, 1994.

Faix RG: Infectious emergencies. In Donn SM, Faix RG (eds): Neonatal Emergencies. Mt. Kisco, NY, Futura Publishing, 1991, pp 209–230.

Feigin RD, Adcock LM, Miller DJ: Postnatal bacterial infections. In Fanaroff AA, Martin RJ (eds): Neonatal-Perinatal Medicine: Diseases of the Fetus and Infant. St. Louis, Mosby, 1992, pp 619–661.

Manroe BL, Weinberg AG, Rosenfeld CR, Browne R: The neonatal blood count in health and disease: I. Reference values for neutrophilic cells. J Pediatr 95:89–98, 1979.

Remington JS, Klein JO (eds): Infectious Diseases of the Fetus and Newborn Infant, 5th ed. Philadelphia, W.B. Saunders, 2001.

Chapter 37

Suprapubic Bladder Aspiration

John D.E. Barks, M.D., and Steven M. Donn, M.D.

I. Indications

Confirmation or diagnosis of urinary tract infection (UTI) in a newborn. "Bag" specimens of urine are notoriously inaccurate (false positives) for culture purposes, especially in females. It is important to be sure of the diagnosis of a UTI in a newborn, since a full diagnostic work-up will be required eventually (e.g., ultrasound, cystogram, intravenous pyelogram, renal nuclear scan) because of the high association with anatomic abnormalities, especially in males.

II. Technique

A. Check with nurse for time of last void.

B. Restrain infant in supine position.

C. Prevent premature voiding by gently pinching penis in males, and by holding knees or labia together in females.

D. Prepare suprapubic region thoroughly with iodine-containing solution.

E. Use a 10-mL syringe with 22-gauge 1″ needle.

F. Palpate (in a sterile manner) the pubic bone and insert needle 1 cm superior to it in the midline, perpendicular to abdominal wall or with a slight (30°) angle cephalad.

G. Aspirate the syringe as needle is advanced.

H. Avoid excessive probing: do *not* change track.

I. If "dry," remove needle and repeat *once* more, entering skin slightly more cephalad.

J. Anticipate postprocedure hematuria.

K. Specimen should be labeled "suprapubic" and transported to laboratory or plated immediately.

Chapter 38

Congenital Infection

Jennifer L. Grow, M.D., and Steven M. Donn, M.D.

I. Definition

Congenital infections are those that are already present at birth. Though congenital infection in the broad sense may also include such overwhelming acute bacterial infections as those caused by group B streptococcus, this section will focus on *chronic* congenital infection. Pathogens responsible for these include, but are not limited to, those that contribute to the acronym TORCH (toxoplasmosis, others [congenital syphilis and virus], rubella, cytomegalovirus, herpes simplex).

II. Importance

A. Frequency—prospective screening studies have identified congenital infection in 0.5–2.8% of all liveborn infants.

B. Potential for mortality and significant neurodevelopmental morbidity

C. Increased appreciation that most congenital infections are asymptomatic in the newborn period, although some of these may become symptomatic with increasing age

D. New epidemiologic data have permitted better understanding of transmission and pathogenesis and, therefore, better opportunities for prevention, early diagnosis, and therapy; if mother is exposed during pregnancy, prophylaxis is available in some circumstances to prevent maternal and hence fetal infection.

E. Much broader range of organisms now included in "others" than previously appreciated

F. New antenatal diagnostic techniques and molecular biologic tools have permitted specific diagnosis in utero and created opportunities for preventing or ameliorating adverse outcomes.

G. Changing characteristics of the reproductive population (e.g., substance abuse, sexual practices, HIV infection) have brought new demographic, diagnostic, and therapeutic difficulties to infections previously thought to be easily treatable or on the wane.

H. Infection control issues

III. Clinical Manifestations

A. Asymptomatic—most common at birth

1. Many remain asymptomatic for life (percentage varies with organism).
2. Some who are asymptomatic at birth subsequently develop problems (e.g., CMV: 10–15% go on to develop sensorineural hearing loss, learning and seizure disorders, dental enamel hypoplasia; toxoplasmosis: chorioretinitis; syphilis: bony, vascular, CNS changes).

B. Symptomatic—only 5–10% of those with congenital infection are symptomatic at birth (percentage varies with organism)
1. Micro/macrocephaly
2. Hepatosplenomegaly
3. Calcifications, intracranial or intra-abdominal
4. Bony lesions
5. Adenopathy
6. Anemia, hemolytic and nonhemolytic
7. Thrombocytopenia
8. Sensorineural deafness
9. Chorioretinitis
10. Cataracts
11. Dermatopathy
12. Hepatopathy
13. Growth restriction
14. Hydrops fetalis
15. Neuronal migration anomaly (e.g., lissencephaly, pachygyria, polymicrogyria, others)
16. Aseptic meningitis
17. Seizures
18. Cardiopathy
19. Others

C. Clinical signs evident at birth may be suggestive of a particular pathogen, but are rarely pathognomonic.

IV. Responsible Agents
A. Classic
1. *Treponema pallidum* (syphilis)
2. *Toxoplasma gondii*
3. Rubella
4. Cytomegalovirus
5. Herpes simplex (usually acquired during birth process and therefore a perinatal pathogen; rarely a cause of true congenital infection)

B. Others

1. Enterovirus
2. Hepatitis B (also often a perinatal pathogen)
3. Parvovirus B19
4. Varicella-zoster virus
5. Human immunodeficiency virus (HIV)
6. Mycobacterium tuberculosis
7. Epstein-Barr virus (?)
8. Plasmodia (malaria)
9. Trypanosomes
10. Others

V. Importance of Knowing Which Specific Infectious Agent Is Responsible

A. Specific treatment is available for some (e.g., syphilis, toxoplasmosis). Specific therapy may not reverse injury that has already occurred, but may ameliorate further injury.

B. Prognosis varies with organism and degree of involvement.

C. Follow-up and rehabilitation may be markedly influenced since natural history varies with pathogen (e.g., serial audiologic evaluation for CMV; serial ophthalmologic assessment for toxoplasmosis).

D. Infection control issues—universal precautions may limit horizontal transmission for many of these infections. Specific immunization of nonimmune caretakers should be provided for those diseases for which a vaccine exists (e.g., hepatitis B, rubella).

VI. Diagnosis

A. Selection of tests will be influenced by maternal history, demographic/lifestyle factors, and physical and laboratory findings as well as infant findings and any fetal testing that may have been performed.

B. Classic tests
1. VDRL (qualitative and quantitative), FTA-ABS on maternal and infant serum
2. Long bone films
3. Darkfield microscopy of suspicious lesions or placenta on mother and/or infant
4. CSF VDRL, cell count, and biochemical studies
5. Viral cultures of urine, mouth, conjunctiva, CSF, rectum, depending on likely organism, obtained within first week of life, if possible
6. Careful placental examination (gross and microscopic)
7. IgM-specific antibody titers against suspect organisms (up to

two-thirds of culture-proven congenital infection may not have IgM-specific antibody detected, depending on technique used; rheumatoid factor may cause false positives.)

8. Total IgM (very nonspecific and insensitive)
9. Serial IgG-specific antibody titers against specific organisms
   a. Single titers are not helpful, because this often reflects passive transfer of maternal antibody.
   b. If antibody actively produced by the infant, titers that do not steadily decline by 6 months are quite suspicious; fourfold titer rises or newborn titer fourfold or more higher than maternal at birth are diagnostic; it is critical that the same laboratory test all sera, preferably simultaneously.
10. Neuroimaging tests
11. Biopsy of specific lesion with culture, microscopy, other organism detection tests

C. Newer tests (variable availability)
   1. Specific monoclonal antibodies that allow detection of miniscule quantities of pathogen with/without culture
   2. Polymerase chain reaction-based assays that may allow diagnosis even if only a single molecule of organism-specific DNA or RNA is present
   3. Modifications of conventional culture techniques for more rapid results (e.g., "shell vial" techniques with centrifugation of specimen, pretreatment of tissue culture with dexamethasone, availability of tissue culture rather than animal inoculation studies for toxoplasma).
   4. Harvesting of neonatal lymphocytes for in vitro detection of specific antibody production or antigen-specific DNA proliferation

D. Nonspecific testing
   1. Complete blood count with differential, reticulocyte count, platelet count
   2. Liver function tests
   3. Audiometric evaluation
   4. Ophthalmologic examination

VII. Treatment

A. Specific (be certain to treat mother as well, when appropriate)
   1. Syphilis—parenteral penicillin G as appropriate for stage and severity of disease; may require 10 days for initial course
   2. Toxoplasmosis—pyrimethamine and sulfadiazine with folinic acid for up to 1 year; spiramycin is available through CDC for selected circumstances.

3. Herpes simplex—acyclovir or vidarabine for 14–21 days; equally effective, although acyclovir easier to administer
4. Others as indicated for specific organism; utility of some agents and indications for their use remains controversial (e.g., ganciclovir for congenital CMV)
5. Effective, safe antimicrobial agents are not available for all organisms; therefore, symptomatic and rehabilitative therapies may be all that are possible.
6. Be certain to assure adequate follow-up with appropriate serologic and/or other tests to assess cure or need for retreatment.

B. Nonspecific
1. Serial neurodevelopmental assessment with appropriate rehabilitative therapy to produce improved outcome
2. Serial audiometric and ophthalmologic assessment
3. Others as indicated by clinical manifestations and responsible organism

Suggested Reading

American Academy of Pediatrics Committee on Infectious Diseases: Red Book 2000, 25th ed. Elk Grove Village, IL, AAP, 2000.

Greenough A, Osborne J, Sutherland S (eds): Congenital, Perinatal and Postnatal Infections. Edinburgh, Churchill Livingstone, 1992.

Grose C, Itani O: Pathogenesis of congenital infection with three diverse viruses: Varicella-zoster virus, human parvovirus, and human immunodeficiency virus. Semin Perinatol 13:278–293, 1989.

Hohlfeld P, Daffos F, Thulliez P, et al: Fetal toxoplasmosis: Outcome of pregnancy and infant follow-up after in utero treatment. J Pediatr 115:765–769, 1989.

Ikeda MK, Jenson HB: Evaluation and treatment of congenital syphilis. J Pediatr 117:843–852, 1990.

Kinney JS, Kumar ML: Should we expand the TORCH complex? A description of clinical and diagnostic aspects of selected old and new agents. Clin Perinatol 15:727–744, 1988.

Remington JS, Klein JO (eds): Infectious Diseases of the Fetus and Newborn Infant, 5th ed. Philadelphia, W.B. Saunders, 2001.

Chapter 39

Candida Infection

Jennifer L. Grow, M.D., and Steven M. Donn, M.D.

I. Importance

A. *Candida* species are frequent pathogens in VLBW infants (< 1500 g) with late-onset nosocomial infection in many NICUs.

B. Mortality and morbidity may be substantial, especially since these infections tend to occur primarily in the most compromised infants.

C. Difficulty of making diagnosis

1. Cultures of blood, CSF, or other body fluids may be sterile despite histologically proven infection because of sequestered site of infection, tissue binding, inadequate sampling or handling of specimen, or time at which specimen is obtained.

2. Cultures, even when positive, may take > 72 hours for growth to become evident.

3. May occasionally be a contaminant of cultures, but this conclusion should be based on a process of rigorous exclusion. *Recovery of* Candida *from a normally sterile site should not be assumed to be a contaminant.*

D. Therapeutic difficulties

1. Available effective antifungal agents often have potential for significant toxicity.

2. Penetration of agents into such common infected sites as the central nervous system, eye, liver, spleen, kidney, and focal deep abscesses in multiple loci is often problematic.

3. Resistance to available agents

II. Diagnosis

A. Clinical setting

1. Signs of late-onset infection in VLBW infant or infant with congenital or acquired abnormality of GI or GU tract

2. Prior history of mucocutaneous candidiasis in VLBW infant

3. Prolonged broad-spectrum antibiotic therapy

4. Chronic instrumentation of mucoepithelial surfaces

5. Presence of an indwelling vascular catheter

6. New-onset dermatitis

7. Long-term glucocorticoid therapy

B. Hematologic findings

     1. Usually neutrophilic with left shift
     2. More than 50% (up to 90% has been reported) will have platelet counts $< 150,000/mm^3$.
     3. Yeast occasionally seen on blood smear

C. Cultures/direct microscopy
     1. Blood (at least 1.0 mL)—peripheral and from indwelling catheters; limited data suggest arterial blood may yield positive cultures more frequently than venous blood; grows best with aerobic incubation; usually grows well with standard bacteriologic processing.
     2. CSF—important because CNS involvement is frequent (up to 67% in some reports) and may be the only site that is culture-positive; CSF inflammation with negative culture has been reported on multiple occasions in patients found to have diffuse *Candida* infection of the CNS at postmortem examination.
     3. Urine—preferably suprapubic aspirate; frequent colonization or local infection of the perineum and genitalia by *Candida* makes urine specimens obtained by bagging or even catheterization suspect.
     4. Surgical tissue or sterile aspirates of suggestive lesions.
     5. Gram stain/direct microscopy of CSF, urine, other normally sterile body fluids are very important, because culture may take up to 7 days for growth to be detected, while stain/wet prep may be positive immediately.
     6. Tests for *Candida* antigens and/or host antibodies directed against *Candida* antigens suffer as yet from lack of sensitivity and specificity, although recent studies of enolase and *Candida*-specific DNA as a marker of infection are promising.

III. Management/Treatment

A. Amphotericin is currently the agent most commonly used for treatment of invasive candidiasis in NICU infants. The combination of amphotericin B and flucytosine (*see* pages 98 and 102 for doses) is recommended by many to facilitate CNS penetration (a frequent site of occult infection) and offer additive/synergistic antifungal effects; some authors recommend only amphotericin B if there is no evidence of CNS involvement. Flucytosine should not be used as monotherapy because of frequent resistance.

B. Fluconazole, a newer agent, has been used successfully in NICU infants. Limited data suggest excellent activity against *Candida* strains with good CSF penetration and bioavailability with both PO and IV formulations and the potential for greatly reduced toxicity compared to amphotericin B and/or flucytosine. There are, however, several reports of resistant infections that responded once therapy was changed to a regimen including amphotericin. Comparative data for fluconazole versus amphotericin in NICU infants are sparse.

C. Possible utility of itraconazole and liposomal amphotericin B in newborns has not been systematically addressed. Both miconazole and ketoconazole have serious limitations.

D. Monitor hepatic (ALT; bilirubin, conjugated and unconjugated), renal (creatinine), and hematopoietic (leukocyte, platelet, and reticulocyte counts) function before therapy and then weekly; serum potassium and magnesium should be assessed before therapy and then every 2 to 3 days; modification of dosing regimen may be mandated by toxicity.

E. Test flucytosine susceptibility of the isolate, if that agent is used in therapy; assess flucytosine serum concentrations weekly, if possible. (Concentrations > 60 μg/mL have been associated with bone marrow suppression.)

F. Remove or replace indwelling vascular catheters.

G. Reculture infected body fluids at frequent intervals (at least weekly) to assure sterilization; strongly consider doing this for at least 2 weeks after cessation of therapy (since late recurrence and recrudescence are well-known complications).

H. Ophthalmology evaluation for endophthalmitis

I. Strongly consider serial cranial, cardiac, and abdominal sonography to assess fungus ball uropathy, aqueductal stenosis, ventriculitis, deep abscesses, and other complications, especially if cultures of normally sterile sites are persistently positive.

J. Careful serial examination for local suppurative foci that might require drainage or topical therapy

K. Nystatin 0.5 mL to each side of mouth by swab four times daily to reduce mucosal organisms; topical to other sites as needed (some investigators have reported oral nystatin to be effective prophylaxis for *Candida* infection; others have noted the development of disseminated infection despite nystatin.)

L. Treat with systemic antifungals for 2 weeks or more after sterilization of infected body fluid. (Limited evidence suggests that infants with isolated UTIs and other well-localized infections may respond to shorter courses of therapy and may do well with only amphotericin; further data are needed before this can be routinely recommended.)

Suggested Reading

Baley JE, Kliegman RM, Fanaroff AA: Disseminated fungal infections in very-low-birth-weight infants: Clinical manifestations and epidemiology. Pediatrics 73:144–152, 1984.

Baley JE: Neonatal candidiasis: The current challenge. Clin Perinatol 18:263–280, 1991.

Butler KM, Rench MA, Baker CJ: Amphotericin B as a single agent in the treatment of systemic candidiasis in neonates. Pediatr Infect Dis J 9:51–56, 1990.

Faix RG: Systemic *Candida* infections in infants in intensive care nurseries: High incidence of central nervous system involvement. J Pediatr 105:616–622, 1984.

Faix RG, Kovarik SM, Shaw TR, et al: Mucocutaneous and invasive candidiasis among very low birth weight (<1,500 g) infants in intensive care nurseries: A prospective study. Pediatrics 83:101–107, 1989.

Miller MJ: Fungal infections. In Remington JS, Klein JO (eds): Infectious Diseases of the Fetus and Newborn Infant, 5th ed. Philadelphia, W.B. Saunders, 2001, pp 813–854.

Rowen JL, Atkins JT, Levy ML, Baer SC, et al: Invasive fungal dermatitis in the ≤1000-gram neonate. Pediatrics 95:682–687, 1995.

Sims ME, Yoo Y, You H, et al: Prophylactic oral nystatin and fungal infections in very-low-birth-weight infants. Am J Perinatol 5:33–36, 1988.

Chapter 40

Intrapartum Chemoprophylaxis of Group B Streptococcal Infection and Management of the Newborn

Robert E. Schumacher, M.D.

I. Background

A. Because of the frequency and severity of early-onset group B streptococcal infection in newborn and peripartum women, strategies have been developed (and are continuing to evolve) to prevent or ameliorate these infections.

B. Most prominent strategies:

1. Targeted antibiotic therapy during labor and delivery to reduce transmission of group B streptococcus (GBS) from the colonized or infected mother to the infant.

2. Initiate transplacental therapy of incipient fetal/neonatal infection.

C. Conflicting recommendations by the American Academy of Pediatrics and the American College of Obstetricians and Gynecologists in 1992 have recently been supplanted by consensus recommendations from the Centers for Disease Control (CDC), developed with input from both specialty organizations as well as many others.

D. While it is recognized that the CDC guidelines are imperfect and will likely undergo modification as further research is reported and incorporated, it appears that the recommended strategies (as well as others) are associated with reductions in perinatal group B streptococcal disease.

E. Failure to adopt any strategy because of continuing uncertainty as to which is the best strategy will likely not be acceptable policy. It will be incumbent on each institution involved in perinatal health care delivery to consider and implement an institution-specific strategy for prevention of group B streptococcal disease.

F. The guidelines currently used by the University of Michigan for management of the mother and infant are outlined below, although it is highly likely that changes will be implemented as knowledge and the state of the art evolves.

II. Guidelines

A. For women with a history of GBS bacteriuria during the pregnancy or a previous newborn infant with GBS infection, administration of intrapartum antimicrobial prophylaxis (IAP) is definitely recommended.

B. For other women, the CDC guidelines have recommended either screening the vagina and rectum for GBS at 34–36 weeks' gestation (using selective media) *or* the use of clinical risk factors to determine which mothers should receive IAP.

C. Our institution has adopted the preferential use of risk factors rather than routine screening for perineal carriage of GBS as the strategy of choice.

    1. If the maternal carriage status is known, for whatever reason, within 6 weeks of delivery, that information is used to facilitate making decisions about IAP.

    2. If IAP is indicated, intravenous penicillin G is the agent of choice (5 million U initially, then 2.5 million U every 4 hours).

    3. For women with penicillin allergy, clindamycin or vancomycin are acceptable alternatives. We have not included erythromycin as an alternative because of unreliable penetration into cord blood and the amniotic cavity.

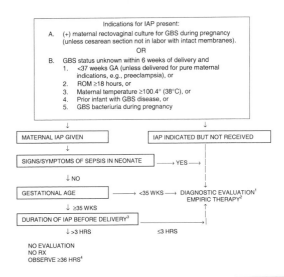

Figure 6. Guidelines for the management of a newborn born to a mother who qualifies to receive intrapartum antimicrobial prophylaxis for prevention of early-onset GBS disease.

    4. Women who are being treated for other infectious problems (e.g., chorioamnionitis) and receiving other regimens that include agents effective against streptococci do not need penicillin G added to the regimen.

D. The guidelines for management of the infant born to a mother who qualifies to receive IAP are summarized in Figure 6.

    1. This diagram was developed with the knowledge that our particular institution would be emphasizing the use of risk factors, so that it would be unlikely to encounter a woman known to be colonized with GBS who did not also have clinical risk factors.

    2. These guidelines may not be appropriate for other institutions that have opted to use routine perineal culture for GBS in all pregnant women as their primary tool for making decisions about IAP.

Chapter 41

Necrotizing Enterocolitis

Jennifer L. Grow, M.D., and Steven M. Donn, M.D.

I. Importance

A. Characterized by diffuse or patchy gastrointestinal injury which may progress to frank necrosis accompanied by systemic derangements

B. Frequency: 2–5% of all infants (10–20% of VLBWs) admitted to NICUs will develop this disorder.

C. Mortality/morbidity: of those that develop necrotizing enterocolitis (NEC), 10–15% will die and another 10–20% may develop significant complications.

II. Clinical Manifestations

These are variable and may be subtle initially.

A. Early
1. Poor feeding
2. Apnea
3. Gastric retention
4. Diarrheal stool (often positive for heme and reducing substances)
5. Vomiting (may be bilious)
6. Abdominal distention
7. Jaundice
8. Ascites

B. Later findings, often more dramatic
1. Increasing lethargy
2. Pallor and shock
3. Oliguria
4. Blood-streaked or grossly bloody stools, sometimes with necrotic mucosal debris
5. Peritonitis (cellulitis of anterior abdominal wall, exquisitely tender abdomen, bluish discoloration of anterior abdominal wall)
6. Temperature instability
7. Coagulopathy
8. Respiratory failure

III. Laboratory Manifestations

A. Hematologic
1. Marked neutrophilia or neutropenia; many immature forms may be present

      2. Thrombocytopenia

      3. Abnormal coagulation profile

      4. Hemolysis

  B. Metabolic

      1. Sudden hyponatremia

      2. Hypoproteinemia

      3. Metabolic acidosis

      4. Hyperglycemia (without change in previously tolerated glucose load)

  C. Radiographic

      1. Dilated, edematous bowel loops

      2. Intramural gas (pneumatosis intestinalis)

      3. Portal system gas

      4. Pneumoperitoneum (with perforation)

      5. "Triangle sign" on lateral projection of abdomen

      6. Ileus

      7. Hepatic microbubbles on sonography

  D. Infectious—positive blood and/or CSF culture, positive peritoneal fluid culture or Gram stain

IV. Typical Demographic Profile

  A. Prematurity (especially < 1500 g; up to 90% patients are low birthweight)

  B. Previous asphyxia, hypoxia, acidosis, shock, or other process that may induce an enteric insult

  C. Prior feedings, usually of commercial formula

  D. Most infants with these risk factors will not develop NEC; conversely, some with NEC may not have any of these identified prior to onset.

  E. In epidemics of NEC, none of these factors may be present.

V. Pathogenesis

  A. Appears to be multifactorial; there is no single identified necessary and sufficient factor. NEC appears to require concurrent presence of mucosal injury and colonization of the gut with pathogenic flora, both of which may be facilitated by provision of appropriate intraluminal substrate, e.g., enteral feedings.

  B. Enteric mucosal injury

      1. Ischemia

         a. Asphyxia—possible manifestation of the "diving seal" reflex in human newborns

         b. Polycythemia

    c. PDA, especially if significant retrograde diastolic flow. Also associated with indomethacin treatment.

    d. Low-output congenital heart disease

    e. Exchange transfusion

    f. Umbilical artery catheter

    g. Other low-output states

  2. Osmotic injury

  3. Diarrhea

  4. Hypoxia

  5. Cold stress

C. Colonization of gut with pathogenic flora

  1. Gram-negative bacilli, including anaerobes such as *Escherichia coli, Klebsiella pneumoniae,* and *Enterobacter cloacae* type 3305573

  2. Viruses, including rotavirus, adenovirus, coronavirus, and enterovirus,

  3. Enterotoxins from both gram-positive and gram-negative organisms

  4. Others

D. Intraluminal substrate (commercial formula associated with much higher risk than breast milk)

VI. Treatment

A. Medical

  1. NPO

  2. Decompress (NG or OG) with suction, intermittent if single-lumen tube, continuous if sump tube

  3. Sepsis work-up

    a. Blood culture, aerobic, and anaerobic

    b. Consider lumbar puncture, if condition permits.

    c. Consider urine culture by suprapubic aspiration or catheterization.

    d. Consider peritoneal fluid culture.

    e. Stool culture recommended by some, especially if NEC epidemic is present

  4. Parenteral antibiotics for likely gram-positive and gram-negative aerobic and facultative anaerobic organisms. (Gentamicin and vancomycin are agents of choice in our NICU. The further addition of clindamycin was not found to be helpful for medical NEC. There are no data regarding the advisability of routine empiric inclusion of metronidazole during the medical phase of NEC.) Use of clindamycin or metronidazole may be warranted if perforation

or intestinal gangrene develops, or if cultures yield an organism that requires their addition.

5. If patient develops NEC while receiving antibiotics, consider additional antibiotic(s) and/or change.
6. Total parenteral nutrition
7. Insure adequate oxygenation, perfusion.
8. Blood component therapy as needed
9. Remove UAC if possible.
10. Paracentesis may be considered in individual cases for culture and Gram stain, especially if intestinal gangrene is suspected.
11. Parameters to follow
    a. Abdominal radiographs to assess for perforation and/or intestinal gangrene; initially may need to assess every 6–8 hr, less frequently as condition improves. Crosstable lateral for "triangle" sign may be particularly useful.
    b. Transillumination of abdomen to assess for perforation. Visualization of falciform ligament or hyperlucency of entire abdomen suggests pneumoperitoneum.
    c. Abdominal examination, including girth (measured at umbilicus)
    d. Urine output, blood pressure
    e. Blood pH, PaO_2, and $PaCO_2$
12. Some recommend enteric isolation/precautions for all afflicted infants to minimize risk of NEC "epidemic."

B. Surgical
1. If not already obtained, consultation should be sought at time of definitive diagnosis (e.g., pneumatosis intestinalis)
2. Indications for surgery
    a. Perforation
    b. Intestinal gangrene
    c. Deterioration despite aggressive medical management
    d. Post-NEC obstruction
3. Procedures
    a. Resection and enterostomy
    b. "Second look" procedures to maximize preservation of questionable bowel
    c. Peritoneal lavage and drainage for infants too unstable for resection
    d. Others

C. Cessation of therapy
1. May discontinue OG suction when distention is resolved. Leave tube to chimney.

2. Stop antibiotics after 7–14 days if clinically well (longer duration may be warranted depending on culture results and/or presence of focal suppurative complication).
3. Feeding may be resumed cautiously after antibiotics are stopped and infant is stooling (note—there may be some residual heme in stools).
4. Some clinicians prefer to restart enteral feedings with a formula that is lactose-free and of reduced osmolality (e.g., half-strength Pregestimil).
5. Observe closely for relapse.
6. Ultimately, advance to breast milk or lactose-containing formula.

VII. Complications in Survivors
A. Adhesions and obstruction from strictures (two thirds in colon; remainder in small bowel, especially terminal ileum).
B. Complications associated with gut resection and/or ostomy formation
C. Complications associated with long-term TPN with cholestasis
D. Intra-abdominal abscess
E. Short-gut syndrome (up to 25%)
F. Enteric fistulas
G. Acquired Hirschsprung's disease
H. Developmental delay (not known to be a direct sequela)

VIII. Differential Diagnosis
A. Malrotation with volvulus
B. Toxic megacolon/Hirschsprung's disease
C. Intestinal stenosis/atresia
D. Other causes of acute mechanical obstruction
E. Gastritis/peptic ulcer disease
F. Spontaneous gastric or bowel perforation
G. Sepsis/meningitis
H. Inborn errors of metabolism
I. Pneumoperitoneum associated with pulmonary air leak
J. Enteric vascular accidents
K. Milk protein intolerance
L. Pseudomembranous enterocolitis
M. Low-output congenital heart disease

IX. Prevention
A. Remains controversial
B. Suggested strategies with varying empirical support

1. Antenatal/postnatal glucocorticoids
2. Human breast milk feedings
3. Oral feeding of IgG-IgA, other Ig preparations
4. Cautious feeding regimens
5. Enteral nonabsorbed or minimally absorbed antimicrobials
6. Intentional gut colonization with low virulence organisms
7. Supplemental gastric acid to facilitate gut colonization with less pathogenic organisms

Suggested Reading

Boccia D, Stolfi I, Lana S, Moro ML: Nosocomial necrotising enterocolitis outbreaks: Epidemiology and control measures. Eur J Pediatr 160:385–391, 2001.

Caplan MS, Jilling T: New concepts in necrotizing enterocolitis. Curr Opin Pediatr 13:111–115, 2001.

Faix RG, Polley TZ, Grasela TH: A randomized, controlled trial of parenteral clindamycin in neonatal necrotizing enterocolitis. J Pediatr 112:271–277, 1988.

Holman RC, Stoll BJ, Clarke MJ, Glass RI: The epidemiology of necrotizing enterocolitis infant mortality in the United States. Am J Public Health 87:2026–2031, 1997.

Holton AF, Kovar IZ: Necrotizing enterocolitis: An infectious disease? Curr Opin Infect Dis 2:427, 1989.

Lucas A, Cole TJ: Breast milk and neonatal necrotizing enterocolitis. Lancet 336:1519–1523, 1990.

Moss RL, Dimmitt RA, Henry MC, et al: A meta-analysis of peritoneal drainage versus laparotomy for perforated necrotizing enterocolitis. J Pediatr Surg 36:1210–1213, 2001.

Stoll BJ, Kliegman RM (eds): Necrotizing Enterocolitis. Clinics in Perinatology, vol. 21, no. 2. Philadelphia, W.B. Saunders, 1994.

Uauy RD, Fanaroff AA, Korones SP, et al: Necrotizing enterocolitis in very low birth weight infants: Biodemographic and clinical correlates. J Pediatr 119:630–638, 1991.

Chapter 42

Neonatal Acquired Immunodeficiency Syndrome

Jennifer L. Grow, M.D., and Steven M. Donn, M.D.

I. Epidemiology

It is estimated that 280–370 infants in the USA are infected perinatally with human immunodeficiency virus (HIV) each year. An estimated 96–128,000 HIV-infected women of childbearing age reside in the USA. Perinatal use of zidovudine (ZDV) has decreased transmission of HIV to infants from ~16–25% to ~5% and < 1% in mothers with undetectable viral loads. Combination antiviral therapy and use of cesarean section have aided with the dramatic decline of transmission. 30% of infant cases of HIV occur prior to delivery; 70% occur during the delivery. Of these perinatal cases, ~2/3 occur during the 2 weeks prior to delivery.

II. Detection of Disease in Infants

Disease in infants < 18 months of age includes recovery of HIV from culture of blood or tissues; detection of P24 Ag in infant serum; detection of HIV viral-specific DNA in infants lymphocytes by polymerase chain reaction (PCR); or positive antibody to HIV in serum of an infant who also has clinical signs of disease meeting the CDC definition of acquired immunodeficiency syndrome (AIDS). Seropositive status alone in an infant < 18 months of age does not confirm the diagnosis.

III. Transmission

HIV has been recovered from cord blood, amniotic fluid, breast milk, tears, and vaginal secretions of HIV-positive mothers. Perinatal transmission is now estimated at ≤ 11% in the USA and Western Europe.

A. Acquisition may occur via multiple routes, but vertical transmission from mother to baby accounts for 95% of pediatric AIDS in the USA.

    1. Intrauterine—cellular mechanisms for transmission have not yet been elucidated. HIV can be acquired transplacentally. The infection has been seen in first trimester abortuses, but the actual timing of infection is usually unknown.

    2. Intrapartum—transmission may arise from infected maternal

blood or vaginal secretions. Although an unproven risk, it appears advisable to avoid intrapartum procedures that expose the infant to maternal blood (e.g., scalp electrodes, scalp blood sampling).

3. Peri/postnatal—acquisition after birth is primarily via infected breast milk. Studies have shown that women in the acute phase of infection are more likely to transmit the virus in their breast milk.

B. Factors that may influence the transmission of virus to the fetus include the following:

1. Cesarean section has been shown to possibly reduce the risk of transmission to infants if mothers do not receive antiviral therapy antepartum. There are concerns regarding increased maternal morbidity in mothers who receive cesarean sections, such as postpartum fever.

2. Approximately 15–40% of infants born in the USA to HIV-positive mothers who are not receiving antiretroviral therapy will acquire true infection.

3. Increased risk for transmission is associated with clinical AIDS in the mother, low maternal CD4 counts, P24 antigenemia in maternal serum, histologic chorioamnionitis, POL/PROM, STDs. Increased risk factors for perinatal transmission are maternal–fetal blood exchange, breastfeeding within the first few months of life, advanced maternal HIV disease, maternal high plasma viral load, preterm delivery, no perinatal antiviral treatment, prolonged rupture of membranes > 4 hr, maternal STD, and chorioamnionitis.

4. Decreased risk for transmission is associated with a positive maternal serum antibody to HIV protein gp120 and good prenatal care.

5. Prenatal ZDV therapy. (Vertical transmission was decreased from 20% to 8% with prenatal ZDV therapy in the Pediatric AIDS Clinical Trials Group Protocol 076 study.)

6. Prenatal exposure to ZDV therapy has not been associated with increased risk of congenital anomalies, preterm delivery, or low birthweight.

IV. Diagnosis

Diagnosis is difficult to establish clearly in newborns. Postnatal evaluation of infants at risk for HIV infection begins immediately after birth. Infants need to be diagnosed early, since perinatally infected infants may easily succumb to *Pneumocystis carinii* pneumonia, a fatal opportunistic infection.

A. The diagnosis in children is most frequently suspected based on the knowledge that the parents are HIV positive.

1. Antibody to HIV—maternal anti-HIV antibody is acquired transplacentally from the 27th week of gestation on, and may persist in infant serum up to 15 months postnatally. As above, an isolated positive Ab test at birth does not denote infection. These standard antibody assays are less useful for the diagnosis of infants < 18 months. Mothers transmit passive antibody and many infants may test antibody passive until 18 months regardless of true infectious status.

   a. ELISA (enzyme-linked immunosorbent assay) is a highly sensitive assay that has a moderate false-positive rate (e.g., there is a cross reactivity with Abs from other immune-mediated diseases). It cannot distinguish passively acquired maternal Ab from actual infant-generated Ab. Repeatedly positive tests over time are very reliable for diagnosis. Documentation of rising Ab titers in an infant is also indicative of infection.

   b. Western blot—a highly specific and sensitive immunofluorescent Ab test used to identify specific Ab against HIV proteins separated by electrophoresis. Used at most centers to confirm a positive ELISA test.

2. HIV culture—technically difficult in newborns, but diagnostic for infection; send infant blood (not cord blood) or tissue for viral culture (a send-out study at many institutions, requiring 10–12 days for results); very specific, but there are a high number of false negatives in newborns.

3. HIV P24 antigen—send infant serum (also often a send-out study, requiring 10–12 days for results); very specific, but again sensitivity is low in newborns. There is a risk of false-positive results within the first month of life. Not recommended.

4. HIV viral-specific DNA detected in infant lymphocytes by PCR—again, technically difficult in a newborn, but a positive test is diagnostic (also often a send-out study, requiring 10–12 days for results); very specific, sensitive in newborn.

5. RNA PCR is not recommended for diagnosis in infants < 18 months because of high rate of false-negative results. This may be a useful test to quantify the amount of virus present to measure disease progression.

B. Other markers for infection

1. CD4 (T helper) cell count (decreases with disease progression)
2. Quantitative serum immunoglobulins. (There is often a

hyperproduction of nonspecific and dysfunctional immunoglobulins, especially IgG.)

C. Negative serology, culture, and assays do not exclude HIV infection.
The immature neonatal immune system may not mount an antibody
response to infection. As above, yield for positive culture and PCR is
low in newborns for reasons that are not yet clearly understood.

D. To establish clearly the diagnosis in the newborn, two or more of
the following must be positive with two separate specimens:
   1. HIV culture
   2. HIV P24 Ag
   3. HIV viral-specific DNA identified by PCR. Umbilical cord
   blood is NOT recommended, because of risk of contamination.
   DNA PCR is highly recommended within the first 48 hours of
   life, so as to initiate recommended therapy. The second test is
   performed at 1–2 months of age; the third test is performed at
   36 months of age.

E. Infants born to HIV-positive mothers, who demonstrate none of
the above at birth, must be followed with serial investigations and
close clinical follow-up until at least 24 months of age.

V.   Clinical Features

A. 2000 CDC classification system
   1. **P0**—asymptomatic infants up to 18 months of age in whom a
   definitive diagnosis of HIV has not yet been made
   2. **P1**—asymptomatic infants and children regardless of age in
   whom the diagnosis of HIV infection has been established by
   HIV P24 Ag or HIV culture with or without evidence of immunodeficiency
   3. **P2**—symptomatic HIV-infected child (further subdivided into
   subclasses A through F based on disease manifestations)

B. Manifestations in infants less than 1 year of age (clinical signs
may not be prominent in the newborn)
   1. CNS—signs of CNS disease are associated with a poor prognosis; roughly 50% of HIV-infected children who develop AIDS
   demonstrated neurologic signs prior to death.
      a. Acute meningoencephalitis
      b. Seizures
      c. Brain atrophy or microcephaly
      d. Loss of, or failure to attain milestones
      e. Acute encephalopathy
      f. Coma
      g. Behavior changes

2. Respiratory
   a. Lymphoid interstitial pneumonitis (very common)
   b. Recurrent pneumonia (especially pneumococcal)
   c. Recurrent sinusitis
3. Hematologic
   a. Anemia
   b. Neutropenia
   c. Thrombocytopenia
   d. Bleeding diathesis
4. Gastrointestinal
   a. Infections/ulcerations of the oral mucosa, esophagus, stomach, and small intestine
   b. Infectious colitis
   c. Primary HIV hepatitis
   d. Chronic malnutrition
   e. Recurrent diarrhea
   f. Splenomegaly
5. Renal—roughly 3–4% of infants and children who are HIV positive manifest glomerulonephritis that progresses to renal failure.
6. Cardiac—cardiomyopathy is rare.
7. Others
   a. Lymphadenopathy
   b. Hepatosplenomegaly
   c. Chronic, painless swelling of the parotid gland
   d. Failure to thrive
   e. Weight loss
   f. Recurrent fever
   g. Malignancies (very common in this population)

C. Many infants and young children will manifest infection with increased incidence of sepsis, chronic and recurrent otitis, sinusitis, or pneumonia.

D. Common opportunistic pathogens
   1. *Pneumocystis carinii*—most common in the first few months of life
   2. *Candida albicans*—may manifest as nonresponsive thrush, severe diaper dermatitis, or esophagitis
   3. CMV—roughly 50% of children with HIV infection are co-infected with CMV at birth
   4. *Mycobacterium tuberculosis*—the incidence is still low in infants and children

E. Survival
   1. Mean survival increased to 82 months in 1993 for congenitally

infected babies. 15–20% of untreated infants die before 4 years of age, with a mean age of 11 months at the time of death.

2. Median survival of congenitally infected infants is 75–90 months based on recent estimates.

VI. Management

A. Infection control—these babies do not require isolation. Universal body substance precautions must be taken when caring for the infant. Gloves and protective wear are not necessary for some routine care (e.g., holding and feeding). Breastfeeding should be avoided as the virus may be transmitted in breast milk of infected mothers.

B. Baseline laboratory studies should include CBC with platelet count and differential, infant blood for HIV culture or PCR, and baseline ELISA; consider CD4 and CD8 counts, quantitative immunoglobulins, type and screen of baby's blood, and urine for CMV. Babies do not routinely require bacterial culture of blood or CSF unless clinically warranted.

C. Treatment
   1. Antiretroviral therapy
      a. ZDV/AZT—first line drug used in newborns, and is usually very well tolerated by this population. Oral ZDV should be administered as soon as baby can tolerate enteral feeds. The dose is 2 mg/kg/dose every 6 hr for the first 6 weeks of life, with the first dose given within 8–12 hr of birth. Premature infants may need dosing of 2 mg/kg every 12 hr then every 8 hr after 2 weeks of age. The intravenous dose of ZDV is 1.5 mg/kg/dose infused over an hour, given every 6 hr; the first dose is given within the first 8–12 hours of birth. Side effects of ZDV include profound anemia and neutropenia in some children. It may also cause significant gastrointestinal upset. ZDV is the best drug for treatment of CNS disease. Blood levels may be increased if used in combination with methadone.
      b. Didanosine (DDI)—used in children who cannot tolerate ZDV, or in whom disease progresses despite ZDV therapy. Felt to be effective in combination therapy with ZDV. Well tolerated by infants.
      c. Zalcitabine (DDC)—a third-line drug used when other therapy fails (not yet approved for use in children). Often used in combination therapy.
      d. Lamivudine (3TC)—another antiviral drug well tolerated by

infants and children used in combination therapy. Currently in clinical trials in neonatal infants.

2. *Pneumocystis carinii* pneumonia

   a. TMP/SMZ is the drug of choice

   b. All perinatally exposed infants at ages 4–6 weeks until infection status determined need to be receiving PCP prophylaxis (2000 CDC guidelines). Prophylaxis should be discontinued for infants in whom HIV has been excluded.

3. Intravenous immunoglobulin therapy (IVIG)—this therapy is usually reserved for older infants and children in whom chronic bacterial infections are recurrent and difficult to treat (e.g., recurrent sinusitis and pneumonias). Given in addition to anti-retroviral therapy.

4. Immunizations

   a. Asymptomatic HIV positive (or suspected HIV positive): all routine immunizations including IPV should be administered; MMR is safe; administration of yearly influenza vaccine should start at 6 months of age; pneumococcal vaccine should be given at 2 years of age; BCG is safe for asymptomatic children, and should be given in areas where tuberculosis is endemic.

   b. Symptomatic HIV infection: in these patients, BCG vaccines should be avoided; MMR is safe and necessary; all other routine vaccines should be given; again, yearly influenza vaccine should be given, starting at 6 months of age; pneumococcal vaccine should be administered beginning at 2 years of age.

   c. Passive immunoprophylaxis is recommended for symptomatic children exposed to any vaccine-preventable disease regardless of vaccine history (e.g., VZIG, tetanus IG).

   d. Infants and children who live with an HIV-positive person who is immunocompromised should be given IPV, and MMR is safe.

5. The HIV-positive infant, or any infant in whom HIV infection is suspected, should be referred to an infectious disease or other specialist familiar with the care of infected children for close, serial follow-up and management.

Suggested Reading

Boyer PJ, Dillon M, Navaic M, et al: Factors predictive of maternal-fetal transmission of HIV-1: Preliminary analysis of zidovudine given during pregnancy and/or delivery. JAMA 271:1925–1930, 1994.

Centers for Disease Control and Prevention: Revised recommendations for HIV screening of pregnant women. MMWR Morb Mortal Wkly Rep 50:63–85, 2001.

Connor EM, Sperling RS, Gelber R, et al: Reduction of maternal-infant transmission of human immunodeficiency virus type 1 with Zidovudine treatment. N Engl J Med 331:1173–1180, 1994.

Connor EM, Mofenson L: Zidovudine for the reduction of perinatal human immunodeficiency virus transmission: Pediatric AIDS clinical trials group protocol 076—results and treatment recommendations. Pediatr Infect Dis J 14:536–541, 1995.

Evans HE (ed): Perinatal AIDS. Clinics in Perinatology, vol. 21, no. 1. Philadelphia, W.B. Saunders, 1994.

Fernandez AD, McNeeley DF: Management of the infant born to a mother infected with human immunodeficiency virus type 1 (HIV-1): Current concepts. Am J Perinatol 17:429–436, 2000.

Krivine A, Firtion G, Cao L, et al: HIV replication during the first few weeks of life. Lancet 339:1187–1189, 1992.

Mofenson LM: A critical review of studies evaluating the relationship of mode of delivery to perinatal transmission of human immunodeficiency virus. Pediatr Infect Dis J 14:169–177, 1995.

Mueller BU, Pizzo P: Acquired immunodeficiency syndrome in the infant. In Remington JS, Klein JO (eds): Infectious Diseases of the Fetus and Newborn Infant, 5th ed. Philadelphia, W.B. Saunders, 2001, pp 447–476.

Newell ML, Dunn D, Reckham C, et al: Risk factors for mother-to-child transmission of HIV-1. European Collaborative Study. Lancet 339:1007–1012, 1992.

Pickering LK (ed): 2000 Red Book: Report of the Committee on Infectious Diseases, 25th ed. Elk Grove Village, IL, American Academy of Pediatrics, 2000.

Chapter 43

Immunization

Jennifer L. Grow, M.D., and Steven M. Donn, M.D.

I. Background

A. A period of physiologic hypogammaglobulinemia may occur from 2 to 6 months of postnatal age as transplacental maternal antibody wanes.

B. Premature infants often have lower immunoglobulin (Ig) levels because of decreased transplacental transport of maternal IgG during their shortened gestation.

C. Both term and preterm infants are capable of responding to antigenic challenge and can synthesize antigen-specific immunoglobulin if large quantities of maternal antibody are present. However, maternal Ig may bind the antigen and block recognition and endogenous Ig production by the infant.

II. Active Immunizations

A. The long-term goal of immunization is eradication of disease among the population; the immediate goal is to prevent disease in individuals.

B. Active immunization involves inducing an immunologic response in an individual by the administration of a microorganism (or modified product of the microorganism) in such a manner as to not pose risk to the individual.

C. Some vaccines confer complete protection for life (e.g., oral polio vaccine [OPV]), while others provide partial protection requiring boosters (e.g., tetanus).

D. Vaccines can be of several types:
   1. Live (activated)—patient may shed live virus after immunization (e.g., OPV)
   2. Live (attenuated) (e.g., measles, mumps, rubella vaccine [MMR])
   3. Killed (inactivated) (e.g., IPV)

III. Implications

A. If not hospitalized, all infants should receive standard immunizations at 2 months of age (diphtheria-pertussis-tetanus [DPT], OPV, *Haemophilus influenzae* b conjugate vaccine [HbCV]) when passive protection by maternal antibody is abating.

B. If still hospitalized, standard non-live vaccines (DPT and HbCV) should be administered at two months of age; live vaccine (e.g., OPV) may be administered at discharge to minimize potential infection of other nursery infants who may be immunocompromised, or alternatively, killed vaccine (inactivated polio vaccine [IPV] can be administered at the usual intervals.)

C. Immunization should not be delayed in premature infants. They are capable of mounting an adequate immune response in most cases.

D. Both premature and low birthweight infants should receive the usual dose of vaccine. Use of half-dose regimens may result in inadequate antigenic stimulation and inadequate immunization.

E. Although breast milk contains substantial amounts of IgA, which could theoretically interfere with polio or other live virus immunization, significant interference has not been demonstrated clinically.

F. Common sites for injection (IM or subcutaneous) in children include the anterolateral aspect of the upper thigh, or the deltoid area of the arm. In infants 1 year or younger, the thigh is the preferred site as it is the largest muscle. The upper outer aspect of the buttock is NOT preferred in an infant because the gluteal region remains mostly fat until the child has been walking for some time.

G. Vaccines with adjuvants (DPT, DTaP, DT, TD, Recombivax or HbCV) must be given deep into muscle to avoid local irritation, inflammation, granuloma formation, and necrosis; it is acceptable to administer two injections in the same extremity at two different sites if muscle mass allows.

IV. Practice

A. Hepatitis B

1. All infants (preterm, low birthweight, and term) born to mothers who are positive for hepatitis B surface antigen should routinely receive hepatitis B immune globulin (HBIG) within 12 hours of life (0.5 mL IM). Hepatitis B vaccine (HBV) also should be given as soon as possible after birth (0.5 mL IM). These agents should be given at separate sites, using different syringes. If the vaccine cannot be administered to a term infant shortly after HBIG, it must be given in the first 7 days of life. For premature infants or sick, low birthweight infants in whom the vaccine cannot be given after HBIG, it must be given within the first month of life. The remaining two doses of the vaccine series should then be administered 1 and 6 months after the first dose of vaccine is given.

2. For infants born to hepatitis B surface antigen-negative mothers:

   a. Term: should receive the first vaccine by 2 months of age;
      the second vaccine should be given 1–2 months after initial
      vaccine; the third and final vaccine is given 6 months after
      first vaccine.
   b. Preterm: the optimal time to initiate the hepatitis B vaccine
      in preterm infants < 2 kg has not been determined because
      studies of these infants have shown decreased seroconver-
      sion rates. For preterm infant of hepatitis B surface antigen-
      negative mothers who weighs < 2 kg, it may be advisable to
      delay initiation of the vaccine series until the infant weighs 2
      kg, or until the infant is 2 months old and ready for other
      routine immunizations.
3. In the USA, the hepatitis B vaccine is synthesized using recombinant DNA techniques and does not contain human plasma; it
   does not contain live virus, and its use is completely safe. The
   most commonly reported side effect is pain at the injection site.

B. DPT
   1. 0.5 mL IM should be administered at 2, 4, 6, 15–18 months,
      and 4–6 years.
   2. Common side effects (usually attributable to the pertussis com-
      ponent) include localized edema, irritation, fever, drowsiness
      and irritability; persistent crying for over 1 hour occurs in ap-
      proximately 3% of children.
   3. More severe, but rare side effects to pertussis vaccine include
      convulsions or hypotonic-hyporesponsive episodes.
   4. Administration of diphtheria-tetanus (DT) vaccine and avoidance
      of the pertussis component may be considered for infants with:
      a. A progressive neurologic disorder associated with develop-
         mental delay and/or neurologic findings
      b. An active seizure disorder
      c. A neurologic condition that predisposes a child to seizures
         or neurologic deterioration (e.g., tuberous sclerosis)
      d. A documented adverse event to a prior dose of pertussis vac-
         cine
         i. Encephalopathy within 7 days
         ii. Convulsion within 3 days
         iii. Persistent severe inconsolable screaming, high-pitched
              crying for 3 hours or more
         iv. Hypotonic-hyporesponsive episode within 48 hours
         v. Temperature of 40.5°C or more within 48 hours that is
            otherwise inexplicable
         vi. Immediate allergic reaction to vaccine

5. Pertussis may cause significant morbidity in infants, which can lead to secondary bacterial pneumonia, seizures, encephalopathy, apnea, hypoxemia, intracranial hemorrhage, and death. The immunization should be given whenever possible. Local reactions, low-grade to moderate fevers ($< 40.5°C$) following previous doses, family history or severe DPT reaction, mental retardation, controlled seizures, prematurity, and allergies are not valid contraindications to the pertussis vaccine.

6. Infants and children may be premedicated with antipyretics (e.g., acetaminophin 10 mg/kg) prior to administration of whole-cell pertussis vaccine.

7. Acellular vaccine is not currently recommended as first dose in infants < 15 months old.

C. Polio

1. Mild-type polio is a highly contagious virus, transmitted via fecal-oral route, with seroconversion rates as high as 90% seen in unimmunized household contacts.

2. The advantages of OPV include:
   a. Does not require an injection
   b. Both mucosal and humoral immunity conferred with vaccine
   c. High rate of efficacy (nearly 100%)

3. The new improved IPV was approved for use in the USA in 1988, and now also has much improved efficacy (nearly 100%). However, while OPV confers lifetime immunity, the duration of immunity with IPV is less certain. Therefore, IPV recipients may require boosters. However, IPV has no risk of vaccine-associated polio, a rare complication that can occur with OPV.

4. OPV is usually deferred in hospitalized infants until discharge to minimize cross infection. A repeat dose of OPV may be given at discharge to facilitate assumption of the routine vaccine schedule. Routine OPV schedule requires administration at 2 and 4 months, with the third dose at 18 months (an additional dose at 6 months is optional in endemic areas). These are followed by a booster at 4–6 years of age. ***Do not*** use OPV if there is an immunocompromised member of the nuclear family.

5. IPV may be administered during hospitalization. Doses are given at 2, 4, and 18 months. A booster is given at 4–6 years. The vaccine of choice if there is an immunocompromised family member.

6. Some investigators propose a combined regimen for both IPV and OPV, but such a schedule is not currently recommended.

D. *Haemophilus influenzae* b conjugate vaccine (HbCV)

1. *Haemophilus influenzae* type b (Hib) is the most common cause

of meningitis in children aged 2 months to 5 years; the bacteria may also cause other serious infections including pneumonia, sepsis, osteomyelitis, epiglottis, and pericarditis, among others.

2. All children should be considered for Hib immunization unless they are older than 5 years of age and healthy.

3. There are currently four immunization preparations available in the USA:

   a. HBOC: links the subunit of the Hib polysaccharide with diphtheria toxoid, and is approved for use in children 2 months of age and older; given in four doses at 2, 4, and 6 months, and again at 12–15 months.

   b. PRP-OMP: contains the Hib PRP which is conjugated with the protein of the outer membrane of Neisseria meningitidis group B; it is given at 2, 4, and 12 months of age.

   c. PRP-T: links the Hib PRP with the tetanus toxoid; given in four doses at 2, 4, and 6 months, and again at 12–15 months of age.

   d. PRP-D: not approved for use in children younger than 12 months of age.

4. Tetramune is the first combined vaccine containing HbCV and DPT components, and can be given when both vaccines are needed.

5. Contraindication to HbCV administration is prior anaphylactic reaction.

6. Adverse reactions include mild fever and local erythema or tenderness at the injection site.

E. Influenza

1. The vaccine is available to help prevent disease caused by influenza types A and B.

2. It is recommended for anyone older than 6 months of age who is at high risk for complications due to influenza:

   a. Any infant with chronic lung disease

   b. Any infant with significant cardiovascular disease

   c. Any infant who is immunocompromised

3. The vaccine can be administered safely to hospitalized infants

4. Only the split virus or purified surface antigen preparations should be given to those younger than 13 years of age.

5. Children younger than 3 years old get 0.25 IM; it is best given mid-October through mid-November. Protective antibody is detectable about 2 weeks after immunization.

6. The vaccine is contraindicated in children with egg protein allergy.

7. The most common side effect is pain and tenderness at the injection site, but occasionally, patients may experience mild fever, malaise, and myalgia.
F. Varicella
   1. This is a live attenuated vaccine given to children 12 months and older who have not yet had chicken pox.
   2. Administration is optional.
   3. Dose is 0.5 mL IM.
   4. The vaccine is contraindicated in immunocompromised children, and children with immunocompromised household contacts.
   5. Side effects include low-grade fever and vesicular rash.

V. Summary
   A. Birth: HBV #1
   B. 1–2 months: HBV #2
   C. 2 months: DPT, HbCV, OPV (IPV)
   D. 4 months: DPT, HbCV, OPV (IPV)
   E. 6 months: DPT, HbCV, influenza vaccine for those with chronic disease
   F. 6–18 months: HBV #3, OPV (IPV)
   G. 12 months: varicella (optional)
   H. 12–15 months: HbCV, MMR
   I. 15–18 months: DTaP

Suggested Reading

Committee on Infectious Diseases: Recommended childhood immunization schedule—United States, 2002. Pediatrics 109:162, 2002.

Edwards KM: Pediatric immunizations. Curr Prob Pediatr 23:186–209, 1993.

Pickering LK (ed): 2000 Red Book: Report on the Committee on Infectious Diseases, 25th ed. Elk Grove Village, IL, American Academy of Pediatrics, 2000.

Zimmerman RK, Burns IT: Childhood immunization guidelines: Current and future. Prim Care 21:693–715, 1994.

Section VII.   DISORDERS OF RESPIRATORY CONTROL

Chapter 44

Apnea

Mohammad A. Attar, M.D., and Nancy A. McIntosh, R.N., Ph.D.

I. Definitions

A. Apnea—cessation of respiratory airflow. The respiratory pause may be central or diaphragmatic (e.g., no respiratory effort), obstructive or mixed. Short (< 15 sec) central apnea can be normal at all ages.

B. Pathologic apnea—a respiratory pause is pathologic if it is prolonged (20 sec) or associated with cyanosis; abrupt, marked pallor or hypotonia; or bradycardia.

C. Periodic breathing—a breathing pattern in which there are three or more respiratory pauses of greater than 3-seconds' duration with less than 20 seconds of respiration between pauses.

D. Apnea of prematurity (AOP)—pathologic apnea in a preterm infant, the result of the immature regulation of breathing. Apnea of prematurity usually ceases by 37 weeks' postconceptional age but occasionally persists to several weeks past term.

E. Apparent life-threatening event (ALTE)—an episode that is frightening to the observer and characterized by some combination of apnea (central or occasionally obstructive), color change (usually cyanotic or pallid, but occasionally erythematous or plethoric), marked change in muscle tone (usually severe limpness), choking, or gagging. In some cases, the observer fears that the infant has died. Previously used terminology such as "aborted crib death" or "near-miss SIDS" should be abandoned because it implies a possibly misleading close association between this type of spell and SIDS.

F. Apnea of infancy (AOI)—an unexplained episode of cessation of breathing for 20 seconds or longer, or a shorter respiratory pause associated with bradycardia, cyanosis, pallor, and/or marked hypotonia. The terminology "apnea of infancy" generally is reserved for infants who are greater than 37 weeks' postconceptional age at onset of pathologic apnea. AOI should be used for those infants for whom no specific cause of ALTE can be identified. In other words, these are infants whose ALTE was idiopathic and believed to be related to apnea.

G. The multichannel study (MCS)—a physiologic study used in the management of apnea in infants and young children. It is a continuous and simultaneous recording of the respiratory waveform, heart rate, oxygen saturation, and airflow, usually conducted over a minimum of 8–12 hours. It may also include pH probe, end-tidal CO_2, or QRS complex. This test does not include measures to allow sleep staging and cannot be substituted where polysomnography (PSG) is indicated.

II. Apnea as a Sign

A. Apnea, with or without bradycardia and oxygen desaturation, is a frequent occurrence in premature infants and may be central, obstructive, or mixed. Apnea spells may accompany:

1. Systemic infections, e.g., sepsis
2. Localized infection, e.g., meningitis, NEC, pneumonia
3. CNS disorders, e.g., seizures, IVH, PVL, encephalopathy, congenital central sleep hypoventilation syndrome
4. Metabolic disorders, e.g., hypoglycemia, hyperammonemia, inborn errors
5. Hyperthermia, hypothermia
6. Drug-induced problems
7. Airway obstruction which may be anatomic, functional, positional, or secondary to secretions
8. Circulatory changes, e.g., PDA, hypotension, and anemia
9. Intrinsic pulmonary disease
10. Infection with respiratory syncytial virus (RSV)

B. Each apneic infant must be evaluated for specific causes after his/her first spell. To diagnose or rule out many of these explanations for apnea, the following information or tests should be obtained after a thorough physical assessment:

1. Complete blood count
2. Sepsis evaluation
3. Chest radiograph
4. Blood gas determination
5. Electrolytes, blood glucose
6. Cranial sonogram

III. Bradycardia

Heart rates vary greatly in premature and sick infants. Sudden drops to below 90 bpm are considered bradycardia. Causes include:

A. Apnea or other respiratory disturbances ("A and B spells"). Evaluation and treatment as for the primary respiratory events.

B. Sinus arrhythmia, e.g., heart rate fluctuation within physiologic limits, albeit sometimes exaggerated in frequency and rate. This is often seen in infants with a low baseline heart rate. No intervention is required unless there is associated hypoxemia.

C. Pathologic arrhythmia (including congenital heart block) is somewhat rare. Evaluate with ECG (including single lead printout from monitors).

D. Isolated bradycardia should not be treated with methylxanthines.

IV. Oxygen Desaturation and Hypoxemia

A. Normal baseline oxygen saturation in room air in the healthy premature infant as measured by pulse oximetry is > 94%.

B. Desaturation episodes accompany many acute illnesses (*see* II, A, above) and resolve as these problems are addressed.

C. In addition to these situations, desaturation episodes are seen frequently in convalescing infants.

1. As acute desaturations, synchronous with respiratory events (e.g., apnea; periodic or disorganized breathing), with a return to a normal baseline. Treat the respiratory events. Occasional brief dips into the 80% range require no supplemental oxygen.

2. As low baseline saturation, < 93%, with or without further desaturation episodes. Start continuous oxygen at ¼ LPM by nasal cannula, especially while asleep. Adjust liter flow as needed.

3. Infants with persistent or progressive need for oxygen supplement may need to be evaluated for other causes of hypoxemia such as increased pulmonary edema or pneumonia.

D. Many growing premature infants have clinically unrecognizable hypoxemia. As a result of differences in recording parameters, hypoxemia may not be noted on NICU pulse oximeters but be apparent on MCS.

V. Apnea of Prematurity

A. *AOP is a diagnosis of exclusion.* The apnea may be central, obstructive, or mixed. The incidence of AOP increases with decreasing gestational age.

B. Apnea from other causes and AOP may overlap in a patient. *Keep looking for underlying causes.*

C. In most instances AOP will disappear after about 36 weeks, but final resolution may not occur until 44–46 weeks' postconceptual age.

D. Treatment

1. Nonpharmacologic measures
   a. Prone positioning
   b. Tactile stimulation
   c. Increase FiO_2 slightly, monitor blood gases, or use pulse oximeter

  d. CPAP, delivered by nasal prongs, nasopharyngeal tube, or face mask

  e. Mechanical ventilation may become necessary.

 2. Methylxanthine therapy

Both theophylline and caffeine have been shown to be effective in the treatment of AOP in many infants. The drugs have different kinetic properties resulting in a substantial difference between the dosing schedule and need for drug monitoring. Caffeine offers a number of advantages over theophylline, including a higher therapeutic index and once-a-day dosing. The commercial preparation of caffeine is more expensive than theophylline and this may be a consideration when an infant is to be discharged on a methylxanthine.

  a. Theophylline and caffeine dosage (*see* pages 79 and 94)

  b. Special considerations

   i. Watch for signs of toxicity (e.g., excessive tachycardia, vomiting, jitteriness, seizures, hyperglycemia, hyponatremia, hypokalemia, hypotension, increased gastroesophageal reflux, gastrointestinal bleeding).

   ii. When used to facilitate extubation, aminophylline or theophylline should be discontinued when the planned 4-day periextubation course is completed.

   iii. By 36 weeks' postconceptional age, theophylline should be discontinued as a trial to see if maturation of breathing has occurred.

   iv. Methylxanthine therapy may cause an increase (~20%) in metabolic rate and oxygen consumption.

VI. Periodic Breathing

 A. Periodic breathing (PB) occurs in premature infants so commonly that it is considered a physiologic marker of immature respiratory control. Typically the incidence of PB will decrease to less than 10% by term although normative data on this respiratory pattern are not available. "Excessive" periodic breathing above this amount may persist in some cases for many weeks.

 B. In some cases, periodic breathing may be associated with significant drops in oxygen saturation (below 90%). In these cases, periodic breathing may need to be suppressed with either methylxanthines and/or oxygen.

VII. Discharge Planning for Infants with AOP and/or Persistent Hypoxemia (Figure 7)

 A. AOP may persist in an infant who is otherwise ready for discharge

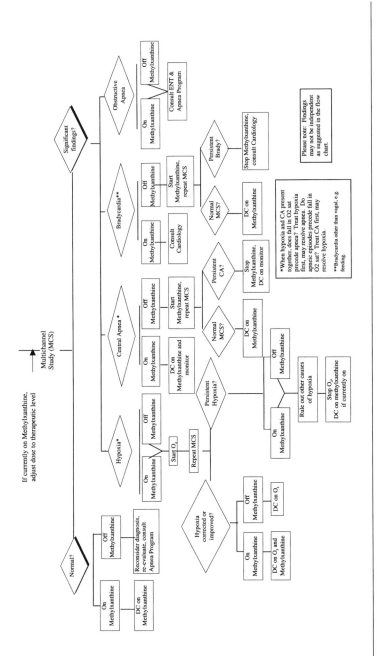

Figure 7. Management for preterm infants with clinically apparent episodes of apnea within the previous 7 days but otherwise ready for discharge.

(e.g., no clinically apparent episodes of apnea within the previous 7 days). Thus, short-term outpatient management, usually not past 44–46 weeks' postconceptional age, may be necessary.

B. Methylxanthines, cardiorespiratory monitoring, and oxygen may be used either individually or in some combination to manage infants with AOP after discharge. The choice of these should be based on information obtained from a MCS. A repeat MCS may be necessary to establish the effectiveness of the selected intervention(s).

C. Infants who are receiving a methylxanthine at a therapeutic level for AOP and who have been asymptomatic by documented monitoring in the previous 7-day period may be discharged on this drug without further studies. If optimal period of documented monitoring is not available, an MCS should be considered before discharge.

D. Select the treatment interventions
1. Methylxanthines
   a. When effective in eliminating or significantly reducing pathologic central apnea, with or without bradycardia. When desaturation episodes precede central apnea on MCS, the treatment of the hypoxia may resolve the apnea.
   b. If methylxanthine reduces but does not eliminate pathologic apnea, add cardiorespiratory monitoring.
2. Cardiorespiratory monitoring (*see* page 242)
   a. Indicated for AOP when methylxanthines are ineffective or contraindicated
   b. Cardiorespiratory monitoring is not a treatment for AOP per se; it is prescribed to help the caregiver recognize when the infant is apneic and may need stimulation or other interventions to limit the episode.
3. Supplemental oxygen
   a. Prescribed where MCS documents low baseline saturation or significant desaturation episodes and these problems respond to the use of supplemental oxygen. Note that when central apnea precedes desaturation on the MCS, the successful treatment of the apnea with a methylxanthine may resolve the hypoxia.
   b. Use enough oxygen (¼–½ LPM) via nasal cannula.
   c. Home pulse oximetry is not indicated for this situation.

E. Discuss the diagnosis and treatment plan with the parents. Identify the typical endpoint of treatment (44–46 weeks' postconceptional age). Do not anticipate a specific discharge date, which is dependent upon a number of factors.

F. Advise the nursing staff of the patient's diagnosis and your management plan. They will provide discharge teaching following established protocols for this population.

G. If a methylxanthine is ordered, write the discharge prescription before discharge so the medication can be available in the NICU prior to discharge.

H. If a home cardiorespiratory monitor is indicated, *see* Chapter 45.

I. If supplemental oxygen at home is indicated, contact the discharge planning service to arrange.

J. Referrals for community health nursing, monitoring, parent support groups, etc., for further education and family support, should be initiated per the health care team's assessment.

K. Schedule follow-up medical care for AOP either with the infant's primary care physician or an apnea clinic. Return visit should occur within 2–3 weeks of discharge.

L. Arrange for the first outpatient theophylline or caffeine level to be drawn within 2 weeks either at the private physician's office or an apnea clinic.

M. Include in the discharge summary:
1. Patient's diagnosis and the usual endpoint for treatment (44–46 weeks' postconceptional age)
2. Theophylline or caffeine dose, the most recent trough level, and when the next level should be measured
3. Monitor alarm settings, if monitor prescribed, and, if known, name of medical equipment company

Chapter 45

Home Cardiorespiratory Monitors

Mohammad A. Attar, M.D., and Nancy A. McIntosh, R.N., Ph.D.

I.   Function
   A. The home cardiorespiratory monitor is designed to detect episodes of central apnea as well as episodes of bradycardia or tachycardia as defined by preset limits within the monitor.
   B. Home cardiorespiratory monitors utilize an indirect measure of respiration, transthoracic impedance.

II.   Limitations
   A. False apnea alarms arising from poor electrode placement, shallow breathing by the infant, or the combination of the two
   B. Failure to alarm for true apnea because the monitor may interpret motion, electrical noise, or cardiogenic artifact as breathing
   C. Impedance pneumography technology cannot detect obstructive apnea because it senses chest wall movement rather than airflow. Although prolonged obstructive apnea may trigger a bradycardia alarm, significant hypoxia may already be present.

III. Monitor Types
   A. Basic cardiorespiratory monitors
      1. Produce audible and visual alarm signals when preset limit of bradycardia, tachycardia, or apnea delay is exceeded
      2. Additional alarm signals indicate equipment conditions such as low battery power and loose leads.
      3. Equipped with rechargeable batteries
      4. Do not have oscilloscope screens
   B. Enhanced monitors (memory monitors, documenting monitors)
      1. Extend the capabilities of the basic monitor by providing for the storage and later retrieval of information on monitor use and alarms
      2. Depending on the manufacturer, reports generated from the retrieved information may be in either tabular format alone or tabular with waveforms.
      3. Monitors allow the clinician to elect a second set of thresholds for apnea, bradycardia, and tachycardia, which when exceeded will trigger a recording but not an alarm.

4. A pulse oximeter, either in the alarm or no alarm mode, can be used in conjunction with many manufacturers' monitors.

IV. Standard Monitor Settings (Table 36)

TABLE 36
Standard Monitor Settings

	Alarm Settings	Event-Logging Settings
Apnea delay	20 secs	15 secs
Bradycardia		
Birth to 1 month	80 bpm	90 bpm
1–3 months of age	70 bpm	80 bpm
> 3 months of age	60 bpm	70 bpm
Tachycardia alarm	Off*	Off

*If tachycardia is related to the problem for which the infant is at risk, then 225 bpm for an infant is suggested.

V. Cautions

A. A home cardiorespiratory monitor should only be prescribed for a specific indication. It is important to define the endpoint for its use and to identify follow-up resources in the community. The process of successfully weaning an infant from the monitor begins when the monitor is ordered.

B. A monitor should not be prescribed or continued when it cannot or is not being used.

VI. Arranging for Home Monitoring at the University of Michigan Health System

A. General comments
1. The process may take at least 2–3 days.
2. Thorough instruction in the use of the home monitor, assessment of the infant, and cardiopulmonary resuscitation is mandatory.
3. Both parents are expected to participate in the discharge teaching.
4. A single parent must designate a backup caregiver.
5. There should be a telephone in the home to which the infant is to be discharged.

B. Physician responsibilities
1. Review diagnosis with parents, discuss why you are prescribing monitoring, and establish their acceptance of the proposed treatment and follow-up plan.
2. A consult is sent to discharge planning services to request the

delivery of the home cardiorespiratory monitor. Include the diagnosis for which the monitor is being ordered. Alarm settings will be as indicated above. Monitors are ordered from community medical equipment providers. The *initial* monitor prescription should be written for no longer than a 2-month period. The primary care physician is responsible for renewing this prescription where indicated.

3. A consult is sent to Respiratory Care to request infant CPR instruction for the parents.
4. The unit nursing staff is notified of the patient's diagnosis and management plan. They are accountable for providing the balance of the discharge teaching. Written handouts will accompany verbal instruction.

VII. Conditions that Are *Not* Indications for Home Cardiorespiratory Monitoring

A. Cardiac arrhythmias
B. Seizures
C. Irreversible or terminal conditions
D. Congenital heart defects, with or without associated arrhythmias
E. Distant family history of SIDS
F. Family history of monitor use
G. Severe disability/multiple handicaps
H. Infant of substance abusing mother, if infant has no signs of apnea
I. Asymptomatic sibling of infant with a history of AOI, ALTE, or monitor use
J. Asymptomatic twin of infant with AOP, AOI, ALTE

Suggested Reading

Baird TM, Martin RJ, Abu-Shaweesh JM: Clinical associations, treatment and outcome of apnea of prematurity. Neoreviews 3:66, 2002.

Beckerman RC, Brouillette RT, Hunt CE (eds): Respiratory Control Disorders in Infants and Children. Baltimore, Williams & Wilkins, 1992.

Brooks J (ed): SIDS. Pediatr Ann 24:345, 1995.

Darnall RA, Kattwinkel J, Nattie C, Robinson M: Margin of safety for discharge after apnea in preterm infants. Pediatrics 100:795–801, 1997.

Hageman J (ed): Update on Neonatology. Pediatric Clinics of North America, vol. 40, no. 5. Philadelphia, W.B. Saunders, 1993.

Hunt CE (ed): Apnea and SIDS. Clinics in Perinatology, vol. 19, no. 4. Philadelphia, W.B. Saunders, 1992.

Michigan Association of Apnea Professionals: Consensus Statement on Infantile Apnea, 4th ed. Lansing, MI, MAAP, 1999.

Poets CF, Samuels MP, Southall DP: Epidemiology and pathophysiology of apnoea of prematurity. Biol Neonate 65:211–219, 1994.

Poets CF, Stebbens VA, Richard D, Southall DP: Prolonged episodes of hypoxemia in preterm infants undetectable by cardiorespiratory monitors. Pediatrics 95:860–863, 1995.

Razi NM, Humphreys J, Pandit PB, Stahl GE: Predischarge monitoring of preterm infants. Pediatr Pulmonol 27:113–116, 1999.

Chapter 46

Sudden Infant Death Syndrome

Mohammad A. Attar, M.D., and Nancy A. McIntosh, R.N., Ph.D.

I. **Definition**

Sudden infant death syndrome (SIDS) is defined as the sudden death of an infant less than 1 year of age that unexplained after the performance of a complete case investigation, including autopsy, death scene examination, and review of the case history.

II. **Epidemiology**

  A. In 1999, the CDC found that the incidence of SIDS in the USA was 0.65 per 1000 live births.

  B. SIDS is the single largest cause of postneonatal infant mortality.

  C. SIDS is rare in the first week of life, and 95% of the deaths from this diagnosis occur before 6 months.

  D. The peak occurrence age is 2–4 months. The cause (or causes) of SIDS remains unknown.

  E. Apnea of prematurity is not a risk factor for SIDS; however, there is a higher likelihood of SIDS among premature and low birth-weight infants.

III. **Siblings of Infants Who Died from SIDS**

  A. The risk of sudden infant death syndrome for subsequent siblings has not been clearly established.

    1. Determination of the risk of recurrence is problematic because SIDS is a relatively infrequent event, and a subsequent event in a sibling is extremely rare.

    2. Various studies have found the risk for siblings to range from no additional risk to as much as a fivefold increase over the background risk of SIDS.

  B. At present there are no screening studies available for SIDS.

IV. **Prevention**

  A. Sleep position

    1. In 1994, the United States Public Health Service initiated a national "Back to Sleep" educational campaign in collaboration with the American Academy of Pediatrics and the SIDS Alliance.

The campaign advocated placing a healthy infant to sleep on his/her back or side to reduce the risk for SIDS.

2. In 1996, the recommendation was revised, and subsequently the supine sleeping position was recommended as the best position.

3. By 1998, the incidence of SIDS had decreased by 42%. That decrease was attributed to the change in infant sleep position recommendations.

B. Other recommendations to parents

1. Keep the infant in a smoke-free environment before and after birth.

2. Breastfeed if possible.

3. Keep the temperature of the room the baby sleeps in at a comfortable level and do not overdress the baby.

4. Have the baby sleep on a firm, flat mattress with a tightly fitted sheet.

5. For premature infants with respiratory distress, significant gastroesophageal reflux, or certain upper airway anomalies, the prone position may well be the position of choice. However, when these problems resolve, the infant should be put in a supine position to sleep.

Chapter 47

Sudden Infant Death Syndrome Siblings

Mohammad A. Attar, M.D., and Nancy A. McIntosh, R.N., Ph.D.

I. **Prenatal Counseling**

   A. Prenatal counseling is recommended for expectant parents who have lost an infant to SIDS. This counseling should be family oriented.

   B. Parents who have had prenatal counseling should be reinterviewed in the immediate postpartum period to reassess their feelings and understanding of the new infant's risk status.

   C. Families should be referred for counseling early in the pregnancy.

   D. Many apnea programs provide this counseling and accept referrals from physicians, midwives, and parents.

II. **Hospital Evaluation**

   A. There are no known predictive physiologic or other tests available for SIDS.

   B. If a subsequent sibling of an infant who died from SIDS becomes symptomatic, the evaluation of this infant should proceed as the clinical presentation indicates.

III. **Discharge Planning**

   A. *Home monitors are not considered a standard of care for this population.* However, monitoring may be appropriate for family management or coping in some cases. The efficacy of home monitors in the prevention of SIDS has not been established. Infants have died while being monitored.

   B. Once parents have made a decision to monitor or not monitor their infant, the decision should be supported.

   C. If home monitoring is chosen, parents of SIDS siblings should receive thorough education in the use of the monitor and assessment of the infant and should be trained in CPR. Referrals for community health nursing, monitoring, parent support groups, and an apnea program consultation for further education and support should be initiated per the health care team's assessment.

IV. **Management of SIDS Siblings at the University of Michigan Health System (UMHS)**

   A. *The Apnea Program (Pediatric Pulmonology) requests a consult on all infants with a family history of SIDS born at UMHS.* This consult should be sent within 24 hours of the infant's birth.

B. A clinician from the Apnea Program will meet with the family, review the evidence for the diagnosis of SIDS in a previous sibling, provide information about SIDS recurrence risk, and discuss options for the new infant. The Apnea Program may already be aware of some families from a past pregnancy or as a result of a prenatal referral during the current pregnancy.

C. Arrangements for home monitoring, when this is the parents' informed choice, will be initiated directly by the Apnea Program.

D. Because these infants have a minimal risk for SIDS during the first week of life, the Apnea Program protocol provides for the home monitor to be set up at the home after discharge. Education of the family in the use of the home monitor will be provided through the medical equipment provider, the community health nursing agency, and the Apnea Program staff.

Section VIII. RESPIRATORY CARE

Chapter 48

Oxygen and Continuous Positive Airway Pressure

Michael A. Becker, R.R.T., and Steven M. Donn, M.D.

I. **Oxygen Therapy, Resuscitation Bag, and CPAP**
   A. Infant hood
      1. Accurately delivers FiO_2 of 0.21–0.90
      2. Provides heated, humidified, blended gas; temperature maintained within $2°$ of incubator temperature
      3. Flow rate of gas: 10 LPM or greater to prevent rebreathing and maintain stable oxygen concentrations
      4. Temperature and FiO_2 analyzed every 4 hr
   B. Oxygen to incubator
      1. Only recommended when infant requires less than 0.30 FiO_2. Higher concentrations difficult to maintain because of intermittent opening of incubator doors.
      2. Heated, humidified, blended gas provided at flows greater than 10 LPM
      3. Temperature and FiO_2 analyzed every 4 hr
   C. Nasal cannula
      1. Nasal cannula oxygen therapy is indicated for infants requiring low concentrations of supplementation oxygen; cannulas come in two sizes, premie and infant.
      2. Recommended for infants needing oxygen for prolonged periods of time; provides greater mobility and is the preferred choice for home oxygen therapy.
      3. Delivers humidified oxygen at flow rates of 0.03–1.0 LPM; the oxygen concentration varies, dependent on liter flow, infant size, respiratory rate, and tidal volume (minute ventilation).
      4. An oxygen saturation monitor is necessary for determining appropriate liter flow.
      5. If oxygen saturations are higher than desired at the lowest possible flow rates, a blender may be used to provide finer control of oxygen delivery.

II. **Resuscitation Equipment**
   A. Self-inflating resuscitation bags are available in delivery rooms and treatment areas for manual ventilation. They are also available

251

at the bedside of all intubated infants. Other infants may have bag-mask devices at the bedside when indicated and ordered by the physician (e.g., apneic episodes, seizures).

B. The resuscitation bags are equipped with reservoirs for delivery of 100% oxygen and pressure relief valves ("pop-offs"). The preset relief valves will open at pressures in excess of 35–40 cm H_2O. The pressure relief valve may be inactivated with a metal clip if a ventilation pressure of greater than 40 cm H_2O is desired.

C. On intubated infants, in-line manometers are attached for pressure monitoring. Optimal ventilator settings may be determined by observing rates and pressures required with the resuscitation bag.

D. PEEP attachments are available for all intubated infants.

E. A properly fitting mask should be available at the bedside in the event of accidental extubation; if the infant is not intubated, the mask should be attached to the bag.

F. Resuscitation bags are routinely attached to a 100% oxygen source; another alternative is to blend the gas flow to the bag for a variable FiO_2. Infants who are in hoods, receiving CPAP, or breathing room air should have their bags placed outside the incubator.

III. Continuous Positive Airway Pressure (CPAP)

Maintains alveolar stability and prevents atelectasis in spontaneously breathing infants. This may decrease intrapulmonary shunting and improve ventilation-perfusion relationships.

A. Indications
1. $PaO_2 < 50$ mmHg on $FiO_2 > 0.50$ with acceptable ventilation
2. Periodic breathing (stimulates pressure receptors within the lung, which may improve regularity of respirations)
3. Prevention of postextubation atelectasis
4. Stabilization of upper airway

B. Effect
1. Improved oxygenation at lower FiO_2
2. Increased alveolar distending pressure
3. May lower respiratory rate and decrease work of breathing

C. Potential complications
1. Barotrauma
2. Decreased venous return or increased pulmonary vascular resistance
3. Increased work of breathing and carbon dioxide retention
4. Occlusion of tubes
5. Nasal irritation and erosion

6. Agitation; inability to secure device
7. Abdominal distension (place OG tube) and feeding intolerance
D. Recommended parameters
1. CPAP: 4–8 cm H_2O
2. FiO_2: variable, but usually unchanged from previous requirements
E. Methods of delivery
1. Nasal cannula CPAP—easiest to set up and secure and best tolerated delivery method. At flow rates of 1–2 LPM, a level of CPAP is delivered, but the actual pressure is not measured. The nasal cannula needs to be the infant size and should be set up with a blender for optimal control of oxygen concentration.
2. Nasal CPAP—delivered by a CPAP device (generator) through either nasal prongs or mask. Alternating the prongs and mask may decrease the skin and nasal irritation from constant pressure that is associated with long-term use of nasal CPAP delivery system. The physical principle used to produce CPAP may differ from one circuit to another but all have the ability to adjust and monitor positive airway pressure and FiO_2. Many sizes of prongs and masks are available.
3. Nasopharyngeal CPAP (NPCPAP)—route of delivery is through an endotracheal tube placed in one naris and positioned behind the uvula. The tube must be suctioned frequently to prevent occlusion.
4. Endotracheal CPAP (ETCPAP)—may be tried for a short time prior to extubation. It is usually not tolerated for extended periods because of increased resistance and work of breathing.
F. Suggested weaning sequence
1. Decrease FiO_2 to < 0.3.
2. Decrease CPAP to 4 cm H_2O.
3. Place on a low-flow nasal cannula.

Chapter 49

Neonatal Blood Gases

Steven M. Donn, M.D., and Michael A. Becker, R.R.T.

I. **Blood Gas Assessment**
   A. Patient considerations
      1. Sample size
      2. Observation of patient
      3. Comparison to other gases (trends)
   B. Sampling considerations
      1. Excess heparin may decrease pH.
      2. A sample taken too soon after $NaHCO_3$ is given may have an increased pH and $PaCO_2$.
      3. TPN/lipids in sample may decrease pH.
      4. Air in sample will elevate PaO_2 (unless patient has $PaO_2 > 160$ mmHg) and lower $PaCO_2$.
   C. Interpretation
      1. Evaluate pH, $PaCO_2$, and HCO_3^-
      2. Determine primary abnormality by matching pH with PCO_2 or HCO_3^-

	Respiratory	*Metabolic*
Acidosis	↑ PCO_2	↓ HCO_3^-
Alkalosis	↓ PCO_2	↑ HCO_3^-

        a. Combined respiratory and metabolic problems may exist (mixed acidosis).
        b. pH may be normalized when compensation occurs (3–4 days).
      3. Evaluate oxygenation (PaO_2 and saturation).
   D. Ranges of blood gases (Table 37)
   E. Flow diagram to assist in blood gas interpretation (Figure 8)
   F. Capillary blood gases
      1. Capillary-to-arterial correlations
           a. pH: small difference
           b. PCO_2: 8–10 mmHg higher
           c. PO_2: 17–20 mmHg lower (higher capillary PO_2 values correlate poorly and lower values correlate more closely)
      2. Factors affecting correlations
           a. Technique
           b. Response of patient

TABLE 37
Acceptable Newborn Ranges of Blood Gases

	Arterial	Capillary	Venous
pH	7.30–7.45	7.25–7.35	7.25–7.35
PCO_2 (mmHg)	35–45	40–50	40–50
PO_2 (mmHg)	50–70	35–50	35–45
HCO_3^- (mEq/L)	20–24	18–24	18–24
SaO_2	92–96%	70–75%	70–75%

    c. Acidosis
    d. Hypoxia
    e. Hypotension/perfusion
    f. Bruising/acrocyanosis
    g. Temperature
G. Electrolytes/co-oximetry
    1. Whole blood electrolytes can be obtained with blood gas measurements. Values for sodium, potassium, and ionized calcium are available, as well as conductivity hematocrit.
       a. Sample size should be 0.3 mL, drawn into a lithium heparin syringe.
       b. Numerous comparison studies have shown acceptable correlation.
    2. An analyzed breakdown of the different forms of hemoglobin can be obtained through a co-oximeter. Measured values of oxyhemoglobin, carboxyhemoglobin, and methemoglobin are available. A sample size of 0.3 mL is required.

II. Continuous Monitoring
Recent advances in technology have led to the ability to continuously monitor oxygenation and ventilation noninvasively. All infants requiring mechanical ventilation or oxygen therapy benefit from some form of continuous monitoring.
A. Methods
    1. Pulse oximetry continuously monitors oxygen saturation with a sensor wrapped around the hand or foot.
    2. Transcutaneous monitoring monitors oxygenation and ventilation; an electrode attached to the skin surface estimates partial pressure of oxygen and carbon dioxide by measuring diffusion through a semipermeable membrane.
    3. Capnometry (end-tidal CO_2) monitors exhaled carbon dioxide at the endotracheal tube.
B. Clinical applications

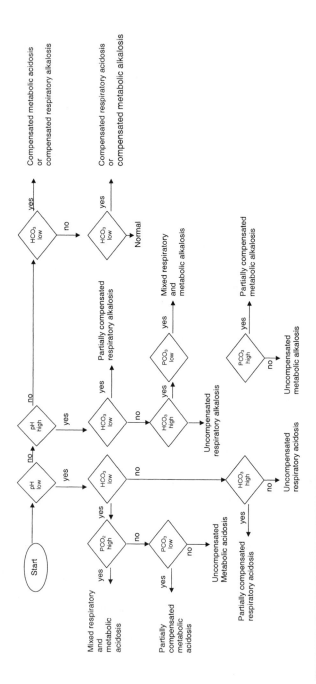

Figure 8. A flow diagram to assist in blood gas interpretation. (From Carlo WA, Chatburn RL (eds): Neonatal Respiratory Care, 2nd ed. Chicago, Year Book, 1988, p 56, with permission.

1. Evaluation of oxygenation and/or ventilation trends
2. Avoidance of prolonged episodes of hypoxemia or hyperoxia
3. Guide for ventilator adjustments and responses
4. Establishing "window orders" for weaning
5. Decreasing the frequency of blood gas sampling

C. Oxygen saturation monitoring
   1. Mechanism
      a. An infrared light and a photodetector are positioned over an artery; the more oxygenated the blood, the greater the amount of light which is transmitted back to the photodetector. The microprocessor-based unit calculates this light into percent oxygen saturation.
      b. Saturation monitors usually correlate well with an arterial sample, but if there is a discrepancy, a co-oximeter analysis should be obtained.
      c. Saturation levels of 92–96% will result in an acceptable PaO_2 in most infants.
   2. Specific indications
      a. More reliable indication of tissue oxygenation, since the hemoglobin carries more oxygen to the tissues than that dissolved in the plasma.
      b. An understanding of oxygen transport and the oxyhemoglobin dissociation curve is essential in the clinical application of saturation monitoring.
   3. Factors affecting accuracy
      a. Perfusion (acidosis, hypotension, hypoxia, temperature)
      b. Accuracy of pulse detection
      c. Motion
      d. Light interference (e.g., phototherapy)
      e. Probe site and placement (lateral aspect of foot or hand; avoid wrist)

D. Transcutaneous monitoring
   1. Mechanism—diffusion of oxygen and carbon dioxide through the skin to a heated electrode
   2. Specific indications
      a. When partial pressure of oxygen is a more reliable indicator than saturation, such as with hyperoxygenation
      b. Diagnosis and monitoring of right-to-left extrapulmonary shunting with pre- and postductal sites (PPHN)
      c. When monitoring of ventilation is important, including establishing optimal ventilator parameters, weaning, hyperventilation, and high-frequency ventilation

3. Factors affecting accuracy
   a. Perfusion (e.g., acidosis, hypoxia, hypotension)
   b. Condition of site (bruising or edema)
   c. Shunting
   d. Temperature of electrode
   e. Pharmacologic agents
   f. Site location and placement
4. Complications
   a. Reversible erythema is normal and usually resolves within 24 hours.
   b. Frequent site changes (every 2–3 hr) are necessary to avoid blistering.
   c. Damage to skin from adhesives

E. Capnography (end-tidal CO_2 monitoring)
1. Mechanism
   a. Analyzes exhaled carbon dioxide at the airway
   b. The level of carbon dioxide at the airway is dependent upon patency of the airway, ventilation and perfusion within the lung, and metabolism.
2. Specific indications
   a. A measurement of lung function (e.g., quality of perfusion and/or ventilation of alveolar units); prediction of severity and recovery of lung disease may be made.
   b. Evaluates effectiveness of mechanical ventilation and spontaneous breathing
   c. Facilitates weaning from mechanical ventilation and assesses ability to tolerate changes
   d. Has been used to verify endotracheal intubation
3. Factors affecting accuracy
   a. In lungs that are poorly perfused and/or ventilated, carbon dioxide at the airway will be low.
   b. Lung disease will result in a wide gradient between arterial PCO_2 and expired CO_2; the gradient may be > 20 mmHg, but as lung function improves, there will be an improvement in correlation, with gradients of < 10 mmHg. When no lung disease is present, the gradient is < 5 mmHg.

Chapter 50

Mechanical Ventilation: General Principles

Michael A. Becker, R.R.T., and Steven M. Donn, M.D.

I. Indications

A. Apnea

B. Ventilatory failure (increase in $PaCO_2$)

C. Unresponsive hypoxia ($PaO_2 < 50$ mmHg with $FiO_2 > 0.5$)

D. Infants < 900 g (relative indication)

E. Obstructive airway anomalies (e.g., choanal atresia)

F. Clinical deterioration

II. Patient Variables

A. Compliance (mL/cm H_2O): volume change per unit pressure change

    1. Chest wall

    2. Lungs

B. Resistance (cm H_2O/L/sec): characteristics of air flow

    1. Airway

    2. Endotracheal tube

C. Time constant (compliance $\times$ resistance)

    1. Time necessary for the lungs to fully inflate and deflate

    2. Decreased in diseases with low compliance and resistance

    3. Increased in diseases with high compliance and resistance

    4. Time constant should be considered when making adjustments in ventilatory rate and inspiratory and expiratory times.

III. Ventilator Parameters

A. Flow

    1. Continuous

        a. Flow delivered throughout the full ventilatory cycle

        b. Used in time-cycled, pressure-limited ventilation (3–10 LPM range for infants) and CPAP

    2. Inspiratory

        a. Flow delivered only during the inspiratory phase

        b. Seen in volume ventilation; flow determines inspiratory time.

    3. Demand

        a. Variable inspiratory flow determined by patient effort

        b. Seen in pressure control and pressure support ventilation

B. Tidal volume (V_T)
1. Primary parameter adjusted in volume ventilation
2. Tidal volume is a variable value in pressure-limited ventilation.

C. Peak inspiratory pressure (PIP): the highest inspiratory pressure delivered for each mechanical breath
1. Primary parameter adjusted in pressure-limited ventilation. The PIP to PEEP difference (delta P or amplitude) determines tidal volume delivery in pressure-limited ventilation.
2. Monitoring of tidal volume and real-time graphics, evaluation of chest wall movement, auscultation of breath sounds are all important assessments.
3. PIP is a monitored vaariable and is determined by the selected tidal volume, patient compliance, and resistance in volume ventilation.

D. Positive end-expiratory pressure (PEEP)
1. Baseline pressure at end expiration
2. Prevents alveolar collapse and improves ventilation/perfusion abnormalities
3. Minimum "physiologic" PEEP is 2–3 cm H_2O

E. Frequency (rate)
1. Mandatory (control) rate delivered by ventilator
2. Assist rate triggered by patient during assist/control ventilation
3. Alters minute ventilation ($V_T \times$ frequency = minute ventilation)

F. Inspiratory time (T_i)
1. Length of the inspiratory phase
   a. Inspiratory time is controlled by the cycling mechanism. The cycling mechanism determines when the ventilator ends inspiration and starts expiration, and vice versa.
   b. Cycling mechanisms
      i. Time
      ii. Flow
      iii. Volume
      iv. Pressure
2. With very rare exceptions, inspiratory time should never be longer than expiratory time in infant ventilation.

G. FiO_2
1. The concentration of inspired oxygen
2. Adjusted to maintain the appropriate PaO_2 and oxygen saturation
3. Prolonged concentrations of > 0.6 may be more likely to result in oxygen toxicity.

IV. Monitored Parameters

    A. Mean airway pressure (Paw)

        1. Composite of all pressure transmitted to the airway and reflects the area under the curve of pressure vs. time

        2. Changes in PIP, PEEP, inspiratory time, and frequency all affect the Paw.

        3. Paw correlates directly with oxygenation.

        4. High Paw (> 10–12 cm H_2O) may be associated with increased incidence of barotrauma and chronic lung disease.

        5. Change in PEEP results in a corresponding identical change in Paw.

    B. Tidal volume: a monitored value in pressure-limited ventilation

    C. Minute ventilation

        1. Monitored in all modes

        2. Normal values: 240–360 mL/kg/min

    D. PIP: monitored value in volume ventilation

    E. Inspiratory time: monitored value in flow-cycled ventilator modes

V. Classifying Modes of Mechanical Ventilation

    A. Control variables: in all modes of conventional ventilation bulk volumes of gas are delivered with an active inspiratory phase and a passive expiratory phase. The choice of what is controlled (pressure or volume) is by the clinician.

        1. Pressure: when pressure is the controlled variable, tidal volume will vary with changes in patient compliance and resistance.

            a. Advantages

                i. Maximum airway pressure is limited

                ii. Flow (either continuous or demand) is available.

            b. Disadvantage: changes in compliance and resistance will affect the tidal volume delivery.

        2. Volume: when volume is the controlled variable, the pressure will vary with changes in the patient compliance and resistance.

            a. Advantages

                i. A set tidal volume is delivered from the ventilator.

                ii. Compliance and resistance changes do not significantly change the tidal volume delivery. The tidal volume change that may be observed is attributed to the compressible volume lost in the circuit.

            b. Disadvantage: the flow rate is adjusted by the clinician to control the inspiratory time and may not meet the needs of the patient.

    B. Triggering mechanisms (start the inspiratory phase)

1. Flow
    a. Triggering by changes in airway flow. Ideally (in infant ventilation) detected at the proximal airway.
    b. Two common methods of flow triggering
        i. Hot wire anemometer (temperature differential)
        ii. Pneumotachometer (pressure differential)
    c. Advantages
        i. Tidal volume monitoring possible
        ii. May allow triggering of both inspiratory and expiratory phases
        iii. "No fault" sensor placement
        iv. Ability to adjust sensitivity for triggering and leaks
    d. Disadvantages
        i. Weight and dead space of the flow sensor
        ii. Possible autocycling
2. Pressure
    a. Pressure below the baseline pressure initiates the breath
    b. Advantages
        i. Requires no additional sensor for triggering
        ii. No sensor placement concerns
    c. Disadvantages
        i. May need an additional sensor to monitor proximal tidal volume
        ii. May not be a sensitive enough for low birthweight infants
3. Abdominal impedance
    a. A sensor is positioned on the abdomen, detects abdominal wall movement, and triggers a mechanical breath.
    b. Advantages
        i. No weight or dead space concerns with sensor
        ii. No autocycling from an airway leak
    c. Disadvantages
        i. No tidal volume monitoring
        ii. Sensor placement is critical
        iii. No sensitivity adjustment
        iv. False trigger from movement artifact
4. Chest wall impedance
    a. Triggering from the respiratory signal of the cardiorespiratory monitor
    b. Advantages
        i. No weight or dead space concerns associated with a sensor
        ii. No autocycling from an airway leak
        iii. Expiratory synchronization

    c. Disadvantages
      i. No tidal volume monitoring
      ii. Sensor placement is critical
      iii. No sensitivity adjustment
      iv. Depends on the reliability of cardiorespiratory monitor

C. Cycling Mechanisms
  1. Time
    a. A set time for inspiration ends the breath.
    b. An example is pressure control.
  2. Flow
    a. A decrease in the inspiratory flow ends the breath.
    b. Two examples are pressure support and flow-cycled pressure-limited ventilation.
  3. Volume
    a. A set volume delivery ends the breath.
    b. An example is volume-targeted ventilation.
  4. Pressure: a set pressure is achieved and the ventilator ends the breath.

VI. Neonatal Pulmonary Mechanics

Pulmonary mechanics monitoring is available for all mechanically ventilated infants. The VIP Bird Gold ventilator measures three signals at the proximal airway with each ventilator breath: pressure, flow, and volume. Graphic waveforms of each of these signals, as well as pressure-volume and flow-volume loops, can be displayed.

A. Procedure
  1. Mechanically ventilated infants can be studied continuously and without interruption of ventilation.
  2. If the graphic monitor is used to study the effects of treatment, suctioning should be preformed 15–30 minutes prior to testing

B. Data analysis
  1. Tidal volume/minute ventilation
  2. Pulmonary compliance
  3. Pulmonary resistance
  4. Peak flow rate

C. Indications: Evaluation of optimal ventilator mode and parameter settings
  1. Mode
  2. Pressure
  3. PEEP
  4. Flow

     5. Tidal volume

     6. Frequency

  D. Comparison of values (Table 38)

TABLE 38
Pulmonary Mechanics Values

	Normal (Full Term)	RDS	BPD
Tidal volume (mL/kg)	6–8	4–7	5–7
Minute volume (mL/kg/min)	240–360	200–280	200–280
Compliance (mL/cm H_2O)	2.25	< 0.8	> 1.0
Resistance (cm H_2O/L/sec)	300–700	< 1000	> 100

  E. Types of monitors

     1. Intermittent use

     2. Continuous use: most ventilators provide basic pulmonary
       graphic monitoring with each unit

Chapter 51

Conventional Mechanical Ventilation

Michael A. Becker, R.R.T., and Steven M. Donn, M.D.

The VIP Bird Gold Infant–Pediatric Ventilator (Bird Products Corporation, Palm Springs, CA) is a neonatal and pediatric ventilator that offers synchronized ventilation in both pressure and volume modes. It is described in detail because it is the infant ventilator of choice in the neonatal intensive care unit at the University of Michigan Health System.

I. **Features**
   A. Flow triggering available in all modes
   B. Neonatal sensor: at the patient connector (proximal)
   C. Pediatric sensor: close to the exhalation valve or distal
   D. Proximal tidal volume measurement with the neonatal sensor
   E. The pediatric sensor provides distal flow triggering and monitoring.
   F. Volume-targeted ventilation with a minimum tidal volume of 10 mL
   G. Rise time inspiratory flow pattern adjustment in both pressure control and pressure support ventilation modes.
   H. Inspiratory and expiratory hold
   I. SIMV/CPAP/PS and assist control (A/C) are available in all modes
      1. SIMV/CPAP/PS: a preset number of synchronized mandatory breaths are delivered. Additional spontaneous breaths are supported by either pressure support or flow (continuous or demand).
      2. A/C: a preset number of synchronized mandatory breaths are delivered (control). Additional spontaneous breaths are supported by another identical breath.
   J. Alarm/limits
      1. Volume
      2. Pressure
      3. Rate
   K. Manual breath
   L. Monitoring
      1. Breath rate
      2. Inspiratory time (T_i)
      3. Inspiratory to expiratory (I:E) ratio
      4. Peak inspiratory pressure (PIP)
      5. Positive end-expiratory pressure (PEEP)

6. Mean airway pressure (Paw)
7. Proximal inspiratory and expiratory tidal volumes (V_T)
8. Proximal expiratory minute ventilation (VE)

II.   Bird Graphic Monitor
   A. Waveforms (displays any 2 of 3 at the same time)
     1. Flow
     2. Volume
     3. Pressure
   B. Loops (mechanics)
     1. Pressure–volume loop
     2. Flow–volume loop
   C. 24-hour trend monitoring
   D. Pulmonary mechanics calculations
     1. Compliance
     2. Resistance

III.   Pressure-limited Modes of Ventilation
   1. Pressure-targeted ventilation: pressure is controlled; the volume varies with changes in patient compliance, resistance, and breathing pattern.
     1. Time-cycled, pressure-limited (TCPL)
       a. Time or flow-triggered
       b. Pressure-limited
       c. Continuous flow
       d. Time- (or flow-) cycled
     2. Pressure control (PC)
       a. Time or flow-triggered
       b. Pressure-limited
       c. Variable flow
       d. Time-cycled
     3. Pressure support (PS)
       a. Flow-triggered
       b. Pressure-limited
       c. Variable flow
       d. Flow-cycled
     4. Initial setup of pressure-limited ventilation
       a. Mode: assist/control
       b. Rate: 30–60 bpm
       c. T_i setting: 0.3–0.4 seconds
         i. PC: T_i is set by the clinician.
         ii. TCPL: with termination sensitivity on, the T_i is a limit.

      iii. TCPL: with TS off, the T_i is set.

      iv. PS: the T_i is a limit

  d. PIP: set at the same PIP that is noted on the manometer of the resuscitation bag.

  e. PEEP: 4–6 cm H_2O

    The difference between the PIP and PEEP (delta P) determines the tidal volume. When the infant is placed on the ventilator, note the inspiratory tidal volume. Make adjustments to deliver 4–7 mL/kg of tidal volume.

  f. FiO_2: set for appropriate oxygen saturation level

  g. Rise time: adjust the flow pattern for PC and PS breaths

      i. Level 1: fastest flow

      ii. Level 7: slowest flow

  h. Weaning pressure-limited ventilation

      i. Rate: decrease rate until the infant is initiating most, if not all, of the breaths.

      ii. Inspiratory time should require no change.

      iii. PIP-PEEP (delta P): as compliance changes take place, make adjustments to continually deliver 4–7 mL/kg of tidal volume.

      iv. FiO_2: make adjustments to obtain appropriate saturation level.

      v. Other considerations and options: switching to SIMV/PS

        (a) A set number of control breaths (TCPL or PC) will be delivered; additional spontaneous breaths are supported by PS. The PS breaths may be at a lower pressure level and deliver tidal volume of 4–6 mL/kg.

        (b) Wean ventilation by decreasing the number of control breaths to zero and consider extubation from either PS or CPAP.

IV. Volume-targeted Ventilation

Volume is controlled; the pressure varies with changes in patient compliance, resistance, and breathing pattern.

  A. Volume control

    1. Time or flow-triggered

    2. Volume-targeted

    3. Square or decelerating flow

    4. Volume-cycled (fixed T_i determined by the flow pattern and flow rate)

  B. Initial setup of volume-targeted ventilation

    1. Mode: assist/control

    2. Tidal volume: set at approximately 10–12 mL/kg to deliver 4–7 mL/kg at the proximal airway. (There is compressible volume loss in the circuit. Know tubing compliance.)

    3. Rate: 30–60 bpm

    4. Waveforms
      a. Square
      b. Decelerating

    5. Flow rate
      a. Flow rate and waveform determine inspiratory time.
      b. Set flow waveform and then adjust flow to give an inspiratory time between 0.3 and 0.4 seconds.

    6. PEEP: 4–6 cm H_2O

    7. FiO_2: set for appropriate oxygen saturation level.

C. Weaning volume-targeted ventilation
    1. Rate: decrease rate to < 40 bpm.
    2. Change to SIMV/PS; set PS level to deliver 4–6 mL/kg.
    3. Wean ventilation by decreasing the number of control breaths to zero and consider extubation from either PS or CPAP.
    4. PEEP: wean PEEP to 4 cm H_2O before considering extubation.
    5. FiO_2: make adjustments to obtain appropriate saturation level.

IV. Volume Assured Pressure Support (VAPS)

A combination mode of ventilation. The breath begins as a pressure support breath. At a set flow rate the delivered tidal volume is measured. If the minimum assured volume is delivered, the breath ends and is flow-cycled. If the minimum tidal volume is not delivered, it transitions to a volume-targeted breath. The minimum tidal volume or the maximum inspiratory time limit will end the breath.

A. VAPS
    1. Time or flow-triggered
    2. Pressure-targeted
    3. Variable flow
    4. Check of tidal volume
      a. Minimum tidal volume is delivered: flow-cycled
      b. Minimum tidal volume is not delivered: volume or time-cycled

B. Available in both assist/control and SIMV/PS modes

C. Weaning VAPS
    1. Clinical use of this mode is still under investigation.
    2. Suggested weaning sequences
      a. Weaning pressure
      b. Weaning tidal volume
      c. Switching to SIMV/PS

Chapter 52

High-frequency Ventilation

Michael A. Becker, R.R.T., and Steven M. Donn, M.D.

I. **Indications**
   A. Intractable air leaks
   B. Respiratory failure unresponsive to conventional ventilation
   C. The use of high-frequency ventilation (HFV) is preferred by some as a primary strategy.

II. **Successful Applications**
   A. Pulmonary interstitial emphysema (PIE)
   B. Respiratory distress syndrome (RDS)
   C. Persistent pulmonary hypertension of the newborn (PPHN)
   D. Meconium aspiration syndrome (MAS)
   E. Tracheoesophageal fistula (TEF)
   F. Respiratory syncytial virus (RSV) pneumonia
   G. Congenital diaphragmatic hernia (CDH)

III. **Classification**
   A. High-frequency positive pressure ventilation (HFPPV): ventilation at rapid rates (60–150 bpm) using conventional ventilators
   B. High-frequency jet ventilation (HFJV): ventilation with small pulses of gas under pressure at rapid rates, delivering very small tidal volumes (less than dead space). Inspiration results in a flutter or vibration of the chest wall, while the expiratory phase is passive; rates range from 240–660 bpm.
   C. High-frequency oscillatory ventilation (HFOV): ventilation with small volumes of gas moving in and out of the airways; both inspiration and expiration are active, resulting from piston-generated action; rates range from 3 to 15 Hz (1 Hz = 60 cycles/min).

IV. **Mechanisms of Gas Exchange**
   A. Bidirectional (coaxial) flow results in inspiratory gases moving down the center of the airway while expiratory gases move along the wall.
   B. Enhanced diffusion may occur from high-velocity gas flow, which results in increased molecular movement of gas.
   C. Resonant frequency—the lungs have an optimal frequency or rate

of breaths that optimizes ventilation. At the resonant frequency, less pressure is required to ventilate.

V.   Benefits
A. Optimization of Paw and lung volume
B. Reduction in air leaks; resolution of PIE
C. Improvement in hemodynamic function
D. Improvement in ventilation and oxygenation

VI.   Complications
A. Mucus plugging of airways and endotracheal tubes (avoidable with good humidification system), which may result in "super PEEP." This should be suspected if *both* PaO_2 and $PaCO_2$ are elevated.
B. Necrotizing tracheobronchitis (NTB): tracheal and bronchial inflammation, necrosis, and erosion, which may be the result of poor humidification and trauma from the high-velocity gas flow; this has also been found in infants treated with conventional mechanical ventilation; diagnosis is made with bronchoscopy (or at autopsy). Its incidence has dropped dramatically.
C. Recurrence of air leaks
D. HFJV may be delivered with a triple lumen "jet" endotracheal tube (jet, pressure, and main lumens), but this requires reintubation, which is not without risk in the severely compromised infant. A proximal adapter is available, which is placed in a standard endotracheal tube, and there is now no need for reintubation.

VII.   Clinical Assessment
A. Observe chest wall vibration frequently; decreased vibration could result from secretions, obstruction, misplaced endotracheal tube, or pneumothorax.
B. Breath sounds have a "jack-hammer" quality and are usually high pitched; low-pitched sounds may result from pneumothorax or atelectasis; musical squeaks may occur from secretions. Determine if breath sounds are equal on both sides.
C. Heart sounds and precordial activity are very difficult to assess; placing the high-frequency ventilator in standby may be necessary.

VIII.   Sensormedics 3100A High-Frequency Oscillator
A. Time-cycled, piston-driven high-frequency ventilator that delivers small volumes of gas, actively, on inspiration and expiration. Optimum lung expansion is maintained through a continuous flow of gas and resistance to an expiratory diaphragm.

B. Operates independently without the need for tandem conventional ventilation

C. Ventilator parameters/monitoring
   1. Mean airway pressure (Paw) adjust: 3–45 cm H_2O
   2. Delta P: variable (approx. 0–100 cm H_2O)
   3. Inspiratory time: 30–50%
   4. Frequency: 3–15 Hz
   5. Bias flow: 0–40 LPM
   6. Mean pressure limit: 10–45 cm H_2O

D. Alarms include maximum/minimum Paw

E. Clinical management for HFO
   1. Ventilation is provided through a conventional endotracheal tube.
   2. Both oxygen saturation and transcutaneous CO_2 monitoring are recommended.
   3. Frequent chest radiographs are needed to assess lung volumes.
   4. Initial settings for HFO
      a. High-volume strategy
         i. Paw: 1–2 cm H_2O higher than conventional; optimum inflation should show radiographic expansion to ninth rib.
         ii. Delta P: 25–50 cm H_2O (adjust for "chest wiggle factor")
         iii. Inspiratory time: 33%
         iv. Frequency: 8–12 Hz
         v. Wean by lowering FiO_2, then Paw unless the chest radiography indicates a greater than nine rib expansion.
      b. Low-volume strategy
         i. Paw: same as conventional; lower lung volumes should be maintained.
         ii. Delta P: 25–30 cm H_2O (adjust for chest wiggle factor)
         iii. Inspiratory time: 33%
         iv. Frequency: 12–15 Hz
         v. Wean by lowering Paw to decrease lung volumes, then FiO_2.
   5. Adjustments in HFO
      a. PaO_2 is dependent on Paw and FiO_2.
      b. $PaCO_2$ is dependent on delta P and frequency.
      c. Increasing the frequency will increase $PaCO_2$ and decreasing the frequency will decrease $PaCO_2$.
   6. Suctioning
      a. Suctioning should be performed as necessary; vibration of the chest wall may result in the need for more frequent suctioning. Suctioning is indicated for decreased chest wall movement or increase $PaCO_2$.

b. Suctioning may be performed through an inline suction adapter during HFO, or the patient may be manually ventilated during the suction procedure.

IX. **Bunnell Life Pulse High-Frequency Jet Ventilator**
   A. First FDA-approved jet ventilator
   B. Time-cycled, pressure-limited, flow interruption jet ventilator that includes ventilator with humidifier, patient circuit, and "patient box"
      1. Ventilator circuit consists of humidifier cartridge, which delivers heated humidity to incoming gas, and a heated inspiratory line; the distal end of the inspiratory line has a segment of silicon tubing, which inserts into the jet valve and connects to the proximal jet adapter or the jet lumen of the triple lumen jet endotracheal tube.
      2. "Patient box" is a small box that lies in the bed with the baby; it consists of a pinch valve (jet valve) that occludes the silicon tubing intermittently and delivers pulsations of gas down the endotracheal tube through the jet adapter port (or the jet lumen of the triple lumen tube). The pressure transducer is also in this box; it connects to the pressure line of the jet adapter (or the monitoring lumen of the triple lumen tube). A purge valve is also part of this box and keeps the pressure monitoring lumen clear of secretions and moisture.
      3. The Life Pulse is operated in tandem with a conventional ventilator, which attaches at the main opening of the jet adapter (or triple lumen tube), through which exhalation of gas occurs. Tandem ventilation is necessary for delivery of PEEP and conventional sigh breaths.
      4. Ventilator parameters
         a. Peak inspiratory pressure (PIP): 8–50 cm H_2O.
         b. Rate: 240–660 bpm
         c. Jet valve "on" time (inspiratory time): 0.02–0.034 seconds (20–34 msec)
      5. Monitoring includes PIP, PEEP, delta P, servo pressure (driving pressure [PSI] required to maintain PIP), and Paw.
      6. Alarms include power failure, low gas inlet pressure, high and low peak, mean, and servo pressures, and electronic and mechanical failures.
      7. Clinical management for HFJV
         a. Approved by the FDA for RDS complicated by PIE or other air leaks and failure to respond to conventional ventilation
         b. If a triple lumen jet tube is used, it is important to be aware that this tube has a half size larger outer diameter than the

standard endotracheal tube (e.g., 2.5-mm jet tube has the same outside diameter as a 3.0-mm conventional tube).

c. Both oxygen saturation and transcutaneous CO_2 monitoring are recommended during HFJV.

d. Initial settings for HFJV
   i. Rate: 400 bpm
   ii. PIP: same or slightly lower than conventional PIP
   iii. Inspiratory time: 0.02 sec

e. Initial conventional mechanical ventilation tandem settings
   i. Rate: 0–10 bpm
   ii. PIP: 5 cm H_2O lower than HFJV
   iii. Inspiratory time: 0.3–0.4 sec
   iv. PEEP: same as with conventional (3–6 cm H_2O)

f. Adjustments in HFJV
   i. $PaCO_2$ is dependent on delta P (PIP-PEEP) and rate (to a lesser extent).
   ii. PaO_2 is dependent on Paw and FiO_2

g. Adjustments in conventional mechanical ventilation
   i. With PIE, no conventional mechanical ventilation rate is best initially.
   ii. Conventional mechanical ventilation rate should be increased for atelectasis and when other attempts to improve oxygenation fail.
   iii. Conventional mechanical ventilation pressures should be adjusted so that the jet breaths are not interrupted (exception: at low jet PIPs, conventional mechanical ventilation PIP should not be lowered to < 15–18 cm H_2O for effective "sigh").

h. Weaning strategy
   i. Weaning pressure in treating air leaks is critical.
   ii. At low HFJV settings, conventional rate may be increased as the "jet" settings are further decreased.

i. Suctioning
   i. Suctioning should preferably be done as needed or at a minimum of every 8 hr. Secretions can decrease the effectiveness of the jet causing inadequate ventilation; an increase in measured PEEP (inadvertent PEEP) may be noted when there is a need for suctioning.
   ii. Suction is applied *continuously* (insertion and withdrawal) to prevent pressure buildup.
   iii. Jet ventilation may be continued during the suction procedure.

Chapter 53

Surfactant Replacement Therapy

Steven M. Donn, M.D., and Michael A. Becker, R.R.T.

I. Indications

A. Surfactant replacement therapy is indicated in infants with respiratory distress syndrome (RDS), where the normal production of surfactant is delayed because of pulmonary immaturity.

B. Newborns may be given surfactant as soon as the diagnosis of RDS has been confirmed by radiologic examination and intubation has been performed.

C. In very low birthweight infants, it may be beneficial to administer the surfactant as soon as possible after intubation.

II. Benefits

A. Improved oxygenation with ability to lower FiO_2 requirements

B. Improved compliance that results in increased tidal volumes and ability to ventilate at lower peak inspiratory pressures

III. Complications

A. Oxygen desaturation and bradycardia secondary to airway occlusion during administration

B. Rapid change in compliance resulting in hyperventilation, overdistention, and potentially air leaks

IV. Types of Surfactant

A. Modified natural surfactant

   1. Survanta is a surfactant that combines natural bovine lung extract with artificial substances including DPPC, palmitic acid, and tripalmitin. Each vial contains 8 mL of suspension that needs to be stored refrigerated and warmed to room temperature before administration.

   a. Dosage/frequency: 4 mL/kg every 6 hr; four doses is a standard course.

   b. Delivery is via direct instillation at the tip of the endotracheal tube with a 5 F catheter.

   c. Survanta is given in four aliquots with a different patient position for each portion.

   2. Other modified natural surfactants include Curosurf (porcine

lung extract), Infasurf (calf lung lavage), and Surfactant-TA (minced bovine lung).

B. Artificial surfactant

1. Exosurf Neonatal is a protein-free artificial surfactant. The major component of Exosurf is DPPC, which is formulated with cetyl alcohol, tyloxapol, and sodium chloride. Exosurf is stored as a powder and is reconstituted with 8 mL of sterile water to become a milky white solution. The reconstituted drug can be stored in a syringe at room temperature for 12 hours.

   a. Dosage/frequency: 5 mL/kg every 12 hr. Two doses is standard, but a third or fourth may be given for persistent respiratory distress.

   b. Delivery is via direct instillation into an endotracheal tube with a side port adapter.

   c. Exosurf is given in two aliquots with positioning side-to-side between each portion.

Chapter 54

Ventilatory Management of Specific Respiratory Disorders

Steven M. Donn, M.D., and Michael A. Becker, R.R.T.

I. **Respiratory Distress Syndrome (RDS)**

A. Pulmonary immaturity associated with surfactant deficiency leads to diffuse atelectasis and decreased lung compliance. The disease is complicated by mechanical considerations, such as very small lung volumes and a compliant chest wall, as well as an increased incidence of PDA.

B. Prematurity is the single most important factor. Others include asphyxia, infant of a diabetic mother, and delivery by cesarean section. The incidence is higher in males and the second-born twin.

C. Infants present with multiple signs of respiratory distress (cyanosis, nasal flaring, tachypnea, grunting, and retractions) within the first few hours of life. Chest radiographic findings show lung fields with a ground glass (reticulogranular) appearance and air bronchograms.

D. Early initiation of therapy is most effective in infants with signs of respiratory distress, because the disease is progressive. Mechanical ventilation is usually required when signs of respiratory distress are present. Surfactant replacement therapy is indicated to decrease the severity of the disease.

E. Synchronized ventilation in either a pressure or volume mode is desirable. This may decrease the incidence of barotrauma caused by the infant "fighting the ventilator," reduce the amount of sedatives needed, eliminate the need for skeletal muscle relaxants, and decrease the length of time mechanical ventilation is required.

F. Peak inspiratory pressure should be adjusted so that good air exchange is auscultated with the ventilator cycles. When volume monitoring is available, tidal volume should be maintained at 4–8 mL/kg, depending on the size of the baby.

G. FiO_2 and PEEP should be adjusted for optimum oxygenation.

H. Another strategy for infants requiring higher conventional ventilatory support is high-frequency oscillation (HFO).

I. Watch very closely for signs of recovery from RDS (e.g., diuresis and improved compliance). Weaning ventilator support as tolerated and avoiding overdistention may reduce complications associated with mechanical ventilation.

II. Pulmonary Interstitial Emphysema (PIE)

A. PIE is a major complication of mechanical ventilation. It primarily occurs in small premature infants who are ventilated using large tidal volumes and associated with high PIP and Paw. Small air leaks from the alveoli or small airways dissect into the perivascular tissues causing compression atelectasis of the adjacent alveoli. This necessitates a further increase in ventilator pressure, thus promoting more escape of air into the interstitial tissues. PIE also compresses the pulmonary and lymphatic vessels, causing decreased pulmonary blood flow and increased lung water.

B. High-frequency ventilation (HFV) is indicated to provide adequate ventilation at lower Paw. HFV has been successful in the management of infants with RDS complicated by PIE. It is recommended that, when the PIE has been resolved, the HFV be continued for at least 24 hours to prevent recurrence. High-frequency jet ventilation (HFJV) or HFO using a low lung volume strategy may be used.

C. Weaning strategy should include reduction in Paw before lowering the FiO_2.

D. Permissive hypercapnia (higher $PaCO_2$) may facilitate a reduction in Paw.

E. If the PIE is unilateral, place the infant with the affected side down to compress that side. Also, if the PIE is on the left, right main bronchus intubation may be considered.

F. If HFV is not an available option, inspiratory time should be lowered to 0.2 seconds, even if increased frequency and pressure are necessary.

III. Persistent Pulmonary Hypertension of the Newborn (PPHN) (*see also* Chapter 79)

A. Increased pulmonary vascular resistance causes right to left shunting through the foramen ovale and ductus arteriosus. It is clinically manifested as severe hypoxemia.

B. PPHN is most often seen in term or post-term infants who have more mature muscularization of the pulmonary vessels. It is also associated with hypoxic episodes *in utero*. Diagnosis can be made by obtaining pre- and postductal blood samples, using transcutaneous monitoring (pre- to postductal gradient > 20 mmHg), dual site pulse oximetry (gradient $> 10\%$), or by echocardiography.

C. Considerations for ventilatory management include attempts to optimize pulmonary blood flow, sometimes accomplished by hyperoxygenation and hyperventilation, through maximal ventilatory support, or alternatively achieved by using least possible ventilatory pressures ("conservative" ventilation), or somewhere in the middle.

D. Administration of sodium bicarbonate or THAM may facilitate alkalinization.

E. Continuous monitoring of oxygenation and ventilation with transcutaneous PO_2/PCO_2 and pulse oximetry monitors may provide useful trends.

F. Volume ventilation has been successful in improving oxygenation, especially in infants with PPHN secondary to pulmonary disease.

G. A trial of low PEEP (2–3 cm H_2O) may be attempted, because higher PEEP may increase pulmonary vascular resistance in an infant with compliant lungs.

H. Monitoring of blood pressure and fluid status is extremely important. Increased systemic pressure may improve pulmonary blood flow and decrease shunting.

I. Inhalational nitric oxide is FDA approved for use with infants demonstrating hypoxemic respiratory failure secondary to PPHN.

J. Weaning should be done *very slowly*.
1. FiO_2: decrease 1–2% every 30–60 min
2. PIP: decrease 1–2 cm H_2O per change
3. Rate: decrease 1–2 bpm per change

K. Transitional disease
1. Occurs on day 3 or 4
2. Lability decreases; there is less responsiveness to ↓ pH, ↑ $PaCO_2$ and ↑ PaO_2
3. Normalize blood gases, pH

L. Management of infants with PPHN is very controversial. Direct comparisons by randomized, controlled clinical trials are lacking. Among commonly used treatments are:
1. Hyperventilation
   a. Alkalosis
   b. Hypocapnia ↓ pH → higher PaO_2.
2. Conservative ventilation with permissive hypercapnia
3. High-frequency ventilation
   a. HFJV
   b. HFOV
4. Volume-targeted ventilation
5. Vasodilating drugs (e.g., tolazoline, chlorpromazine, magnesium sulfate)
6. Inhaled nitric oxide

IV. Meconium Aspiration Syndrome (MAS)

A. If meconium passage is noted during labor, after the infant is born, direct laryngoscopy with endotracheal intubation and suctioning through the endotracheal tube is performed when the infant is depressed.

B. Other than PPHN (which frequently develops with meconium aspiration), several respiratory problems can develop. An obstructive problem occurs from meconium, which may result in a ball valve mechanism that allows air to pass into the alveoli during inspiration but does not allow air outflow during expiration. This can cause air trapping and hyperinflation. Meconium can also cause alveolar-capillary block as a result of inflammation, atelectasis, and infectious or chemical pneumonitis. Ventilation-perfusion mismatch and air leaks occur frequently. Meconium appears to inactivate surfactant.

C. Oxygenation should be continuously monitored for evidence of sudden deterioration, possibly from a pneumothorax or PPHN.

D. Volume-targeted ventilation may facilitate a more even distribution of ventilation. Slower rates and longer expiratory times may reduce the risk of air trapping.

E. When diffuse lung disease is present, HFO may be beneficial.

F. With MAS, hyperventilation may be indicated when PPHN is present (*see* page 410), but avoid air trapping.

G. Optimal humidification is extremely important. If tolerated, vigorous percussion, vibration, and suctioning should be performed frequently, as necessary.

H. Surfactant therapy either as a single dose or lavage remains investigational.

V. Congenital Diaphragmatic Hernia (CDH)

A. Caused by a failure of the posterolateral portion of the diaphragm to close properly (most commonly on the left). Clinical signs of CDH include scaphoid abdomen, diminished breath sounds on the affected side, and shift in heart sounds. Diagnosis is confirmed by chest radiography, which reveals bowel in the chest cavity.

B. Cardiopulmonary problems associated with a diaphragmatic hernia include uneven ventilation; one lung is hypoplastic and difficult to ventilate, while the functional lung may potentially be overinflated. The presence of an underdeveloped pulmonary capillary bed causes high pulmonary vascular resistance and PPHN.

C. The infant should be intubated and ventilated *immediately;* bag and mask ventilation should be avoided because this could increase abdominal distension and further compromise ventilation. An OG tube should be inserted to decompress abdominal contents.

D. The lowest possible ventilating pressure necessary to maintain desired $PaCO_2$ should be used. High FiO_2 is usually necessary; low levels of PEEP (2–3 cm H_2O) are usually effective. Volume-targeted ventilation and HFO are alternative ventilatory strategies.

E. Because of the high incidence of PPHN, weaning should proceed *very slowly.*

F. Continuous monitoring of oxygen saturation and transcutaneous oxygen/carbon dioxide monitoring are suggested.

G. Surgery is usually delayed for several days, until the infant is completely stable and requiring lower ventilatory support and has had an opportunity to "remodel" transitional circulation.

H. ECMO may be necessary for cardiopulmonary failure when conventional management fails.

VI. Bronchopulmonary Dysplasia (BPD)

A. This is the major form of chronic pulmonary disease in newborns. The etiology appears to be ventilatory support with high pressure and FiO_2 for a prolonged period of time. Other contributing factors include air leaks, infection, PDA, and the immaturity of the respiratory system.

B. Oxygen saturations > 90% are important because of the risk of pulmonary hypertension leading to cor pulmonale. Higher levels of $PaCO_2$ are usually tolerated as long as pH is reasonable.

C. Ventilatory management with BPD can be very challenging. Because of variable compliance and high expiratory resistance, fluctuations in tidal volume delivery frequently occur. Volume-targeted ventilation may provide more consistent tidal volume delivery. Additionally, infants with BPD intermittently experience air hunger with acute oxygen desaturations. Pressure support ventilation (PSV), which provides variable demand flow, may alleviate extreme episodes of air hunger.

D. Infants with BPD may have a fixed intrapulmonary shunt and reductions in FiO_2 may not adversely affect the PaO_2.

E. Weaning is usually a very slow process. A team plan should be formulated to assure a certain level of progress is made over a defined period of time. Occasional blood gases should be obtained (every 1–2 days) to monitor weaning progress. Care should be taken not to change too many parameters at one time. Nutrition and weight gain should be monitored closely during weaning.

F. Steroid therapy may help reduce the inflammation throughout the airways and facilitate weaning from mechanical ventilation. However, this is very controversial because of adverse long-term effects. Consult with an attending neonatologist.

G. Airway problems associated with BPD include bronchospasm and tracheobronchomalacia. Bronchospasm may be relieved with bronchodilator therapy via metered dose inhalation (MDI). Response should be evaluated with pulmonary mechanics monitoring. Airway malacia may be detected with pulmonary mechanics monitoring, but is usually confirmed with flexible bronchoscopy. In an infant with bronchomalacia, higher PEEP may help to stint the airways open.

H. Chest physiotherapy to prevent atelectasis and retention of secretions is recommended.

I. If prolonged (> 2–3 months) mechanical ventilation is required, evaluation for tracheostomy should be considered.

VII. Tracheoesophageal Fistula (TEF) and RDS

A. Ventilatory management can often be very difficult in the infant with TEF, especially with prematurity. Repair of the TEF is sometimes delayed because of size and instability. If lung disease, characterized by poor compliance, is present, delivered gas will preferentially go through the fistula, resulting in alveolar hypoventilation and hypoxia.

B. Several techniques to improve ventilation:
   1. Place a gastrostomy tube to water seal at 6–10 cm H_2O
   2. HFJV to reduce flow of gas from the fistula and improve alveolar ventilation
   3. Insertion of a Fogarty catheter into the fistula and inflating it to occlude airflow

Suggested Reading

Donn SM (ed): Neonatal and Pediatric Pulmonary Graphics: Principles and Clinical Applications. Armonk, NY, Futura Publishing, 1998.

Donn SM, Sinha SK: Invasive and noninvasive neonatal mechanical ventilation. Respir Care [in press].

Goldsmith JP, Karotkin EH (eds): Assisted Ventilation of the Neonate, 4th ed. Philadelphia, W.B. Saunders, 2003.

Sinha SK, Donn SM (eds): Manual of Neonatal Respiratory Care. Armonk, NY, Futura Publishing, 2000.

Sinha SK, Donn SM (eds): Newer Concepts in Neonatal Respiratory Care. Seminars in Neonatology, vol. 7, no. 5, 2002.

Wiswell TE, Donn SM (eds): Update on Mechanical Ventilation and Exogenous Surfactant. Clinics in Perinatology, vol. 28. Philadelphia, W.B. Saunders, 2001.

Chapter 55

Inhalational Nitric Oxide Therapy

Steven M. Donn, M.D., and Michael A. Becker, R.R.T.

I. Description

A. Nitric oxide (NO) was identified in 1987 as endothelium-derived relaxing factor.

B. Potent pulmonary vasodilator first used for PPHN in 1992

C. Effect of NO depends on underlying pathophysiology.

II. Mechanism

A. Endogenous NO is synthesized from arginine by NO synthase in the endothelium. NO activates guanylate cyclase to form cGMP to produce smooth muscle relaxation. cGMP is rapidly hydrolyzed by phosphodiesterase enzymes.

B. Inhaled NO diffuses across alveolar membranes and similarly produces vasodilatation without apparent changes in systemic vascular resistance.

C. NO improves V/Q mismatch in some respiratory diseases.

D. In animals, NO does not alter LV output, cerebral blood flow, or cerebral O_2 consumption, despite an increased L→R shunt across the PDA.

E. In adults, NO also reduces PA pressure in primary pulmonary hypertension, ARDS, and after mitral valve replacement. In animals, it is a bronchodilator.

III. Potential Toxicities

A. Inhaled NO forms methemoglobin in the bloodstream. In the clinical arena with proper ventilator techniques, this toxicity is rare.

B. Prolonged bleeding times in animals and humans (presumed to be from platelet dysfunction) have been reported. There is concern about IVH in premature infants.

C. NO is highly reactive with oxygen to form nitric dioxide, NOx, and free radicals. Peroxynitrite may be formed; this raises concerns for membrane integrity and inactivation of surfactant.

D. A rebound "hypoxemia" has been described in patients in whom NO has been abruptly removed. Weaning to 1 ppm may prevent/attenuate this phenomenon.

IV. Clinical Trials

A. Twelve randomized trials of NO use in near-term infants have been reviewed as a part of a meta-analysis.

B. The use of NO at various doses does not improve mortality, but does reduce the need for ECMO. (Number needed to treat is 5.3.)

C. NO improves short-term physiologic measures of illness (oxygenation index, PaO_2) at 30–60 minutes.

D. In controlled trials, infants with congenital diaphragmatic hernias do not seem to benefit from the use of NO.

E. Additional clinical observations suggest the disease process may predict response. Response to NO for PPHN appears best with diffuse homogenous lung disease.

F. Proper lung inflation via the use of high-frequency ventilation may improve the response.

G. A prospective evaluation of dose response found no detectable differences in response from 5–80 ppm. Use lowest efficacious dose, usually $\leq$ 20 ppm.

H. Systematic review of the use of NO in preterm infants fails to demonstrate improvement in clinically meaningful outcomes. Short-term oxygenation may be improved.

V. Management at the University of Michigan Health System

A. Patient selection

  1. Term or near-term with severe respiratory failure (OI > 20, PaO_2 < 100 mmHg on FiO_2 1.0, or lability).

  2. Evidence of PPHN, such as echocardiogram, pre-postductal PaO_2 or SaO_2 gradient, or extreme lability.

  3. Consider use to stabilize transported patient with severe respiratory failure.

B. Optimize ventilator settings using pulmonary graphics monitor to provide adequate lung expansion. Consider trial of high-frequency oscillation, particularly with air leak, homogenous lung disease, MAS, or need for high airway pressure.

C. Proper ventilator setup includes high flow rate, NO inlet at the endotracheal tube, a scavenger system, and monitoring of NO, NO_2, NOx levels in inspired and expired gases.

D. Send baseline methemoglobin level (< 5%). Place pre- and postductal monitors (arterial catheters or pulse oximeters).

E. Begin inhaled NO at lowest efficacious dose. Start at 20 ppm and wean slowly if there is a response. 80 ppm may be attempted, but this is rarely necessary. Remember that inhaled NO causes a corresponding dose-dependent drop in FiO_2.

F. Monitor methemoglobin levels every 12 hr. If $> 5\%$, try to wean NO and if unable, consider methylene blue treatment.

G. Continue close monitoring. Patients who respond to NO may still ultimately require ECMO.

Suggested Reading

Barrington KJ, Finer NN: Inhaled nitric oxide for respiratory failure in preterm infants (Cochrane Review). In The Cochrane Library, Issue 1. Oxford, Update Software, 2002.

Finer NN, Barrington KJ: Nitric oxide for respiratory failure in infants born at or near term (Cochrane Review). In The Cochrane Library, Issue 1. Oxford, Update Software, 2002.

Finer NN, Etches PC, Kamstra B, et al: Inhaled nitric oxide in infants referred for extracorporeal membrane oxygenation: Dose response. J Pediatr 124:302–308, 1994.

Chapter 56

Extracorporeal Membrane Oxygenation

Robert E. Schumacher, M.D.

I.   Definition

Extracorporeal membrane oxygenation (ECMO) is a means whereby an infant with terminal or near terminal, but potentially reversible, lung failure is afforded a period of lung "rest" by use of an artificial lung. Such a period of "rest" may allow for lung recovery and ultimately survival of the infant.

II. ECMO Circuit

A. For venoarterial (VA) bypass, venous blood is passively drained via the right atrium and passed via a roller pump to a venous capacitance reservoir (bladder box), a membrane lung, a heat exchanger, and an arterial perfusion cannula. The right internal jugular vein and common carotid artery are used as access points and are ligated as part of the bypass procedure.

B. For venovenous (VV) bypass, a double lumen cannula is used. Blood is removed from and returned to the right atrium, the remainder of the circuit being the same as in VA ECMO.

C. To prevent thrombotic complications while on ECMO, the patient is treated with heparin to achieve bleeding times above normal.

III. Patient Selection

A. For "standard" neonatal ECMO the patient must:

1. Be ≥ 35 weeks' gestation (intracranial hemorrhage remains a significant concern for premature infants)
2. Have a cranial sonogram with no IVH > grade I
3. Have no major bleeding problem
4. Not have an irreversible condition that is uniformly associated with poor outcome such that attempts to prolong life are futile or not in the best interests of the infant (e.g., pulmonary hypoplasia, trisomy 18)
5. Be < 1 week old (relative contraindication, used as a marker for infants with a significant component of irreversible respiratory failure)
6. Be failing conventional medical management

B. *Failure of conventional medical management is a definition that should be individualized for each ECMO center.*
   1. Guidelines are used but the ultimate decision is up to those caring for the infant.
   2. Oxygenation index (OI) criteria:
      a. Index: $\dfrac{\text{mean airway pressure} \times \text{FiO}_2}{\text{PaO}_2 \text{ (postductal)}} \times 100$

      b. *After* stabilization if the patient has index values ≥ 40 on 3 of 5 occasions (each value separated by > 30 and < 60 min) ECMO criteria have been met (University of Michigan criteria).
      c. VV ECMO *may* not provide the same cardiac support that VA ECMO does.
         (1) ECMO registry data suggest VV ECMO is as "good" as VA at providing total support.
         (2) Because the risk of carotid artery ligation is not present, consideration of VV ECMO is made at lower OI values (25–40).
   3. Other criteria include A-aDO$_2$ values, acute deterioration, intractable air leaks, and "unresponsive to medical management."

IV. Management
A. Initial bypass problems
   1. Hypotension
      a. Hypovolemia: ECMO circuit has high blood capacitance; treat this with volume. The technician will have blood components or colloid available.
      b. Sudden dilution of vasopressors, especially with VV ECMO; treat by having separate pressor infusion pumps to infuse into circuit.
      c. Hypocalcemia from stored blood: circuit can be primed with calcium to prevent this.
   2. Bradycardia: from vagal stimulation by catheter(s)
   3. Consequences of catheter misplacement: correct catheter placement should be documented radiographically.
B. Initial management
   1. VA bypass: wean ventilator rapidly (10–15 min) to rest settings (FiO$_2$ 0.3, pressure 25/4, rate 20, with inspiratory time of 0.5–1.0 sec); use SvO$_2$ as guide. CPAP/high PEEP (10–12 cm H$_2$O) may shorten bypass time. Inotropes can usually be discontinued.
   2. VV bypass: wean with caution, infant is still dependent on

innate myocardial function for O_2 delivery. SvO_2 useful only for trends at same pump flow rate. Innate lung still provides gas exchange. High CPAP with VV ECMO may impede cardiac output; if desired, use $ETCO_2$ to optimize PEEP. Inotropes must be weaned with caution.

3. Infants have self-decannulated; restraints are mandatory.
4. Head position is critical; head turned too far left will functionally occlude the left jugular vein (the right is already ligated).
5. Sedation is usually required. Fentanyl or morphine are used for analgesia; if patient needs additional sedation, benzodiazepines or phenobarbital often work.
6. Heparin management
   a. Load with 100 U/kg prior to cannulation
   b. Drip concentration is 60 U/mL [6 mL heparin (1000 U/mL) in 94 mL D_5W].
   c. Usual consumption is 20–40 U/kg/hr.
   d. Titrate heparin to keep activated clotting time in desired range (usually ~180 sec).

C. Daily management, patient protocols, problems:
1. Chest radiograph: daily
2. Cranial sonogram: obtain the first day after cannulation, after every change in neurologic status, and minimally every third day.
   a. Brain hemorrhage: includes both typical and atypical (including posterior fossa) hemorrhages. If seen and patient is able to come off ECMO, do so. If patient is likely to die if removed from bypass, has stable hemorrhage, or is neurologically stable, consider staying on bypass with strict attention to ACTs, keeping platelets above 125,000/mm^3.
   b. Cranial sonography is not as good as CT or MRI for demonstrating peripheral and posterior fossa lesions.
3. Fluids: follow I/Os, weights; the membrane lung provides an additional area for evaporative losses.
   a. Total body water (TBW) is high: a common problem, etiology probably multifactorial. A problem arises when TBW is high but intravascular volume is low (capillary leak); vigorous attempts at diuresis in this instance can be harmful. Aggressive diuresis may allow for more caloric intake. Some argue that vigorous attempts at diuresis can hasten lung recovery; others state that diuresis is a marker for improvement and attempts to hasten it are of no avail. If diuresis is deemed advisable, use furosemide first, hemofilter last. Expect decreased urine output when a hemofilter is used.

b. K^+: often low, may result from blood bank providing K^+ poor (washed) RBCs; check for alkalosis.

c. Pump is primed with banked blood; ionized Ca^{2+} is initially low; priming the circuit prevents this.

4. Hemostasis/hemolysis

a. Obtain fibrinogen, fibrin split products, serum hemoglobin, and platelet counts daily.

b. Clots are common especially in venous capacitance reservoir (bladder). Pre-lung clots are usually left alone. Post-lung clots are handled by ECMO technician. When clots appear, review factors such as platelet or heparin consumption and FSP.

c. Bleeding

i. From neck wound: treated with cannula manipulation (by surgeon), light pressure, or fibrin glue

ii. Hemothorax/pericardium will present with decreased pulse pressure and decreased pump filling. Treated with drainage first.

iii. A more common problem if previous surgery has been done (CDH, thoracostomy tube).

iv. Treat with blood replacement, keep platelet counts high ($> 125–150,000/mm^3$), lower acceptable ACT values.

5. TPN: a *major* benefit of ECMO can be immediate TPN and adequate caloric/low volume intake (may use high dextrose).

6. Blood products

a. Minimize donor exposures; give only when indicated.

b. Excessive PRBC administration without increasing pump flow leads to lower aortic PO_2 but is similar to greater oxygen delivery.

7. Hypertension is a known complication. The final mechanism by which it is achieved is usually high total body water. It is almost always transient and resolves near the end of a run. A working definition is MAP > 75 mmHg. Initial treatment is with diuretics.

8. WBCs often low

9. Infections not a common problem

10. Bilirubin can be elevated especially with sepsis or long ECMO runs. A cholestatic picture is typical; plastic tubing (phytalate) may be hepatotoxic. Hepatosplenomegaly is common.

11. Cardiac stun: once on ECMO, a dramatic decrease in cardiac performance is seen in up to 5% of patients. It is more common

on VA ECMO and may be VA ECMO-induced from increased afterload. The stun phenomenon usually resolves, but patients with it do have higher overall mortality rates. Treatment is supportive.

D. Circuit problems (selected, more common problems)

1. Air in circuit: treatment depends on location; can often be aspirated.

2. Pump cutouts: kinked tube, malposition, low volume, low filling pressure (pneumothorax, hemopericardium), agitated infant

3. Pump
   a. Electric failure: can be cranked by hand
   b. Occlusion set too loose: false high flow readings. Too tight: hemolysis.

4. Lung pathophysiology: the membrane lung can get "sick" — can have pulmonary embolus, edema, etc. Treatment depends on specific problem.

E. Weaning

1. Easiest to follow SvO_2; technician to wean by preset parameters

2. Chest radiograph is very helpful
   a. Usually shows initial complete opacification
   b. Starts to clear prior to "reventilating" the lungs and serves as a marker for lung recovery

3. Pulmonary mechanics tests: compliance becomes poor hours after going on and improvement is an early marker of lung recovery.

4. $ETCO_2$: increasing expired CO_2 indicative of return of lung function

F. Trial off

1. Lung conditioning: lungs are periodically (hourly) inflated using a long (≥ 5 sec) inspiratory time in preparation for trial off VA ECMO.

2. Simply turning up the ventilator FiO_2 and following SvO_2 will give a feel for whether or not there is effective pulmonary gas exchange.

3. Increased ventilator settings 30–60 min before trial off allows for recruitment of lung units.

4. VA: obtain blood gases every 10 min $\times$ 3, weaning aggressively per pulse oximetry.

5. VV: halt gas flow to membrane lung, keep pump flowing. Since infant is still on bypass but with no effective gas exchange through membrane, use venous line SvO_2 to wean FiO_2, as it is now a true venous saturation.

6. A successful trial off depends upon the individual patient. Patient should be stable on ≤ 0.4 FiO$_2$, settings as per trial off.

G. Decannulation

1. Notify surgeon as early as possible.
2. Infant will be paralyzed to prevent air embolism.
3. Need for repair of carotid artery or jugular vein remains controversial.

V.   Post-ECMO Follow-up

A. Neck: sutures removed in 7 days

B. Platelets will continue to fall post ECMO. Serial counts are necessary until stable (24–48 hr).

C. CNS

1. EEG, if normal on ECMO (if obtained), no need to repeat
2. EEG is a sensitive screening test for problems. Focal abnormality correlates with structural findings, and CT or MRI is needed.
3. CT: obtained because of relative insensitivity of sonography for posterior fossa and peripheral parenchymal lesions.
4. BAER: because of high incidence of sensorineural hearing loss with PPHN, hearing screening is recommended.

D. Airway: vocal cord paresis seen in 5% of infants post ECMO; acute respiratory deterioration has occurred. If persistent stridor is noted, flexible bronchoscopy is required. Paresis has always resolved clinically (days to months).

E. Follow-up: mandatory

1. Neurodevelopmental follow-up: 10–20% of patients show major problems.
2. Medical problems include lower respiratory tract infections in > 50%.

Suggested Reading

Zwischenberger JB, Steinhorn RH, Bartlett RH (eds): ECMO: Extracorporeal Cardiopulmonary Support in Critical Care, 2nd ed. Ann Arbor, MI, Extracorporeal Life Support Organization, 2000.

Section IX. CARDIOVASCULAR DISEASE

Chapter 57

Congenital Heart Disease

John D.E. Barks, M.D.

I. Presentation and Classification

A. Not all congenital heart disease (CHD) manifests clinically in the neonatal period. An isolated ventricular septal defect (VSD) or atrial septal defect (ASD) may present later in infancy or childhood. Not all symptomatic structural heart defects will present with a murmur. Serious disease usually presents one of three clinical patterns. These classic presentations may be attenuated or absent at birth in infants identified antenatally by ultrasound and fetal echocardiography.

   1. Central cyanosis
   2. Poor cardiac output
   3. Congestive failure with respiratory distress

B. Formulating a differential diagnosis (prior to echocardiogram)

   1. Careful physical examination
   2. Arterial blood gases
   3. Chest radiograph (CXR)
   4. Electrocardiogram (ECG)

C. Common lesions and nonstructural differential diagnoses

   1. Central cyanosis

     a. Central cyanosis, decreased pulmonary vascular markings on CXR

       i. Pulmonary or tricuspid atresia
       ii. Severe tetralogy of Fallot
       iii. Critical pulmonic stenosis
       iv. Ebstein's anomaly

     b. Central cyanosis, normal or increased pulmonary vascular markings on CXR

       i. Simple or complex transposition of he great arteries
       ii. Total anomalous pulmonary venous return
       iii. Truncus arteriosus
       iv. Double outlet right ventricle (Taussig-Bing variant)

     c. Noncardiac differential

       i. Parenchymal lung disease
       ii. Persistent pulmonary hypertension of the newborn (PPHN)

        iii. Severe transient myocardial or tricuspid insufficiency (history of birth depression)

  2. Poor cardiac output

    a. Structural cardiac conditions

        i. Hypoplastic left heart syndrome

        ii. Coarctation of the aorta

        iii. Interrupted aortic arch

        iv. Critical aortic stenosis

        v. Anomalous left coronary artery

        vi. Cor triatriatum

    b. Nonstructural differential

        i. Sepsis

        ii. Cardiomyopathy (including infant of diabetic mother)

        iii. Severe transient myocardial insufficiency (birth depression)

        iv. Viral myocarditis

        v. Arrhythmias

  3. Congestive failure and respiratory distress

    a. Structural cardiac conditions

        i. Total anomalous pulmonary venous return (TAPVR)

        ii. Truncus arteriosus

        iii. Endocardial cushion defect

        iv. Absent pulmonic valve

        v. Single ventricle

        vi. Complex transposition

        vii. Other complex lesions

    b. Nonstructural differential

        i. Parenchymal lung disease $\pm$ PPHN

        ii. Severe anemia

        iii. Arteriovenous malformation

II. Diagnostic Tests

A. Blood pressure (all four limbs)

B. Chest radiograph

  1. Heart size and shape

  2. Pulmonary vascular markings

  3. Position of aortic arch

C. Arterial blood gases (and lactate if available)

  1. Determine degree of hypoxia

  2. Estimate of tissue oxygen delivery by degree of metabolic acidosis

  3. Evaluate adequacy of ventilation

D. Hyperoxia test (CHD vs. parenchymal lung disease)
  1. Place infant in FiO_2 of 1.0, 10–15 min.
  2. If $PaO_2 > 150$ mmHg, most cyanotic cardiac defects are ruled out (except TAPVR).
E. Echocardiogram with Doppler imaging—diagnostic modality of choice if clinical findings and tests A through D (above) are suggestive of CHD.
F. Electrocardiogram—relatively nonspecific except for arrhythmias. (Questionable value for Dx of CHD.)
  1. QRS axis
  2. Chamber hypertrophy
  3. Absence of forces
  4. Myocardial ischemia
  5. Arrhythmia
G. Ductal shunt (CHD vs. PPHN)
  1. Simultaneous pre- and postductal ABGs
  2. Right-to-left ductal shunt is usually present if preductal PaO_2 is 15 mmHg greater than postductal PaO_2; suggests increased pulmonary vascular resistance (i.e., PPHN).
  3. With severe hypoxemia, shunting may be present without a gradient.
H. Hyperoxia-hyperventilation test (CHD vs. PPHN)
  1. Hyperoxia test plus hyperventilation ($PaCO_2 = 25$ mmHg)
  2. With most PPHN, rise in PaO_2 will be noted.

III. Stabilization (Prior to Surgery or Transcatheter Intervention)

A. Supportive care
  1. Attempt to provide adequate oxygenation and ventilation.
  2. Maintain oxygen saturation only sufficient to prevent metabolic acidosis (e.g., in mid-70s). Hyperoxygenation is potentially harmful by:
      a. Dilation of pulmonary arteries, which can exacerbate LV outflow obstruction by diverting flow from systemic to pulmonary circuit
      b. Ductal closure
  3. Avoid hyperventilation unless noncardiac PPHN.
  In ductal-dependent LV outflow obstruction lesions, hyperventilation with alkalosis-induced pulmonary vasodilatation is potentially harmful, by diverting blood flow from systemic to pulmonary circuit.
  4. $NaHCO_3$

    a. Partially correct metabolic acidosis.

    b. Assure adequate ventilation.

5. Correct anemia (goal HCT > 40%).

   Note: Use leukocyte-poor irradiated blood and blood products if suspected DiGeorge syndrome, i.e., hypocalcemia or absent thymic shadow and CHD (primarily conotruncal defects, e.g., interrupted aortic arch, tetralogy of Fallot, truncus arteriosus, absent pulmonic valve).

6. Correct metabolic abnormalities (e.g., hypoglycemia, hypocalcemia).

B. Prostaglandin E_1 infusion

1. Maintains ductal patency

2. Use for ductal-dependent lesions, e.g., RV outflow obstruction or transposition of great arteries in central cyanosis group; LV outflow obstruction in poor cardiac output group.

3. Do not use in lesions that are not ductal-dependent (e.g., TAPVR, truncus arteriosus).

4. Trial may be warranted if cardiac diagnosis is unclear in presence of severe hypoxemia and acidosis.

5. Dose: start with 0.03 μg/kg/min (max. dose 0.1 μg/kg/min) as IV continuous infusion (e.g., 500 μg diluted in 80 mL provides 0.03 μg/kg/min at 0.3 mL/kg/hr). Many NICUs have unit-specific dosing nomograms.

6. Indications: suspected ductal-dependent lesion and $PaO_2 \leq 30$–35 mmHg, $SaO_2 \leq 70\%$, metabolic acidosis, hypotension/hypoperfusion.

7. Major side effects

    a. Apnea (12%) (Be prepared to intubate and ventilate.)

    b. Fever (14%)

    c. Seizures (4%)

    d. Flushing (10%)

    e. Bradycardia (7%)

    f. Hypotension (4%)

C. Inotropic therapy—adjunctive therapy for hypotension

1. Dopamine (5–20 μg/kg/min)

2. Dobutamine (5–20 μg/kg/min)

Note: Avoid in hypertrophic cardiomyopathy (e.g., infant of diabetic mother)

D. Congestive heart failure therapy

1. Diuretics (e.g., furosemide, *see* page 85)

2. Digoxin (*see* page 82)

Suggested Reading

Beekman RH: Neonatal cardiac emergencies. In Donn SM, Faix RG (eds): Neonatal Emergencies. Mt. Kisco, NY, Futura Publishing, 1991, pp 345–370.

Brook MM, Heymann MA, Teitel DF: The heart. In Klaus MH, Fanaroff AA (eds): Care of the High Risk Neonate, 5th ed. Philadelphia, W.B. Saunders, 2001, pp 393–424.

Roberts RJ: Drug Therapy in Infants. Philadelphia, W.B. Saunders, 1984, pp 138–156.

Wernovsky G, Rubenstein SD (eds): Cardiovascular Disease in the Neonate. Clinics in Perinatology, vol. 28. Philadelphia, W.B. Saunders, 2001.

Chapter 58

Patent Ductus Arteriosus

John D.E. Barks, M.D.

I. Incidence
A. Inversely related to birthweight or gestational age.
B. Increased incidence associated with respiratory distress syndrome (RDS), asphyxia, high altitude, increased fluid intake.

II. Complications
A. Congestive heart failure (CHF)
B. Hypoperfusion of brain, kidneys, intestine—potentially associated with intraventricular hemorrhage (IVH), acute tubular necrosis (ATN), necrotizing enterocolitis (NEC)
C. Chronic lung disease (BPD)

III. Diagnosis
A. Clinical
  1. Murmur—systolic more common than continuous (10% with large PDA will have no murmur.)
  2. Hyperactive precordium
  3. Bounding pulses, palmar pulsations, and increased pulse pressure (> 20–30 mmHg)
  4. Signs of CHF—tachypnea, tachycardia, edema, hepatomegaly, increasing ventilatory requirement
  5. Occasionally refractory hypotension accompanying some of above signs
  6. Pulmonary hemorrhage (rare)
B. Radiographic
  1. Cardiomegaly
  2. Pulmonary vascular engorgement/pulmonary edema
C. Echocardiographic
  1. Echocardiographic imaging of PDA, with left-to-right shunt documented by Doppler
  2. Dilated LA and LV
  3. Rule out ductal-dependent lesion that would be a contraindication to ductal closure

IV. Management of the Symptomatic PDA
A. Prevention

1. Fluid intake ≤ 20–140 mL/kg/d
2. If infant receiving phototherapy, place opaque patch(es) over precordium

B. Medical

1. Fluid restriction, diuretics
   a. Some will close, transiently or permanently
   b. Disadvantages–decreased caloric intake, electrolyte abnormalities, barotrauma from prolonged ventilatory requirement
   c. May only postpone need for definitive closure
   d. Consider fluid restriction in conjunction with indomethacin therapy.

2. Indomethacin (cyclooxygenase inhibitor, decreases prostaglandin production)
   a. Indication—symptomatic PDA, e.g., ventilator-dependent protracted RDS course, congestive heart failure, persistent hypotension, and/or metabolic acidosis
   b. Dose varies with postnatal age at start of therapy (based on pharmacokinetics).
      Initial dose is 0.2 mg/kg
      i. Age < 48 hours:
         0.2 mg/kg initial dose
         0.1 mg/kg subsequent doses, 12, and 24 hr later
      ii. Age 2–7 days:
         0.2 mg/kg/dose every 12 hr for 3 doses
      iii. Age ≥ 8 days:
         0.2 mg/kg initial dose
         0.25 mg/kg subsequent doses, 12, and 24 hr later
         Caution: do not infuse via umbilical artery catheter
   c. Contraindications
      i. Renal failure: urine output < 1.0 mL/kg/hr; serum creatinine > 1.8 mg/dL
      ii. Thrombocytopenia: platelets < 60,000/mm^3
      iii. Frank renal/GI bleeding (IVH not a contraindication)
      iv. Necrotizing enterocolitis
      v. Ductal-dependent cardiac lesion
   d. Response: about 70% closure of PDA; course may need to be repeated.
   e. Complications: oliguria of variable severity frequently follows indomethacin treatment.
      Note: manage this oliguria by fluid restriction, *not* fluid challenges, because this complication is self-resolving and fluid overload may exacerbate PDA.

C. Surgical ligation
1. Indication: failure of indomethacin or indomethacin contraindicated
2. Immediate closure necessary because of rapid clinical deterioration

Suggested Reading

Bell EF, Warburton D, Stonestreet BS, Oh W: Effect of fluid administration on the development of symptomatic patent ductus arteriosus and congestive heart failure in premature infants. N Engl J Med 302:598–604, 1980.

Clyman RI: Medical treatment of patent ductus arteriosus in premature infants. In Long WA (ed): Fetal and Neonatal Cardiology. Philadelphia, W.B. Saunders, 1990, pp 682–690.

Clyman RI: Recommendations for the postnatal use of indomethacin: An analysis of four separate treatment strategies. J Pediatr 128:601–607, 1996.

Gersony WM, Peckham GJ, Ellison RC, et al: Effects of indomethacin in premature infants with patent ductus arteriosus: Results of a national collaborative study. J Pediatr 102:895–906, 1983.

Huhta JC: Patent ductus arteriosus in the preterm neonate. In Long WA (ed): Fetal and Neonatal Cardiology. Philadelphia, W.B. Saunders, 1990, pp 389–400.

Rosenfeld W, Sadhev S, Brunot V, et al: Phototherapy effect on the incidence of patent ductus arteriosus in premature infants: Prevention with chest shielding. Pediatrics 78:10–14, 1986.

Chapter 59

Neonatal Hypertension

Charles R. Neal, Jr., M.D., Ph.D.

I. Introduction

A. Hypertension, defined in the newborn as systolic and/or diastolic blood pressure greater than 95th percentile for age, sex, and population, is observed in approximately 5% of all newborns. This incidence may be higher in the high-risk population treated in secondary or tertiary centers.

B. This condition in the newborn is worrisome because of limited autoregulation of blood flow to such vital organs as the brain. If blood pressure is outside the range at which autoregulation is possible, overperfusion at high pressures may result in disruption of endothelial integrity and resultant intracranial hemorrhage.

C. End-organ injury of all organ systems is also of major concern if the hypertension is sufficiently acute or long-standing.
  1. Nephropathy
  2. Cardiomyopathy or left ventricular dysfunction
  3. Retinal vasculopathy
  4. Encephalopathy

D. Neonatal hypertension increases risk of adult hypertension and associated complications.

II. Measurement of Blood Pressure

A. Invasive measurement involves direct monitoring of intra-arterial pressure through an indwelling vascular catheter with a calibrated manometer or transducer. Thrombi or fibrin accumulations at the catheter tip interfere with transmission of blood pressure and resultant accuracy.

B. Noninvasive measurements vary in their reliability.
  1. Oscillometry (e.g., Dinamap)
  2. Sphygmomanometry with auscultation is limited by the difficulty distinguishing classic Korotkoff sounds in newborns.
  3. Sphygmomanometry with Doppler detection of blood flow and vessel wall movement is limited by diastolic measurements of questionable accuracy in newborns. Also, systolic pressures average slightly higher (1.7 mmHg) than simultaneous intra-arterial measurements.

   4. Sphygmomanometry with fluids is limited by diastolic pressures that are often not discernible.
C. Factors to consider when measuring and interpreting blood pressure
   1. The transducer or manometer should be at the same level as the tip of the indwelling arterial catheter.
   2. A sphygmomanometer cuff (the inner inflatable bladder) must be wide enough to encircle at least two-thirds of the upper arm and long enough to surround the complete arm circumference.
   3. Individual variability in blood pressure is common.
      a. Blood pressure rises with feeding, upright position, sucking, and agitation.
      b. Diagnosis of hypertension should not be based on a single blood pressure measurement; it should require at least three separate measurements.
D. Several reference ranges have been reported and used for normal standards (see Suggested Reading for reference information). Among those most commonly utilized are:
   1. Term infants
      a. The Brompton study (Table 39): Repeated systolic blood pressure measurements using a Doppler technique in a large population of infants with gestational age of ≥ 38 weeks.

TABLE 39
Mean Systolic Blood Pressure

	4 Days	6 Weeks	6 Months	1 Year
Mean systolic blood pressure + SD (mmHg)				
Awake (no.)	76 ± 10 (174)	96 ± 14 (1131)	93 ± 14 (858)	94 ± 11 (1338)
Asleep (no.)	71 ± 8 (1566)	71 ± 11 (506)		
95th Percentile (mmHg)				
Awake	95	113	113	113
Asleep	86	106		

From DeSwiet M, Fayers P, Shinebourne EA: Systolic blood pressure in a population of infants in the first year of life: The Brompton Study. Pediatrics 65:1028–1035, 1980, with permission.

      b. Adelman: Defines pathologic hypertension as SBP > 90 mmHg or DBP > 50 mmHg in a term infant.
   2. Preterm infants
      a. Hegyi et al: During the first 6 hours of life, SBP and DBP

were measured in a large cohort of premature infants in various disease states.

    b. Adelman: Defines pathologic hypertension as SBP > 80 mmHg or DBP > 50 mmHg in a preterm infant.

    c. Zubrow et al: Collection of follow-up data from 608 infants for 1–99 days after delivery generated 9911 infant-day records and 24,052 individual BP measurements.

III. Possible Etiologic Factors

These are not necessarily in order of frequency of importance. Hypertension is much more likely to have a specific identifiable cause in a newborn infant than in an adult.

A. Primary renal disease
1. Renal dysplasia
2. Obstructive uropathy
3. Polycystic disease
4. Renal insufficiency of many causes
5. Renal tumor

B. Renal vascular disease
1. Renal artery thrombosis (often observed secondary to umbilical artery catheter placement)
2. Renal vein thrombosis (most often seen in infants of diabetic mothers)
3. Renal artery stenosis
4. Renal artery calcification or dysplasia

C. Primary cardiovascular disease
1. Coarctation of aorta
2. Hypoplastic or interrupted aortic arch

D. Umbilical artery catheter
1. Induced aortic thrombosis
2. Induced renal artery thrombosis

E. Intracranial hypertension

F. Endocrine
1. Congenital adrenal hyperplasia
2. Cushing disease
3. Primary hyperaldosteronism
4. Hyperthyroidism

G. Catecholamine-secreting tumor
1. Neuroblastoma
2. Pheochromocytoma
3. Adrenocortical carcinoma

H. Fluid or salt overload

I. Hypertension observed in bronchopulmonary dysplasia is likely caused by abnormalities of angiotensin, vasopressin, or aldosterone.

J. Extracorporeal membrane oxygenation (ECMO). The underlying mechanism of hypertension is unclear.

K. Medications, illicit drugs, or substance abuse
   1. Cocaine
   2. Theophylline
   3. Steroids
   4. Pressors
   5. Pancuronium
   6. Topical ophthalmic phenylephrine or tropicamide

L. Postoperative abdominal wall defect repair

M. Genetic or familial causes

N. Seizures

IV. Diagnosis

A. Pertinent medical history is helpful.
   1. Underlying medical conditions
   2. Maternal and infant drug exposure
   3. Maternal diabetes
   4. Relevant family history
   5. Clinical signs are often nonspecific, mandating a high index of suspicion and longitudinal surveillance of blood pressure in high-risk infants.
      a. Failure to thrive
      b. Tachypnea
      c. Tachycardia/bradycardia
      d. Irritability/seizures
      e. Feeding intolerance
      f. Urine output

B. Physical findings
   1. Blood pressure measurements in all four limbs
   2. Differential pulses and perfusion in all extremities
   3. Nephromegaly or enlargement of other organs or masses
   4. Head circumference, fontanel tension, suture widening
   5. Retinal examination
   6. Signs of increased precordial activity and location of point of maximal impulse
   7. Abnormal genitalia
   8. Pigmentation

C. Diagnostic studies—not all are indicated but should be based on index of suspicion.

1. Complete urinalysis, including microscopic examination, with assessment for protein, glucose, pH, and specific gravity
2. Serum electrolyte panel, including creatinine
3. In selected patients:
   a. Renal and adrenal sonography, with an excretory urogram (VCUG) in selected cases.
   b. Echocardiogram to evaluate cardiac anatomy, particularly the aortic arch and descending aorta. Also study left ventricular function and rule out left ventricular hypertrophy.
   c. Doppler flow studies of renal and other vessels
   d. Renal radionuclide scan
   e. Renal angiography with selective renal vein renin measurements
   f. Cranial sonography
   g. Urine catecholamines and metabolites
   h. Plasma renin activity
   i. Serum aldosterone and cortisol levels
   j. 17-OH-progesterone and other pertinent metabolites from steroid synthetic pathways
   k. Serum thyroxine and TSH
   l. Toxicology screen

V. Treatment

A. Therapy should be directed at primary treatment of the specific underlying cause of the hypertension, if one is identified and specific therapy exists.

B. It is important to avoid medications and dietary factors that may exacerbate renal dysfunction or blood pressure abnormalities.

C. Careful attention must be paid to diet, total fluids, and sodium intake.

D. Specific pharmacologic therapy

1. Life-threatening hypertension
   a. Diazoxide, given at 1–5 mg/kg/dose by rapid IV push. May repeat every 5–15 min until control is achieved, then every 2–4 hr PRN. Watch for hyperglycemia, salt and water retention blood dyscrasia, and fever.
   b. Sodium nitroprusside, given at 0.05–5.0 μg/kg/min by continuous IV infusion. Monitor for thiocyanate toxicity, especially if renal dysfunction is present. Observe for hypotension and metabolic acidosis.
2. If the hypertension is not life-threatening and related to fluid overload, consider a thiazide diuretic for chronic treatment. It should be used in addition to spironolactone to minimize potassium loss.

    a. Chlorothiazide, 20–50 mg/kg/d divided every 6–12 hr.

    b. Hydrochlorothiazide, 2–5 mg/kg/d divided every 6–12 hr. Be aware of the potential for reduced renal blood flow when using this drug.

    c. Spironolactone, 1–3 mg/kg/d divided every 6–12 hr. Monitor for hyperkalemia.

    d. Furosemide may be useful for the short-term, given as 1–4 mg/kg/dose. Long-term use is not recommended, particularly in premature infants and infants with severe bronchopulmonary dysplasia, because it causes significant electrolyte imbalance. Long-term sequelae also include osteopenia and renal calculi.

3. If the hypertension is not life-threatening and not related to fluid overload or not responsive to diuretic therapy alone, consider:

    a. Vasodilator: hydralazine, given at 0.1–0.5 mg/kg dose IV or 0.5–1.0 mg/kg/d divided every 6 hr PO. When giving this drug long term, monitor for tachycardia, salt and fluid retention, and blood dyscrasias.

    b. Beta-adrenergic antagonist: propranolol, given at 0.01–0.15 mg/kg/dose IV or 1.0–4.0 mg/kg/d divided every 6–12 hr PO. Beta-adrenergic antagonists should never be used in the presence of hypoglycemia, diminished cardiac function, or reactive airway disease. Monitor carefully for acquisition of these conditions while on long-term therapy. Concurrent use of a barbiturate or indomethacin may decrease beta-antagonist efficacy, whereas cimetidine or hydralazine may increase it.

    c. The angiotensin-converting enzyme inhibitors include captopril, given at 0.01–0.5 mg/kg/dose TID PO, and enalapril, given at 0.01–0.05 mg/kg/dose. These drugs should not be used in patients with renal artery stenosis. Observe patients carefully for signs of cardiopulmonary compromise, hyperkalemia, or acute agranulocytosis. Drug doses should be adjusted in renal failure.

    d. Calcium channel blocker: nifedipine, given at 0.05–0.5 mg/kg/dose PO or sublingually. This dosage may be repeated every 1–2 hr. Watch for arrhythmias or disturbances in serum calcium and magnesium.

E. Careful follow-up is critical to monitor for any complications of prolonged hypertension or its therapy. Resolution of hypertension should be documented as early as possible and careful cessation of pharmacologic agents expedited to minimize side effects.

Suggested Reading

Adelman R: The hypertensive neonate. Clin Perinatol 15:567–585, 1988.

DeSwiet M, Fayers P, Shinebourne EA: Systolic blood pressure in a population of infants in the first year of life: The Brompton Study. Pediatrics 65:1028–1035, 1980.

Flynn JT: Neonatal hypertension: Diagnosis and management. Pediatr Nephrol 14:332–341, 2000.

Gobel MM, Rocchini AP: Neonatal hypertension. In Donn SM, Faix RG (eds): Neonatal Emergencies. Mt. Kisco, NY, Futura Publishing, 1991, pp 387–405.

Hegyi T, Carbone MT, Anwar M, et al: Blood pressure ranges in premature infants: The first hours of life. J Pediatr 127:627–633, 1994.

Perlman JM, Volpe JJ: Neurologic complications of captopril treatment of neonatal hypertension. Pediatrics 83:47–52, 1989.

Rasoulpour M, Marinelli KA: Systemic hypertension. Clin Perinatol 19:121–137, 1992.

Zubrow AB, Hulman S, Kushner H, Falkner B: Determinants of blood pressure in infants admitted to neonatal intensive care units: A prospective multicenter study. Philadelphia Neonatal Blood Pressure Study Group. J Perinatol 15:470–479, 1995.

Chapter 60

Arrhythmias

Charles R. Neal, Jr., M.D., Ph.D.

I. Fetal Arrhythmias

A. Normal fetal heart rates range from 120 to 160 bpm. Heart rates < 100 bpm are considered bradycardia and rates > 180 bpm are considered tachycardia.

1. Fetal arrhythmias may occur at any time during fetal life after the conduction system has developed.
2. Most commonly, they present after 22 weeks of gestation.

B. Complete congenital heart block

1. Ventricular rate ranges from 50 to 100 bpm; atrial rate is around 140 and regular.
2. Complete congenital heart block may be isolated, with no associated congenital heart disease, in which case it is usually associated with maternal connective tissue disorders.
   a. Approximately half of complete heart block cases are associated with maternal anti-Ro or anti-La titers.
      i. These IgG antibodies readily cross placenta.
      ii. They are not specific for the AV node or conducting system, but for cardiac tissue in general.
   b. Intrauterine hydrops is infrequent.
   c. Maternal therapy, which includes plasmapheresis and steroids, has had debatable success.
   d. If no evident fetal distress is detected, and if there is no hydrops, the fetus will tolerate labor well with a fixed HR.
3. Complete congenital heart block may also result from congenital heart disease.
   a. It accounts for 25–33% of cases of heart block.
   b. Hydrops is common in this condition.
   c. Maternal cardiotonic drugs that increase ventricular rate are not effective.
      i. Early delivery should be considered.
      ii. Prognosis is poor.

C. Atrial/junctional tachycardia

1. Untreated fetal SVT has a 12% mortality rate, especially if the arrhythmia is associated with atrial flutter or fibrillation.

2. With ongoing tachycardia, subsequent left ventricular dysfunction leads to increased end-diastolic dimension.
   a. The sequence of events can lead to cardiomyopathy.
   b. Periventricular leukomalacia may follow *in utero* SVT.
3. The treatment of choice is maternal digoxin therapy or other antiarrhythmic medications.
   a. Verapamil use is discouraged.
   b. The success of converting junctional SVT is 88%, versus 66% for atrial flutter.
   c. Consideration of delivery is warranted if the rhythm cannot be converted.
4. Relapse occurs postnatally in 64% of fetal SVT from atrial flutter and 44% in cases of junctional SVT.

II. Neonatal Arrhythmias

A. Consultation with pediatric cardiologists should be considered in all cases.
B. For tachyarrhythmias that are narrow complex:
   1. If possible, examine an ECG during normal sinus rhythm to uncover evidence of preexcitation, such as Wolff-Parkinson-White (WPW) preexcitation syndrome.
   2. An ECG also allows characterization of arrhythmia onset and termination (abrupt versus gradual).
C. Common pathologic neonatal arrhythmias
   1. SVT (includes atrial and junctional rhythms)
      a. This is the most common abnormal arrhythmia in the first year of life.
      b. Presentation can vary from nonimmune hydrops in the fetus or profound cardiovascular collapse in the newborn to poor feeding, tachypnea, or pallor.
      c. The ECG demonstrates a narrow complex QRS with a 1:1 relationship between P and QRS waves during the tachycardia.
      d. Etiologies include WPW (10–20%), congenital heart disease, and idiopathic (approximately 50%).
      e. Types of SVT
         i. Ectopic or nonreciprocating SVT
            (a) Atrial tachycardia has rate variability with warm-up and cool-down features not usually seen in infants. It is most commonly seen after cardiac surgery with

atrial distortion or in myocarditis. The AV node is not involved.

(b) Atrial flutter is diagnosed by the saw-tooth undulation of the ECG baseline from conduction around a reentry circuit within the atria.

(1) Atrial rates can be 300–600 bpm with irregular or regular ventricular rates. An infant may have a 2:1 or 3:1 AV block, or occasionally 1:1 conduction.

(2) Etiologies include CHD with dilated atria, myocarditis, digoxin toxicity, atrial tumors, or a catheter in right atrium.

(3) Therapy includes cardioversion, overdrive, pacing, digoxin, propranolol, and quinidine.

(c) Atrial fibrillation is diagnosed by chaotic low-voltage fibrillatory waves, with an irregularly irregular ventricular response from disordered atrial activity. Therapy is the same as for atrial flutter.

(d) Presence of either atrial flutter or atrial fibrillation usually indicates some significant cardiac pathology.

2. AV reentry or reciprocating SVT
   a. This is the most common mechanism of SVT.
   b. It has an abrupt onset and termination.
   c. 30–40% of these present in the first few weeks of life and are usually not associated with CHD.
   d. The AV node is an essential limb of this circuit.
   e. Mechanisms of AV reentry SVT
      i. With AV reentry tachycardia, the reentry circuit involves both the AV node and an accessory connection between the ventricle and atrium (e.g., WPW), in which accessory pathways "short circuit" the usual delay of ventricular stimulation at the AV node. This leads to a profound premature ventricular depolarization, creating a delta wave on ECG, with a short PR interval and wide QRS.
      ii. With AV nodal reentry tachycardia, there are two limbs of circuit within the AV node.
      iii. In long R-P tachycardia, a reentry circuit utilizes the AV node and a slow conducting pathway. This leads to a frequent start/stop of the arrhythmia during an ECG. Long R-P interval results from the slow conducting path.
   f. Therapy for SVT

    i. Evaluate for hemodynamic instability, which may develop at any point
- (a) Make sure of the diagnosis of SVT.
- (b) Treating the wrong diagnosis with the wrong anti-arrhythmic drug can be dangerous.

   ii. If hemodynamically unstable:
- (a) Vagal maneuvers
  - (1) Ice to face or immersion of face in ice water for 10–20 seconds
  - (2) Do not use ocular compression.
  - (3) Watch ECG and BP during maneuvers.
- (b) Adenosine
  - (1) Slows AV nodal conduction
  - (2) Dose is 50 μg/kg/dose initially.
  - (3) Onset of action is within 10–20 seconds of rapid injection.
  - (4) Double the dose if no response (up to 300 μg/kg/dose). There are no inotropic negative side effects, so it is safe to use adenosine in hemodynamic compromise.
  - (5) Side effects include acute facial flushing, brief hypotension, and severe bronchospasm that can last up to 30 minutes.
  - (6) Adenosine is effective in 86% of junctional tachycardia using accessory conduction—the AV node part of the circuit.
  - (7) This treatment is an important diagnostic aid in differentiating ventricular tachycardia (VT) from true SVT.
    - (aa) Adenosine will terminate the tachycardia if it is from the AV node part of circuit.
    - (bb) Otherwise, an AV block with adenosine will slow an arrhythmia but not terminate it.
  - (8) Tachyarrhythmias may recur in 30% of cases.
  - (9) Infants receiving methylxanthines may require higher doses.
- (c) Overdrive esophageal pacing
  - (1) Pace at a rate slightly greater than the tachycardia.
  - (2) Can be used when the ventricular function is decreased
- (d) Synchronized DC cardioversion

        (1) Dose is 1–2 watts/kg.

        (2) Can also be used when ventricular function is decreased

     (e) Prior to attempting any other antiarrhythmics, consult a pediatric cardiologist.

   iii. Chronic therapy and evaluation

     (a) Digoxin may be used only if WPW is *not* present.

     (b) Propranolol may be used if WPW is present.

     (c) Electrophysiologic study with surgical ablation of accessory pathways is the treatment of choice for arrhythmias difficult to control medically.

  g. Prognosis for SVT is good for those without CHD and presenting in the first month of life. In this population, 60–90% have no further episodes. If concurrent CHD is present, prognosis is guarded.

2. Other arrhythmias

  a. Tachyarrhythmias with a wide QRS complex (> 0.08 sec), such as VT

    i. Defined on ECG by > 3 successive beats of wide QRS, absence of a 1:1 relationship between P and QRS waves, presence of fusion beats (a QRS wave with features of supraventricular impulse and PVC).

     (a) It is important to differentiate this rhythm from SVT with aberrant conduction.

     (b) Measurement of the QT interval is recommended.

    ii. Etiologies tied to VT include hypoxic-ischemic encephalopathy, hypoglycemia, abnormalities in serum Ca^{2+} or K^+, myocarditis, ventricular hypertrophy, presence of a ventricular catheter, acute infant drug intoxication (isoproterenol or dopamine), maternal drug intoxication (cocaine, heroin, meperidine, or mepivacaine), intracardiac tumors (fibromas, rhabdomyomas, hamartomas), and congenital long QT syndromes (sporadic, AR, AD).

    iii. Evaluation includes 24-hour Holter monitoring to quantify the amount of VT, echocardiography to rule out intracardiac pathology, and cardiac catheterization. Biopsy may be necessary to rule out subtle ventricular functional abnormalities.

    iv. Therapy—paroxysmal VT may deteriorate to sustained VT (risk of sudden death).

     (a) For sustained VT, especially if hemodynamically

unstable, treatment of choice is synchronized DC cardioversion.

(1) This should be followed by IV lidocaine or procainamide therapy.

(2) If it is hemodynamically stable, one may treat with IV lidocaine.

(b) For long QT syndrome, use a beta blocker (such as propranolol), phenytoin, or overdrive pacing.

(c) Various other antiarrhythmic agents may be used (consult cardiology) for this arrhythmia, if it remains refractory to conventional drugs.

(d) If all of the above are unsuccessful and VT recurrent and incessant, an electrophysiologic study followed by surgical ablation is indicated.

v. Prognosis

(a) If the VT rate approximates the atrial rate and there is no hemodynamic compromise, prognosis is good and no therapy may be required.

(b) If the infant is symptom-free with isolated, uniform/multiform PVCs or couplets and no CHD, prognosis is good.

(c) If incessant or frequent episodes of paroxysmal VT occur, it is important to rule out intracardiac tumors.

b. Bradyarrhythmias, such as AV block

i. There are three types of AV blocks

(a) 1st and 2nd degree blocks are also known as Mobitz type I and II heart block.

(b) 3rd degree AV block is also referred to as complete heart block (CHB).

ii. Etiologies

(a) Two-thirds of heart block cases occur in the normal heart, with about one-third of cases occurring with minor or major congenital heart disease. The remaining cases are seen with myocarditis, cardiomyopathy, or digoxin toxicity.

(b) Mobitz type II AV block with $\geq$ 2:1 block may progress to CHB.

(c) A strong association exists between several maternal connective-tissue diseases and complete congenital heart block, with SLE much more so than Sjögren's syndrome, rheumatoid arthritis, and dermatomyositis.

       iii. Risk factors for sudden death in complete heart block
          (a) Low resting heart rate (< 55 bpm)
          (b) Onset in infancy
          (c) QT interval prolongation during bradycardia
       iv. Evaluation is via a 24-hour Holter monitor. It is important to monitor heart rate and occurrence of ventricular ectopy.
        v. Indications for treatment include unstable escape rhythm, hemodynamic instability, fetal hydrops, congestive heart failure, ventricular arrhythmia, or failure to thrive.
          (a) Autonomic drugs (atropine or isoproterenol) are used to increase ventricular rate, and result in modest improvement, but may temporize situation.
          (b) Pacing
             (1) Indications include congestive heart failure in an infant with 3rd or 2nd degree AV block, a ventricular rate < 55 bpm with a normal heart, or a heart rate < 65 bpm with congenital heart disease present.
             (2) Temporary pacing is accomplished via transumbilical, transfemoral, or subclavian routes.
             (3) A permanent pacemaker is placed surgically.
       vi. Prognosis is poorest in infants with ventricular rates < 55 bpm, and those who develop hydrops *in utero*.
  c. Irregular rhythms
     i. Premature atrial contractions (PACs)
       (a) On ECG, a premature P wave of unusual contour is evident which may conduct normally, aberrantly with a wide QRS, or not at all, producing a sinus bradycardia. An incomplete compensatory pause follows a PAC.
       (b) Etiologies include atrial enlargement secondary to congenital heart disease or cardiomyopathy, a venous catheter in the right atrium, and toxic levels of sympathomimetic drugs, such as isoproterenol and dopamine. They are also seen as a normal variant.
       (c) Therapy: usually none. If the PACs are frequent, check a CXR and obtain an echocardiogram to rule out congenital heart disease or cardiomyopathy. Observe the infant for 3–4 days and consider a 24-hour Holter monitor. If no SVT or atrial flutter is detected, no therapy is necessary.

      (d) Prognosis: excellent
  ii. Premature ventricular contractions (PVCs)
      (a) On ECG there is no preceding P wave, with a wide QRS earlier than expected.
      (b) Etiologies for PVCs are broad and include congenital heart disease, prolonged Q-T syndrome, hypoxic-ischemic encephalopathy, electrolyte abnormalities (K^+, Ca^{2+}, and glucose), myocarditis, severe ventricular hypertrophy, ventricular tumors, ventricular catheters, drug intoxication with sympathomimetics such as isoproterenol and dopamine, methylxanthines, and digoxin intoxication. This can also be found as a normal variant.
      (c) It is significant if PVCs are multifocal, especially if in couplets. They are precipitated by or increased with activity. They also occur in or result in hemodynamic instability.
      (d) Therapy is not indicated if the PVCs are benign. If they are significant, various antiarrhythmics can be used, including lidocaine, propranolol, quinidine, phenytoin (Dilantin), and procainamide.
 iii. Sinus pause or arrest
      (a) Defined as a momentary cessation in sinoatrial node activity. Sinus arrest, which is of longer duration, usually leads to an escape beat.
      (b) Etiologies include sick sinus syndrome, hypoxia, increased vagal tone, and digoxin toxicity.
      (c) Therapy is rarely necessary unless the cause is digoxin toxicity or sick sinus syndrome.
 iv. Nodal premature or escape beats
      (a) On ECG there is a narrow QRS, with the P wave absent or inverted, falling after the QRS. A compensatory pause may or may not be complete.
      (b) The etiology is usually idiopathic. Nodal premature or escape beats may also follow heart surgery or digoxin toxicity.
      (c) Therapy is not indicated unless the patient has digoxin toxicity.
  v. Atrial fibrillation (discussed above)
 vi. Ventricular fibrillation usually results from a preceding ventricular arrhythmia. It is treated with asynchronous defibrillation (2 J/kg) and CPR.

Suggested Reading

Davis AM, Gow RM, McCrindle BW, Hamilton RM: Clinical spectrum, therapeutic management, and follow-up of ventricular tachycardia in infants and young children. Am Heart J 131:186–191, 1996.

Ralston MA, Knilans TK, Hannon DW, Daniels SR: Use of adenosine for diagnosis and treatment of tachyarrhythmias in pediatric patients. J Pediatr 124:139–143, 1994.

Rosenfeld LE: The diagnosis and management of cardiac arrhythmias in the neonatal period. Semin Perinatol 17:135–148, 1993.

Ross BA: Congenital complete atrioventricular block. Pediatr Clin North Am 37:69–78, 1990.

Tanel RE, Rhodes LA: Fetal and neonatal arrhythmias. Clin Perinatol 28:187–207, 2001.

Till JA, Shinebourne EA: Supraventricular tachycardia: Diagnosis and current acute management. Arch Dis Child 66:647–652, 1991.

Section X.   HEMATOLOGY-ONCOLOGY

Chapter 61

Anemia

Steven W. Pipe, M.D., and Suzanne H. Butch, M.A., M.T.

I.   Definition
   A. Full-term infant: Hgb $<$ 13.5 g/dL
                                   HCT $<$ 42%
   B. Preterm infant: Hgb $<$ 12.0 g/dL
                                   HCT $<$ 38%

II.   Etiology
   A. Hemorrhage
      1. Fetomaternal or twin–twin transfusion
      2. Fetoplacental transfusion, especially with tight nuchal cord
      3. Obstetric bleeding—abruptio placenta, placenta previa, incision of placenta during C-section, rupture of cord, or anomalous vessels
      4. Internal or external fetal or neonatal hemorrhage—subgaleal, adrenal, splenic, hepatic, or intracranial hemorrhage, cephalo-hematoma. *Always consider underlying coagulation disturbance.*
   B. Hemolysis
      1. Immune—Rh or ABO incompatibility, minor blood group incompatibility, maternal autoimmune
      2. Infection, both bacterial and viral
      3. Microangiopathic—DIC, hemangioma, large vessel thrombus, arterial stenosis (renal, coarctation of aorta)
      4. Hemoglobinopathies and thalassemias
      5. Erythrocyte enzyme and membrane defects (e.g., G6PD deficiency, spherocytosis)
   C. Decreased erythrocyte production
      1. Infection—rubella, CMV, parvovirus
      2. Drug effect
      3. Other—osteopetrosis, Down syndrome, Diamond-Blackfan, congenital leukemia

III.   Diagnosis
   A. History—family, maternal, and obstetric
   B. Findings
      1. Examine placenta

    2. Physical examination: trauma, obvious sites of bleeding, hepatosplenomegaly, petechiae/purpura, physical anomalies, stigmata of congenital infection

C. Laboratory (obtain samples prior to transfusion)
1. CBC with smear and RBC indices
2. Reticulocyte count
3. Blood type and direct antiglobulin test
4. Kleihauer-Betke test on maternal blood
5. Extra purple and red top tubes for further studies of immune etiology
6. Coagulation studies, if indicated
7. Blood cultures, if indicated
8. Serial hematocrit determinations

IV. Treatment (Depends on Etiology) (Table 40)

A. Acute hemorrhage
1. Occurrence of hemorrhage and severity may not be reflected by HCT at birth. Signs of asphyxia (such as pallor, hypoperfusion, or respiratory distress) may mask the early signs of hypovolemia, anemia, or shock. Must treat based on the history, laboratory values, and the clinical condition.
2. If the infant is in shock, immediate volume expansion is indicated with albumin, plasma, or saline, followed by blood if indicated.
3. Red blood cells are used routinely. If coagulation factors are needed, use packed red blood cells and fresh frozen plasma. Preparation of "whole blood equivalent" from red blood cells and plasma will take a significant amount of time.
4. Begin with 20 mL/kg over 30–60 min, although if infant's condition is severe, blood may be given at faster rate by a physician. More may be required, but care must be taken to accurately assess the need for further volume support.
5. Most hospitals keep uncrossmatched O-negative red blood cells in the labor and delivery area. In emergencies, this may be used, but should be replaced immediately afterward by notifying the blood bank.

B. Chronic anemia
1. If infant is severely anemic but is hemodynamically well compensated without findings of hypotension, tachycardia, or poor perfusion, packed red cells should be given without delay; however, the amounts given should be in smaller increments (e.g., 2–3 separate transfusions of 10 mL/kg, preferably blood

TABLE 40
Transfusion Therapy Products

Special Requirements Component	Freshest Available	Leukocyte-reduced or CMV seronegative	Lack Sickle Hgb	Irradiated	Volume to Order
Red blood cells (packed cells)	X	X	X	If directed donor from family	Hemorrhage: 20 mL/kg Chronic anemia: multiple transfusions of 10–15 mL/kg
Platelets	X	X		If directed donor from family	10 mL/kg to maintain greater than 50,000
Cryoprecipitated antihemophilic globulin					1 unit
Plasma					10–15 mL/kg to maintain fibrinogen > 100 mg/dL
Whole blood equivalent for exchange transfusion	X	X	X	X	Double volume exchange based on infant's weight (80–85 mL/kg/vol)

of a single donor that has been leukocyte-reduced or has been found to be CMV seronegative). Irradiation of the blood to prevent graft-versus-host disease is not required of most patients.

2. If the infant is hydropic with severe anemia and variable hemodynamic decompensation, the blood should be given without delay in the form of an isovolemic partial exchange transfusion using packed red blood cells. Giving large amounts of blood to a hydropic infant may result in high output congestive heart failure.

V.   Specific Considerations

A. Decisions to treat anemia should be based on etiology, severity, and condition of infant. Thus, a baby who is acutely ill and requiring mechanical ventilation may be transfused when the HCT is 40%, while another infant who is clinically well may not require a transfusion despite a much lower hematocrit. The diagnosis of anemia does not imply definite need for transfusion.

B. The capillary HCT is quite variable. Diagnosis and treatment should be based on venous or arterial samples. These will vary only slightly compared to capillary samples.

C. A "physiologic anemia" occurs in all infants at about 8–12 weeks of age. The Hgb/HCT values tolerated by the infant at this age without difficulty are lower than those on the first day of life. Transfusions should be curtailed accordingly.

Suggested Reading

Avery GB (ed): Neonatology: Pathophysiology and Management of the Newborn, 5th ed. Philadelphia, Lippincott Williams & Wilkins, 1999, pp 1045–1064.

Nathan DG, Orkin SH (ed): Nathan and Oski's Hematology of Infancy and Childhood, 5th ed. Philadelphia, W.B. Saunders, 1998, pp 29–52.

Zak LK, Donn SM: Feto-maternal hemorrhage. In Donn SM, Faix RG (eds): Neonatal Emergencies. Mt. Kisco, NY, Futura Publishing, 1991, pp 423–430.

Chapter 62

Polycythemia

Robert E. Schumacher, M.D.

I. Definition

A. Venous hematocrit > 65%

B. Incidence: 2–5%

C. Site (capillary vs. venous) and timing of sampling (HCT peaks at 2 hr) may affect HCT. Document both where and when the sample was obtained. Do not make a diagnosis based on capillary HCT alone. A venous HCT should be obtained if the capillary HCT is ≥ 65%.

D. *Polycythemia* and *hyperviscosity* are frequently discussed together, but the terms are not interchangeable. Polycythemia refers to increased RBC mass and hyperviscosity refers to abnormal blood flow kinetics with increased resistance to flow. Whole blood viscosity increases linearly with HCT until HCT = 65%, then exponentially. Not all polycythemic newborns, however, are hyperviscous, and, similarly, not all hyperviscous infants are polycythemic. Although there is a direct correlation between hematocrit and viscosity, blood may be hyperviscous because of other factors including increased plasma proteins (fibrinogen) and decreased RBC deformability.

II. Etiology

A. *Increased intrauterine erythropoiesis:* Fetus responds to chronic intrauterine hypoxia by producing additional erythropoietin in an attempt to maintain oxygen delivery. Common examples include IUGR, maternal smoking, preeclampsia, infant of a diabetic mother, high altitude.

B. *Erythrocyte transfusion:* Additional blood volume may result from delayed cord clamping (unattended delivery) or twin-twin transfusion (mono-mono recipient twin). The associated hypervolemia also contributes to signs.

C. Other causes include chromosomal abnormalities (trisomy 13, 18, 21), congenital thyroid disorders, LGA status, and Beckwith-Wiedemann syndrome.

III. Findings

A. Clinical signs resulting from neonatal polycythemia are *associa-*

tions; for the most part, cause and effect relationships have not been proven. Commonly reported signs may be a reflection of the underlying etiology (e.g., chronic hypoxemia, infant of a diabetic mother) and not directly related to the polycythemia. Reported frequencies of symptomatic polycythemia/ hyperviscosity, and long-term complications are variable. Approximately half are asymptomatic.

B. CNS (most commonly reported)
1. Apnea
2. Agitation/lethargy
3. Tremors, jitteriness
4. Stroke
5. Seizures (rare)
6. Long-term follow-up studies have suggested developmental delays and neurologic abnormalities may also be associated with polycythemia or hyperviscosity at birth.

C. Cardiorespiratory
1. Congestive heart failure
2. Increased pulmonary vascular resistance
3. Cyanosis
4. Tachypnea, tachycardia
5. Hypertension

D. Gastrointestinal
1. Poor feeding
2. Gut ischemia. Polycythemia is frequently reported in term infants with NEC; however, this association may be more related to the treatment of polycythemia (exchange transfusion) than to the condition itself.

E. Genitourinary
1. Oliguria (dehydration, ATN)
2. Renal vein thrombosis
3. Priapism
4. Hematuria

F. Laboratory
1. Hypoglycemia (12–40%)
2. Hypocalcemia
3. Hyperbilirubinemia (increased RBC turnover)
4. Thrombocytopenia (20–30%)

IV. Treatment
A. There are no definitive data indicating significant improvement in either short or long-term outcome with treatment, and treatment itself may increase the risk of some reported complications. Deci-

sions to treat must be made on a case-by-case basis in consultation with the attending neonatologist.

B. Correct metabolic abnormalities, hypoxemia, and assure adequate hydration.

C. Partial exchange transfusion with normal saline or 5% albumin to decrease the HCT may be considered for symptomatic newborns and those with HCT > 70%. Fresh frozen plasma is hyperviscous and promotes hypercoagulability; it should *not* be used.

1. Calculate the volume to be exchanged to decrease the venous HCT to an acceptable level (generally 55%) using the following formula:

$$\text{volume} = \frac{\text{baby's blood volume} \times (\text{observed HCT} - \text{desired HCT})}{\text{observed HCT}}$$

Assume newborn blood volume = 85 mL/kg

2. Perform the partial exchange through an umbilical vein catheter in 10–20-mL aliquots. The catheter may be placed either low (4 cm) or at the RA–IVC junction. Assure that it is not wedged in the liver.

3. The total volume of exchange is usually in the range of 50–80 mL. The volume of exchange should be rechecked if it is outside this range.

4. Obtain central HCT after exchange and again 2–4 hours later.

D. In asymptomatic infants with a borderline hematocrit, IV hydration and continued observation alone may be adequate.

Suggested Reading

Oski FA: Polycythemia and hyperviscosity in the neonatal period. In Oski FA, Naiman JL (eds): Hematologic Problems of the Newborn. Philadelphia, W.B. Saunders, 1982, pp 87–96.

Schumacher RE: Neonatal polycythemia/hyperviscosity. In Donn SM, Faix RG (eds): Neonatal Emergencies. Mt. Kisco, NY, Futura Publishing, 1991, pp 447–460.

Werner EJ: Neonatal polycythemia and hyperviscosity. Clin Perinatol 22:693–710, 1995.

Chapter 63

Coagulopathies

Steven W. Pipe, M.D.

I. Differential Diagnosis of Bleeding in the Newborn (Tables 41 and 42)

TABLE 41
Sick-appearing Infants

Lab Studies			
Platelets	PT	PTT	Likely Diagnosis
D	I	I	DIC*
D	N	N	Platelet consumption (autoimmune thrombocytopenia, NEC, sepsis, thrombosis)
N	I	I	Liver disease, serine protease deficiency C
N	N	N	Compromised vascular integrity (e.g., hypoxia, acidosis, hyperosmolality), catastrophic CNS bleed (consider factor XIII deficiency).

D = decreased; I = increased; N = normal; DIC = disseminated intravascular coagulopathy.
*DIC and liver failure may be difficult to distinguish; detection of fibrin split products (FSP), low factor VIII, elevated D-dimer, and a low fibrinogen support a diagnosis of DIC. Adapted from Glader BE, Buchanan GR: Care of the critically ill child: The bleeding neonate. Pediatrics 58:548–555, 1976.

TABLE 42
Healthy-appearing Infants

Lab Studies			
Platelets	PT	PTT	Likely Diagnosis
D	N	N	Alloimmune thrombocytopenia, occult infection, or thrombosis.
N	I	I	Hemorrhagic disease of newborn (vitamin K deficiency)
N	N	I	Hereditary clotting factor deficiency (hemophilia A and B)*
N	N	N	Bleeding secondary to local factors (trauma, some anatomic abnormality). Qualitative platelet defect (rare).

D = decreased; I = increased; N = normal.
*Individual factor assays facilitate diagnosis of hereditary deficiencies.
Adapted from Glader BE, Buchanan GR: Care of the critically ill child: The bleeding neonate. Pediatrics 58:548–555, 1976.

II. Blood Component Therapy
    A. Platelets (*see* Chapter 64)

    B. Fresh frozen plasma

        1. Definition: plasma frozen within 6 hours of collection. Contains normal concentrations of all clotting factors, including V and VIII.

        2. Dose: 10–15 mL/kg as needed to control bleeding

    C. Fresh whole blood

        1. Definition: whole blood less than 24 hours old is not available routinely because of the need for infectious disease testing. As an alternative, freshest available red blood cells reconstituted with fresh frozen plasma may be used.

        2. Use: for exchange transfusion or to replace large volume losses associated with severe hemorrhage

    D. Packed red blood cells

        1. Definition: red blood cells with 80% of the supernatant plasma removed, or red blood cells with the plasma removed and replaced by 100 mL of a preservative solution. This component contains no platelets and limited or no clotting factors.

        2. Use: when the goal of transfusion is increased oxygen-carrying capacity rather than volume expansion

III. Disseminated Intravascular Coagulopathy
    A. Definition: DIC is a pathologic process in which a generalized activation of the hemostatic system occurs, causing diffuse fibrin formation resulting in microthrombosis and consumption of platelets and clotting factors within the vascular system.

    B. Etiology: a number of "trigger mechanisms" have been implicated, such as hypoxia, acidosis, tissue necrosis, infection, and endothelial injury.

    C. Clinical manifestations: infants with DIC are *sick*. Bleeding, thrombosis with necrosis, and organ dysfunction can occur concomitantly.

    D. Diagnosis

        1. Moderate to severe thrombocytopenia

        2. Prolonged PT and PTT (not responsive to vitamin K)

        3. Decreased fibrinogen

        4. Increased fibrin split products

        5. Decreased factor VIII

        6. Increased D-dimer

    E. Treatment

        1. *Treat the underlying disorder*

2. Platelets: 0.2 units/kg as needed to maintain platelet count > 50,000/mm³ and control bleeding
3. Fresh frozen plasma: 10–15 mL/kg as needed to maintain the fibrinogen > 100 mg/dL and control clinical bleeding
4. Maintain adequate hemoglobin level with packed RBC.
5. If infants continue to bleed despite above therapy consider:
   a. Exchange transfusion—provides some clotting factors if blood is fresh, and also removes fibrin degradation products and perhaps some of the "toxic" factors causing DIC. Also improves oxygenation by increased 2,3-DPG, thereby helping to decrease hypoxic tissue injury.
   b. Heparin—should be considered in infants in whom DIC results in thrombosis and potential loss of digits or limbs. The heparin dose should be titrated to the clinical response. A starting infusion of 10–15 units/kg/h is recommended.
   c. The only controlled trial of DIC treatment in newborns (Gross SJ et al., 1982) concluded that outcome was dependent on success of treating underlying process and aggressive supportive care, but was not altered by therapy specifically directed at the coagulopathy.

IV. Liver Disease

A. May result in inadequate factor production
B. Treat underlying liver disease.
C. Provide appropriate replacement therapy.

V. Factor Deficiency

Clotting factor concentrates—used only for treating specific factor deficiencies, e.g., hemophilia A (VIII), hemophilia B (IX). Use fresh frozen plasma for factor XIII deficiency.

VI. Hemorrhagic Disease of the Newborn

A. Definition: coagulopathy secondary to lack of vitamin K, seen especially in premature infants. Results in marked deficiency of factors II, VII, IX, and X. Other risk factors: lack of vitamin K prophylaxis, breastfeeding, GI disease, use of broad-spectrum antibiotics.
B. Clinical manifestations
   1. Early—occurs within first 24 hrs of life, presents with cephalohematoma or serious internal hemorrhage (intracranial, intrathoracic, intra-abdominal), associated with infants of mothers treated with vitamin K antagonists (e.g., coumarin, hydantoins, phenobarbital)

2. Classic—occurs between days 1 and 7, presents with cutaneous, circumcision, umbilical, or GI bleeding

3. Late—occurs after the first week of life, presents with intracranial, cutaneous, or gastrointestinal bleeding; most typically seen in breastfed infants and aggravated by antibiotics; can occur in infants receiving intravenous alimentation if vitamin K supplements are not added. Infants appear healthy unless massive hemorrhage and shock occur. (Consider differential of other factor deficiency, e.g., VIII, IX, XIII.)

C. Treatment—vitamin K_1, 1.0 mg IM. Response to therapy is heralded by a dramatic cessation of bleeding and correction of laboratory abnormalities in 4–6 hours.

VI. Purpura Fulminans

A. Definition: a unique clinical presentation of extensive thrombosis of the dermis and subdermis occurring within 24 hours of birth. Associated with homozygous protein C or S deficiency and severe sepsis.

B. Clinical manifestations: if untreated, the newborn will develop extensive skin, retinal vessel, CNS, gastric, and renal thromboses.

C. Laboratory: often seen with a prolonged PT, PTT, elevated FSPs but a normal platelet count. Protein C and S antigen and activity assays should be performed based on clinical suspicion prior to transfusion.

D. Treatment: fresh frozen plasma 10 mL/kg every 8 hr until diagnosis established.

Suggested Reading

Goodnight SH, Hathaway WE (eds): Disorders of Hemostasis and Thrombosis. New York, McGraw-Hill, 2001.

Gross SJ, Filston HC, Anderson JC: Controlled study of treatment for disseminated intravascular coagulation in the neonate. J Pediatr 100:445–448, 1982.

McMillan DD: Approach to the bleeding newborn. Paediatr Child Health 3:399–401, 1998.

Nathan DG, Orkin SH (eds): Nathan and Oski's Hematology of Infancy and Childhood, 5th ed. Philadelphia, W.B. Saunders, 1998, pp 123–142.

Chapter 64

Thrombocytopenia

Steven W. Pipe, M.D.

I. Definition
A. Normal (term or preterm): 150,000–450,000/mm^3
B. Abnormal: < 150,000/mm^3

II. Etiology
Underproduction, increased destruction, or sequestration are causes.
A. Most newborns who develop thrombocytopenia are ill, premature, and have other problems that contribute to the thrombocytopenia, such as DIC or sepsis.
B. The frequency of thrombocytopenia in "sick" infants is 15%, with the lowest counts occurring several days after delivery.
C. Severe thrombocytopenia (platelet count < 20,000) is uncommon, occurring in < 0.5% of all newborns.
D. Disorders causing thrombocytopenia in mothers (idiopathic thrombocytopenic pupura [ITP], systemic lupus erythematosus [SLE], hypertension, incidental thrombocytopenia) rarely cause moderate to severe fetal or neonatal thrombocytopenia.
E. The group at highest risk for severe thrombocytopenia and increased morbidity is newborns with alloimmune antiplatelet antibodies.

III. Increased Destruction
A. Alloimmune thrombocytopenia
1. Incidence: 1 in 2000–5000 pregnancies
2. Alloantibodies are formed as a consequence of maternal immunization to a foreign platelet antigen.
3. Unlike Rh disease, first pregnancies are often affected.
4. Risk in subsequent pregnancies is 75–90%, with thrombocytopenia usually more severe than in the first affected child.
5. 25–50% of intracranial hemorrhages occur antenally between 32 and 36 weeks' gestation.
6. Most commonly associated with PL^{A1} (HPA-1a) antigen (2% of Caucasian women are PL^{A1} negative)
7. Clinical presentation: healthy, full-term infant with severe thrombocytopenia < 20,000/mm^3, petechiae, and purpura
8. Diagnosis is confirmed by solid phase, ELISA, MAIPA, flow

cytometry, or PCR. Contact the laboratory for specimen requirements and test details.

9. Platelet therapy: a standard volume order per kilogram, such as 10 mL/kg, is sufficient to increase the platelet count to $> 50,000/mm^3$. A unit of platelets has a volume varying from 45 to 65 mL.

10. Observe for associated hypoglycemia.

B. Autoimmune thrombocytopenia
  1. Associated with maternal autoimmune diseases such as ITP, SLE
  2. IgG antibody with passive placental transfer
  3. *Not* associated with severe neonatal thrombocytopenia
  4. Rarely a cause of neonatal morbidity

C. Other causes associated with increased destruction
  1. Exchange transfusion
  2. Polycythemia
  3. Thrombosis
  4. Infection, bacterial or viral, often in association with DIC
  5. Erythroblastosis

IV. Sequestration

A. Splenic—secondary to viral/bacterial infection

B. Hemangioma (e.g., Kasabach-Merritt) associated with disseminated intravascular coagulopathy (DIC)

V. Production Defects

A. Associated with congenital syndromes (e.g., thrombocytopenia-absent radii, Fanconi's anemia, megakaryocytic thrombocytopenia)

B. Associated with cytogenetic abnormalities (e.g., trisomy 21, trisomy 13, trisomy 18)

C. Congenital leukemia

D. Metastatic marrow disease (e.g., neuroblastoma)

VI. Investigations

These should be tailored to severity of thrombocytopenia and clinical state of newborn.

A. Mild ($> 50,000/mm^3$) in clinically healthy newborn—monitor for recovery

B. Moderate–severe ($< 50,000/mm^3$)
  1. Maternal history/platelet count
  2. Review of drug exposure
  3. Thorough physical exam
  4. Serial platelet counts

5. If clinically indicated:
   a. Sepsis work-up
   b. Platelet typing for alloimmune disease
   c. DIC screen in sick newborn

VII. Treatment: Specific for Underlying Cause

A. Increased destruction
   1. Immune-mediated
      a. Maternal washed irradiated platelets for alloimmune thrombocytopenia
      b. IV IgG
      c. Steroids—controversial
   2. DIC
      a. Treat underlying cause
      b. Transfuse platelets for platelet count $< 50,000/\text{mm}^3$ (0.2 units/kg)
      c. Transfuse fresh frozen plasma to maintain fibrinogen > 100 mg/dL

B. Production defect—platelet transfusions to maintain count $> 50,000/\text{mm}^3$

Suggested Reading

Andrew M, Castle VP, Saigal S, et al: Clinical impact of neonatal thrombocytopenia. J Pediatr 110:457–464, 1987.

Burrows RF, Kelton JG: Fetal thrombocytopenia and its relation to maternal thrombocytopenia. N Engl J Med 329:1463–1466, 1993.

Bussel J, Kaplan C, McFarland J: Recommendations for the evaluation and treatment of neonatal autoimmune and alloimmune thrombocytopenia. The Working Party on Neonatal Immune Thrombocytopenia of the Neonatal Hemostasis Subcommittee of the Scientific and Standardization Committee of the ISH (International Society on Thrombosis and Haemostasis). Thromb Haemost 65:631–634, 1991.

Nathan DG, Orkin SH (eds): Nathan and Oski's Hematology of Infancy and Childhood, 5th ed. Philadelphia, W.B. Saunders, 1998, pp 124–127, 1601–1605.

Chapter 65

Neonatal Thrombosis

Steven W. Pipe, M.D

I. Incidence of Thrombosis

2.4/1000 newborn admissions to NICUs; half are arterial and half are
venous thromboembolism

A. Arterial thromboses

With few exceptions, these are iatrogenic complications, occurring
secondary to arterial catheters.

1. Femoral artery—thrombosis complicating femoral arterial
catheterization occurs in 8% of newborns under 10 kg. Half resolve spontaneously.

2. Umbilical arterial catheterization results in severe symptomatic
vessel obstruction in 1–5% of infants studied. Between 9% and
28% of cases had postmortem evidence of catheter-related
thrombosis. Thirty percent may be clinically silent or associated only with hypertension. Minor thromboses resolve without
therapy. Moderate thromboses resolve with a variety of therapies. Infants with UAC thrombi associated with multiorgan
dysfunction usually die irrespective of therapy.

B. Venous thromboses

1. Central venous line–related. IVC and SVC thromboses are
most commonly associated with indwelling central venous lines
including Broviac and UVC. Forty percent of DVT in children
and 80% in newborns occur in the upper venous system secondary to central catheters. DVT is estimated to complicate 1%
of catheters used for TPN when diagnosed clinically, 35%
when diagnosed by echocardiography, and 75% when diagnosed by venography.

2. Renal vein thrombosis is most prevalent in newborns (65% of
all RVT). Associated with perinatal asphyxia, shock, polycythemia, congenital heart disease, maternal diabetes, dehydration, and sepsis. Present with flank mass, hematuria, proteinuria, and thrombocytopenia.

C. Other sites

Additional sites for thrombotic disease in newborns include pros-
thetic valves, intracardiac patches, and shunts (B-T).

II.   Why Newborns Are at Risk for Thromboembolic Disease

A. Virchow's triad

1. **Abnormalities in blood vessels.** Intravascular catheters, hypertonic solutions, sepsis, and shock all lead to damage of the endothelial wall exposing thrombogenic substances.

2. **Disturbances in blood flow.** Catheters and intracardiac hardware may result in slow or turbulent flow. Increased viscosity secondary to polycythemia, dehydration, or the increased RBC diameter of newborns may lead to sluggish flow. Previously described risks for IDM may be related to their risk of polycythemia. Hypotension and shock may result in poor peripheral perfusion with sluggish flow.

3. **Abnormalities in coagulation**

   a. The newborn's coagulation, anticoagulation, and fibrinolytic systems are qualitatively and quantitatively different from adults, slightly favoring thrombosis.

   b. Vitamin K–dependent factors (II, VII, IX, X) are decreased to 30–50% of normal adult levels in a gestational age–dependent fashion. This is largely balanced by a similar decrease in protein C and antithrombin III. Although an intrinsic defect in neonatal platelets limits degranulation, enhanced vWF activity and larger RBC size lead to normal platelet plug formation.

   c. Newborns have a hypofibrinolytic state. Despite increased concentrations of TPA, newborns have decreased plasma levels and activity of plasminogen and increased concentration of plasminogen activator inhibitors (PAI).

   d. Congenital prothrombotic risk factors include heterozygous deficiencies of proteins C and S and antithrombin III deficiency, prothrombin G20210A, and factor V Leiden (activated protein C resistance) mutations.

   e. Inherited defects (homozygous protein C deficiency, homozygous protein S deficiency, and antithrombin III deficiency) may result in purpura fulminans.

III.   Anticoagulation Therapy

A. Heparin

1. Mechanism of action—unfractionated heparin (average molecular weight 15,000 kDa, mean of 45 saccharide units) binds to antithrombin III, causing a conformational change that makes antithrombin III a potent inhibitor of thrombin and factor Xa.

2. Dosing
   a. Loading dose: 75 U/kg IV over 10 min
   b. Maintenance dose: 28 U/kg/h
3. Monitoring
   a. Obtain CBC, PT, and aPTT prior to initiation of therapy. Draw blood for prothrombotic work-up if indicated.
   b. Obtain a PTT 4 hrs after loading dose and adjust heparin rate to keep aPTT at 60–85 sec (approx. 2 × institutional normal for aPTT).
   c. Monitor platelet counts regularly to monitor for heparin-induced thrombocytopenia.
   d. Avoid IM injections and use prolonged external pressure if arterial punctures are required.
   e. The requirement for excessive doses of heparin to achieve a therapeutic level is most likely the result of binding of heparin to other plasma proteins that neutralize its function and the appearance of heparin resistance.
4. Reversal
   a. Termination of the heparin infusion is usually sufficient from rapid clearance.
   b. If immediate reversal is required, protamine sulfate can be administered at a concentration of 10 mg/mL at a rate not to exceed 5 mg/min. Dose is 1 mg of protamine for every 100 mg of heparin received in the preceding 30 minutes. Neutralization occurs in 5 minutes.

B. Low–molecular-weight heparin (LMWH)
1. Mechanism of action
   a. Prepared from unfractionated heparin to yield fractions with molecular weights of 5,000 kDa and mean of 15 saccharide units. Inhibition of thrombin requires that heparins bind to both antithrombin III *and* thrombin whereas inhibition of factor Xa requires that heparins bind only to antithrombin III. Because of the smaller size, LMWHs cannot bind to both thrombin and antithrombin III and thus preferentially inhibit only factor Xa.
   b. Should be considered for newborns because of reduced risk for hemorrhage, no need for venous access, and reduced monitoring requirements
2. Dosage
   a. Therapeutic: 1.5 mg/kg/dose every 12 hr SC
   b. Prophylactic: 0.75 mg/kg/dose every 12 hr SC
3. Monitoring

    a. Because LMWHs do not inhibit thrombin, the aPTT is not useful for monitoring

    b. An anti-Xa level should be obtained 4 hrs following the second dose and adjusted to a range of:
Therapeutic: 0.5–1.0 U/mL anti-Xa activity
Prophylactic: 0.1–0.3 U/mL anti-Xa activity

    c. Response to LMWHs is more predictable and less affected by other concurrent therapies than unfractionated heparin. Thus, after targeting a therapeutic level, anti-Xa levels need be followed only weekly.

    d. Heparin-induced thrombocytopenia is rarely from LMWHs.

    e. Avoid IM injections and use prolonged external pressure if arterial punctures are required.

  4. Reversal

    a. Termination of the LMWH injections is usually sufficient. A 12–24-hour window from termination will allow proceeding with surgical procedures.

    b. If immediate reversal is required, 1 mg of protamine sulfate IV over 10 minutes will reverse 100 units (1 mg) of LMWH given in the preceding 3–4 hours.

C. Coumadin (warfarin)

  1. Mechanism of action—competitively interferes with vitamin K metabolism resulting in a reduction of vitamin K–dependent coagulation proteins (factors II, VII, IX, X, protein C, and protein S) in the plasma.

  2. Dosing—Coumadin binds to many plasma proteins, it is subject to a host of drug interactions, and there is considerable variation in patient response. Loading dose is 0.2 mg/kg PO as a single daily dose and subsequent daily doses adjusted according to the INR response but on average are approximately 0.1 mg/kg/d. Initiation of coumadinization should be done in conjunction with the institutional anticoagulation service if available.

  3. Monitoring

    a. Obtain PT/INR, aPTT, and liver function tests prior to initiating therapy.

    b. Target ranges vary according to indication but are typically an INR of 2.0–3.0 for the vast majority of patients.

    c. INR should be monitored daily until stable for at least 2 consecutive days then can be done less frequently. INR should be repeated with any change in the infant's clinical status, change in dose, or change in other medications.

    d. Since Coumadin interferes competitively with vitamin K

metabolism, vitamin K in the diet or via parenteral nutrition should be minimized and consistent. Breastfed infants can be supplemented with a small amount of formula (~120 mL) to ensure a consistent vitamin K intake of 1 μg/kg/d.

4. Reversal—guidelines for reversal are dependent on the presence or absence of bleeding and the need for urgent traumatic intervention (e.g., surgery). Vitamin K can be administered 0.5–2 mg SC or IV (not IM) and results in reversal over several hours. If immediate reversal is necessary, 5 mg of vitamin K can be administered IV over 10–20 minutes plus fresh frozen plasma, 20 mL/kg.

IV. Thrombolytic Therapy

A. Plasminogen is a serine protease produced in the liver in an inactive form that is hydrolyzed by activators to a two-chain active protein ("plasmin"). Its primary target is fibrin, but any compound with an available Lys-Arg site can be cleaved, including fibrinogen, factor V, factor VIII, vWF, and platelet glycoprotein 1b.

B. The primary endogenous activators of plasminogen are TPA and urokinase. The primary regulator is α_2-antiplasmin, which blocks plasmin's serine protease active site. *When plasmin is bound to fibrin, however, it cannot be inactivated by α_2-antiplasmin.* There are also two antiactivators called PAI-1 and PAI-2, which inhibit TPA and urokinase. Protein C, on the other hand, inhibits the inhibitors.

C. Plasminogen activators (Table 43)

TABLE 43
Comparison of Thrombolytic Agents

	Streptokinase	Urokinase	TPA
Half-life (plasma)	18–30 min	12 min	4–5 min
Half-life (lytic effects)	82–184 min	61 min	46 min
Fibrin specificity	Minimal	Minimal	Moderate
Antigenicity	Yes	No	No
Load	2000 U/kg	4400 U/kg	
Maintenance	2000 U/kg/h	4400 U/kg/h	0.2–0.5 mg/kg/h*

*Adjust dose for preterm infants.

1. Streptokinase (SK)
   Produced by β-hemolytic streptococci (Lancefield group C), it has a unique mechanism of action. SK forms an equimolar SK-plasminogen complex, which then activates free and fibrin-

bound plasminogen. Decreased plasminogen, as seen in newborns, is a disadvantage. It is the most potent activator known. There is no fibrin specificity and free fibrinogen, factor V, and factor VIII degradation occur. SK is a bacterial product with significant antigenicity resulting in allergic symptoms in 5% of those treated. Its efficacy may be limited by antibody titers to streptococcal antigens. SK has a long half-life (18–30 min plasma half-life but a half-life of lytic effects of 82–184 min) and is removed by immunologic means and the reticuloendothelial system. It is the cheapest. *It is generally not recommended for newborns.*

2. Urokinase (UK)

This is an endogenous enzyme made by renal parenchymal cells. It directly activates plasminogen. Like SK, it has no fibrin-binding domain and, therefore, can lead to systemic fibrinolysis. There are no antigenic or allergic side effects and its half-life is intermediate (12 min in plasma and 61 min for lytic effects). Its effectiveness is still theoretically limited in newborns because of their overall physiologically decreased capacity to generate plasmin.

3. Tissue plasminogen activator (TPA)

Isolated first from human melanoma cells, TPA is now produced by recombinant methods. It is a serine protease endogenously synthesized by endothelial cells and can be activated by plasmin, kallikrein, and factor Xa. There is a fibrin-binding "finger" that allows it "fibrin specificity." TPA is a poor activator of free plasminogen, but is markedly improved (several hundred fold) when bound to plasmin. α_2-Antiplasmin activity does not limit its efficacy. It has a short half-life (4–5 min in plasma and 46 min for lytic effects), no allergic/antigenic effects, but a very high cost. Adult studies have largely failed to show any improved efficacy or safety of TPA over UK following myocardial infarction.

V. TPA for Neonatal Arterial Thrombosis

A. Treatment for neonatal thrombosis is still controversial with little thrombolytic experience. Guidelines are available, but randomized trials are lacking.

B. Literature review of small series and single case reports (Hartmann et al., 2001).

1. Overall patency rate of 94% (79% complete clot dissolution and 14% partial clot dissolution). Higher patency rate with

higher dose regimens (0.1–1 mg/kg/h) versus low-dose regimens (0.02–0.08 mg/kg/h)

2. Most reports describe no bleeding complications or minor bleeding confined to local puncture sites.

3. Reports on major complications differ but overall severe bleeding and particularly intracerebral hemorrhage (ICH) are more common with increasing prematurity. A recent review found that according to the age when thrombolytic therapy was performed, ICH was described in 2/468 children after the neonatal period, in 1/83 term infants; and in 11/86 preterm infants; 10/40 preterm infants who were treated in the first week of life developed ICH (Zenz et al., 1997).

VI. TPA for Neonatal Arterial Thromboses: University of Michigan Experience

A. From 1993 to 1995, 7 newborns were treated for arterial thromboses. Thromboses were documented by Doppler USN in 6/7 and by clinical exam alone in 1. Infants were both term (2/7) and preterm (5/7, 24–36 weeks' GA). The median birthweight was 2400 g (range 543–3289). Treatment occurred between days of life 1 and 33; 6/7 were ≤ 96 hours of age at the time of treatment.

B. The location of the thrombi included: aorta (2), iliac artery (2), femoral artery (1), axillary artery (1), and palmar digital artery (1).

C. Umbilical artery catheterization was associated with only 2/7 and only 1/2 aortic clots. Systemic *Candida* infection was an additional risk factor for the only aortic clot with a UAC in place. Only 1/3 iliac or femoral clots were associated with intravascular catheters. *All three with lower extremity (iliofemoral) thromboses were delivered by cesarean section from breech presentation.* The axillary clot was associated with an ipsilateral brachial plexopathy following a C-section delivery from vertex presentation. In three patients, no risk factor for thrombosis was identified. No patient was polycythemic, and none was born to a diabetic mother.

D. All received rTPA (alteplase) by continuous IV infusion (6/7 PIV, 1/7 Broviac) at a median dose of 0.4 mg/kg/h (range 0.1–0.5 mg/kg/h) for a median duration of 26 hours (range 6–38 hours). Two had received an initial bolus of 0.5 mg/kg. All were receiving concurrent heparin at low doses (0.4–5 U/kg/h) to maintain patency of various lines.

E. Clot resolution was "complete" in 4/7 (57%) and partial in 2/7(28%). One patient with multiple thrombi failed therapy. Two patients in the "complete" group, however, had only minimal or partial lysis at the completion of 38–39 hours of TPA infusion but demonstrated complete lysis by follow-up Doppler USN 4–8 weeks later. The other two complete and one partial responders demonstrated marked improvement in physical findings (pulse/perfusion) within 5 hours of treatment.

F. Complications included oozing from puncture sites (4/7), hematuria (2/7), pulmonary hemorrhage (1/7), and intraventricular hemorrhage (2/7; 1 grade II, 1 grade IV). The most serious bleeding, including both cases of IVH and the case of pulmonary hemorrhage, was seen in the two who received high-dose (0.5 mg/kg/hr) TPA. Both died, and in one the death was in part attributed to bleeding complications associated with TPA.

G. Fibrinogen levels were obtained before and during treatment in 6/7; one patient had no pretreatment level. All demonstrated a modest decrease in fibrinogen (mean 14%) with the initiation of fibrinolytic therapy. Unlike those without significant bleeding complications, both patients with IVH continued to demonstrate declining fibrinogen throughout treatment. Those with IVH ultimately had the lowest absolute fibrinogen levels during treatment (127 mg/dL, 114 mg/dL) as well as the greatest decline in fibrinogen during treatment (26%, 36%). Platelet count, PT, and aPTT were not helpful in identifying bleeding risk.

H. Conclusion: TPA can be used to successfully treat central and peripheral neonatal arterial thromboses. However, both minor and major bleeding complications are seen. Avoiding high-dose infusions (0.5 mg/kg/hr) and closely monitoring the trend in fibrinogen may improve safety.

I. Additional considerations
   1. TPA should be considered initially for *all* arterial thrombi.
   2. Concurrent heparin therapy is recommended for all thrombolytic agents. Do *not* bolus. Infuse at 20 U/kg and maintain PTT at 1.5–2 × control (55–85 sec).

J. Absolute contraindications for thrombolytic therapy:
   1. Active bleeding
   2. Significant potential for local bleeding (e.g., general surgery within previous 10 days; neurosurgery within the previous 3 weeks)

K. Baseline investigations
   1. CBC with platelet count
   2. PT, PTT, fibrinogen
   3. Type and crossmatch

L. Monitoring

    1. Response to thrombolytic therapy is monitored by PT, PTT, and fibrinogen level every 2 hours during infusion and every 4 hours for 12 hours following infusion.

    2. Reevaluate clinical exam and radiographic studies after 5 hours. If no improvement, consider additional course or alternative therapy.

    3. Maintain the fibrinogen > 150 mg/dL. Expect a decrease of 20–50% from baseline. Treat low fibrinogen with cryoprecipitate, 1 unit/5 kg.

    4. Maintain the platelet count > 100,000/mm^3.

M. Complications of therapy

    1. Bleeding

       a. Usually oozing from wounds or puncture sites.

       b. If severe, stop infusion and administer cryoprecipitate, 1 unit/5 kg.

    2. Anaphylaxis

       a. Can occur in 1–2% of patients receiving SK

       b. Treat temperature evaluations with acetaminophen (10–15 mg/kg) and corticosteroid/antihistamines for severe reactions.

Suggested Reading

Andrew M, Monagle PT, Brooker (eds): Thromboembolic Complications during Infancy and Childhood. Hamilton, Ontario, Decker, 2000, pp 277–384.

Hartmann J, Hussein A, Trowitzsch E, et al: Treatment of neonatal thrombus formation with recombinant tissue plasminogen activator: Six years' experience and review of the literature. Arch Dis Child Fetal Neonatal Ed 85:F18–F22, 2001.

Michelson AD, Bovill E, Monagle P, Andrew M: Antithrombotic therapy in children. Chest 114:748S–769S, 1998.

Nowak-Gottl U, Kosch A, Schlegel N: Thromboembolism in newborns, infants and children. Thromb Haemost 86:464–474, 2001.

Schmidt B, Andrew M: Report of Scientific and Standardization Subcommittee on Neonatal Hemostasis Diagnosis and Treatment of Neonatal Thrombosis. Thromb Haemost 67:381–382, 1992.

Zenz W, Arlt F, Sodia S, Berghold A: Intracerebral hemorrhage during fibrinolytic therapy in children: A review of the literature of the last thirty years. Semin Thromb Hemost 23:321–332, 1997.

Chapter 66

Neonatal Neoplasms

Steven W. Pipe, M.D.

I. Incidence

A. Overall, neonatal tumors are rare. About 2.5% of all pediatric neoplasms (benign and malignant) present at the time of birth or within the first month of life. About 42% of those are malignant.

B. The types, incidence, clinical features, and behavior of neoplasms occurring in the newborn are different from those seen in older children and adolescents. In addition, their response to therapy is dissimilar.

C. Most common types of congenital/neonatal tumors (benign and malignant)

1. Teratomas (37.7%)
2. Soft tissue tumors (20.5%)
3. Neuroblastoma (13.9%)
4. Leukemia (10.7%)
5. Brain tumors (4.1%)
6. Mesoblastic nephroma (3.3%)

D. With respect to malignant tumors alone, neuroblastoma is the most frequently seen (33.3%), followed by acute leukemia (25.5%), sarcoma (15.7%), and Wilms' tumor and retinoblastoma (5.9% each).

II. Most Commonly Encountered Neonatal and Congenital Neoplasms

A. Teratomas

1. Definition
   a. Embryonal neoplasms consisting of tissues foreign to the area in which it arises and containing representative tissues from all three main germ cell layers (ectoderm, mesoderm, and endoderm)
   b. Teratomas may be mature (always benign) or immature (with or without malignant germ cell elements).
2. Incidence—the most common solid tumors of the neonatal period
3. Presentation
   a. Teratomas may cause complications during pregnancy (e.g., polyhydramnios, protracted labor).

    b. At the time of delivery, teratomas may present as a mass; the most common sites of occurrence are:
      i. Sacrococcygeal region (80%), head (intracranial and extracranial), and neck (10%)
      ii. Additional sites—mediastinum, retroperitoneum
    c. Sacral teratomas should be suspected if there is variation in the size of the buttocks or perianal area.
4. Diagnosis
    a. Early diagnosis is important, because teratomas may undergo malignant degeneration rapidly (within a few weeks to 6 months). In newborns, 5–10% of seemingly benign teratomas have malignant areas.
    b. Lateral abdominal and pelvic radiographs may show anterior displacement of the rectum and calcification in sacral teratomas.
    c. The differential diagnosis of sacral teratomas should include myelomeningoceles, pilonidal cysts, hemangiomas, and chordomas.
5. Therapy and prognosis
    a. Surgical excision is the major therapeutic modality.
    b. Malignant teratomas do not respond well to radiation therapy; chemotherapy may be helpful.
    c. Prognosis is excellent for teratomas diagnosed and treated (excised) in the first 2–4 months of life.
    d. Poor prognostic factors include malignant histology and unresectable tumors.

B. Soft tissue tumors
1. Definition
    a. Tumors that arise from muscle, connective tissue, supportive tissue, and vascular tissue. The majority (85%) are benign.
    b. Examples of malignant soft tissue tumors include fibrosarcoma, hemangiopericytoma, liposarcoma, and rhabdomyosarcoma.
    c. Malignant soft tissue tumors are highly invasive locally and have a high propensity for local recurrence.
2. Presentation
Soft tissue tumors present as masses in various locations—extremities, trunk, neck, face, retroperitoneal, abdominal, and pelvic areas.
3. Diagnosis requires biopsy.
4. Therapy and prognosis
    a. Therapy consists of surgical excision with or without

        chemotherapy (depending on the histology), or radiation therapy.

    b. Prognosis may be excellent in infants with excision alone.

C. Neuroblastoma

   1. Definition—a tumor that arises from neural crest tissue; therefore, it can occur anywhere along the sympathetic chain.

   2. Incidence

    a. The most common malignant tumor noted at birth and in infancy

    b. It is believed that a number of occult neuroblastomas can occur that are never diagnosed and that regress spontaneously.

   3. Presentation

    a. Usually, neuroblastoma presents as an abdominal mass from an adrenal-retroperitoneal tumor, or hepatomegaly secondary to multiple liver metastases.

    b. Unusual presentations include hydrops fetalis (secondary to placental metastases), paralysis, neurogenic bladder, cardiomegaly, hypoglycemia, bone marrow suppression, massive adrenal hemorrhage into tumor, multiple bluish subcutaneous nodules (cutaneous metastases), congenital Horner's syndrome, or diagnosed from a prenatal ultrasound.

    c. The primary site of involvement is the adrenal gland (70%). Ten percent of tumors arise in the posterior mediastinum, and 20% occur in the neck.

    d. Stage IV-S patients have a unique presentation with a small localized primary tumor that does not cross the midline and have evidence of spread to distant sites that include liver, skin and/or bone marrow. There are no bony metastases. They have an excellent prognosis (overall survival > 75%).

   4. Diagnosis

    a. Obtain 24-hour urine for quantitative catecholamine assay (metanephrine, normetanephrine, homovanillic acid [HVA], vanillylmandelic acid [VMA]).

    b. Urine catecholamines are positive in 95% of neuroblastomas if all metabolites are assayed.

    c. Abdominal radiographs may reveal intra-abdominal calcifications.

    d. The extent of tumor growth or metastases is evaluated with skeletal films, bone scans, bone marrow aspirate and biopsy, CT scan, MRI, and abdominal sonography. Staging of the tumor is based on the results of these studies and the pathologic

assessment of the tumor tissue including assessment of
N-myc DNA amplification.

5. Therapy and prognosis
    a. Spontaneous regression of clinically apparent neuroblastoma occurs, especially in patients < 1 year of age with stage I or IV-S disease.
    b. Complete surgical removal of the primary tumor in stage I and II disease is curative in the majority of patients.
    c. The worst prognosis is in patients with stage IV disease. They require multiagent chemotherapy and radiation treatment.
    d. Stage IV-S patients with massively enlarged livers are at risk for respiratory compromise—a short course of low-dose cyclophosphamide or low-dose radiation can induce a remission.

D. Leukemia
1. Definition
    a. Proliferation of hematopoietic blasts with infiltration of non-hematopoietic organs and resultant bone marrow failure.
    b. More than 80% of neonatal leukemias are acute myelogenous leukemia (AML).
    c. AML and acute lymphoblastic leukemia (ALL) have been associated with Down syndrome. However, the leukemic findings seen in some children with Down syndrome undergo spontaneous remission in later weeks or months and have been termed the *transient myeloproliferative disorder* (or leukemoid reaction) *of Down syndrome*. Congenital leukemia must still be excluded in these patients.
    d. Congenital leukemia has been associated with other syndromes as well (e.g., Turner's syndrome, trisomy 13, Klippel-Feil sequence, Ellis–van Creveld syndrome).

2. Presentation
    a. Cutaneous involvement (leukemia cutis) in the form of palpable maroon or bluish gray nodules is common in newborns. This is never seen in patients with a leukemoid reaction and can be used as a distinguishing clinical finding. Leukemia cutis may antedate identifiable bone marrow involvement.
    b. Other presenting signs include pallor, petechiae, ecchymoses, hepatosplenomegaly, lethargy, and respiratory distress; lymphadenopathy and anemia may not be seen at initial presentation.

3. Diagnosis
    a. Diagnosis may be especially difficult in the newborn because

of the variety of disorders that can lead to leukoerythroblastic (leukemoid) reactions in which immature cells are released into the peripheral blood.

   b. The differential diagnosis for congenital leukemia includes viral and bacterial infections, hypoxemia, and severe hemolysis, all of which can cause a leukemia-like picture.

   c. Three criteria are necessary for the diagnosis of congenital leukemia

      i. Proliferation of immature cells of myeloid or lymphoid series

      ii. Infiltration of these cells into nonhematopoietic tissues

      iii. Absence of any other disease which might result in diagnostic confusion (*see* 3b, above)

4. Therapy and prognosis

   a. Congenital leukemia is usually rapidly fatal secondary to overwhelming sepsis or bleeding. Even with chemotherapy the prognosis is dismal.

   b. Chromosomal abnormalities within the blast cell is a particularly ominous sign that the leukemic findings will progress to leukemia.

   c. Leukophoresis or exchange transfusion may be indicated for WBC $> 100,000/mm^3$ if accompanied by signs of hyperviscosity.

   d. Infants should be placed on a national treatment study protocol, because durable remissions have been achieved with high-intensity multiagent chemotherapeutic regimens.

   e. A major difficulty in treating young infants with chemotherapy is the high toxicity of most agents. Substantial morbidity to growth, nutrition, and the CNS is seen.

E. Renal tumors/Wilms' tumor

1. Incidence

   a. Even though renal tumors per se are rare in the neonatal period, non-neoplastic renal masses are not uncommon (e.g., hydronephrosis, cystic kidney).

   b. Classic metastasizing nephroblastoma (Wilms' tumor) is the second most common malignant abdominal neoplasm in the first year of life.

   c. 1.3% of the total childhood cases of Wilms' tumor occurred in the newborn in one series.

   d. Mesoblastic nephroma is the most common (80% of all renal tumors in the newborn). Although initially thought to be benign, more aggressive behavior of this tumor with local recurrence and metastatic disease has been realized.

e. Wilms' tumor is the most common malignant renal tumor of childhood; 1% of all cases are familial; 12–15% of cases are associated with other congenital anomalies (e.g., aniridia, hemihypertrophy, Beckwith-Wiedemann syndrome, genitourinary tract anomalies).

2. Presentation

a. An abdominal mass is the most common presenting sign.

b. Hypertension may result from elaboration of renin from the tumor or from compression of renal vasculature.

c. Microscopic hematuria (more often than macroscopic) may occur.

d. Polycythemia may result from increased erythropoietin levels.

e. A bleeding diathesis may result from the presence of acquired von Willebrand disease.

3. Diagnosis

a. Evaluation of abdominal mass can be accomplished by plain radiography, sonography, CT scan, and biopsy.

b. Assess renal function; avoid nephrotoxic drugs if renal function is compromised.

4. Therapy and prognosis

a. Newborns with Wilms' tumor have much less favorable outcomes than older children.

b. Treatment involves radical excision followed by chemotherapy and radiation therapy.

F. Retinoblastoma

1. Definition

a. A neuroblastic neoplasm of any of the nucleated layers of the retina.

b. Retinoblastoma is responsible for 5% of childhood blindness.

c. 60% of cases are sporadic; 40% of cases are familial with autosomal dominant inheritance. 30% with bilateral or multifocal unilateral tumors have a negative family history.

d. The retinoblastoma gene has been causally linked to other malignancies. Survivors of childhood familial retinoblastoma have an extremely high lifelong risk of developing second malignancies (predominantly sarcomas and osteosarcomas).

2. Incidence is 1/18,000 live births (as common as hemophilia).

3. Presentation

a. The usual age at diagnosis is 18–21 months; however, in

infants born with a family history of retinoblastoma a thorough evaluation must be done at the time of birth.
  b. The most common signs include leukokoria (white pupillary reflex), strabismus, and a red, painful eye.
  c. Calcification can be seen within the eye in 75% of cases.
  d. Findings on CT scan and sonography confirm the diagnosis.
  e. The differential diagnosis includes persistent hyperplastic primary vitreous.
4. Therapy and prognosis
  a. Curable when diagnosed early. Vision need not be sacrificed even when bilateral disease is present.
  b. Local disease can be managed with chemotherapy in combination with local ophthalmic strategies (e.g., photocoagulation laser therapy or cryosurgery). Enucleation is reserved for those lesions where vision cannot be preserved or those with other adverse prognosis features. External beam radiation therapy is avoided if possible because of the potential for adverse side effects (e.g., secondary nonocular malignancies within the radiation field).
  c. Intraocular retinoblastoma with no extension beyond the eye has an overall survival of 92%. Survival is markedly reduced in disease that has extended beyond the globe.
  d. Visual outcome is affected by the area of retina involved. Visual acuity will be significantly reduced with involvement of the macula. Cataracts may develop with tumors involving the ora serrata.

Suggested Reading

Avery GB, Fletcher MA, MacDonald MG (eds): Neonatology: Pathophysiology and Management of the Newborn, 5th ed. Philadelphia, Lippincott, Williams & Wilkins, 1999, pp 1301–1321.

Friedman DL, Himelstein B, Shields CL, et al: Chemoreduction and local ophthalmic therapy for intraocular retinoblastoma. J Clin Oncol 18: 12–17, 2000.

Isaacs H: Congenital and neonatal malignant tumors: A 28-year experience at the Children's Hospital of Los Angeles. Am J Pediatr Hematol Oncol 9:121–129, 1987.

Lanzkowsky P (ed): Manual of Pediatric Hematology and Oncology. New York, Churchill Livingstone, 2000.

Lukens JN: Neuroblastoma in the neonate. Semin Perinatol 23:263–273, 1999.

Parkes SE, Muir KR, Southern L, et al: Neonatal tumours: A thirty-year population-based study. Med Pediatr Oncol 22:309–317, 1994.

Schlesinger AE, Rosenfield NS, Castle VP, Jasty R: Congenital mesoblastic nephroma metastatic to the brain: A report of two cases. Pediatr Radiol 25:S73–S75, 1995.

Werb P, Scurry J, Ostor A: Survey of congenital tumors in perinatal necropsies. Pathology 24:247–253, 1992.

Chapter 67

Fetomaternal Hemorrhage

Steven M. Donn, M.D.

I. Definition

Loss of fetal blood across placenta into maternal circulation. Also referred to as *transplacental hemorrhage* or *fetomaternal transfusion*.

A. Majority of cases involve < 0.1 mL of blood.

B. Rarely, massive blood loss may occur, either acutely or chronically.

C. Important source for maternal isoimmunization (as little as 0.03 mL)

II. Associated Risk Factors

A. Obstetrical procedures

   1. Amniocentesis

   2. External cephalic version

   3. Induced abortion

   4. Manual removal of the placenta

   5. Delivery, especially cesarean section

B. Trauma

C. Vasa previa

D. Placental ischemia

E. Vigorous labor

F. Maternal immune reactions

G. Placental neoplasms

H. Fetal infection

III. Incidence

A. Increases with advancing gestational age

B. May occur in half of all pregnancies, but usually < 0.1 mL

C. Severe hemorrhage (> 30 mL): 0.3–0.7% of pregnancies

IV. Diagnosis

A. Kleihauer-Betke test performed on maternal blood sample

B. Maternal blood smear stained for presence of fetal hemoglobin

C. Results expressed as percentage of "maternal" cells, which take up stain and are thus of fetal origin

D. Size of bleed can then be calculated (maternal red cell volume is approximately 2400 mL).

V. Manifestations

A. Acute fetomaternal hemorrhage

1. Historical features
   a. Usually not helpful
   b. Sinusoidal fetal heart rate pattern
   c. Decreased fetal movement
2. Physical findings
   a. Hypoperfusion or shock
   b. Tachycardia
   c. Decreased central venous pressure
   d. Tachypnea
3. Laboratory findings
   a. Hematocrit initially normal then falls
   b. Normal reticulocyte count
   c. Positive maternal Kleihauer-Betke test
   d. Unremarkable radiographs
4. Initial management
   a. Respiratory support
   b. Vascular access (umbilical)
   c. Measure hematocrit
   d. Transfuse immediately, using whole blood or equivalent 10–20 mL/kg.
5. Stabilization
   a. Maintain hematocrit at 40–50%
   b. Maintain urine output by providing fluids at 100 mL/kg/d or more

B. Chronic fetomaternal hemorrhage

1. Historical features
   a. Polyhydramnios
   b. Sinusoidal fetal heart rate pattern
   c. Decreased fetal movement
2. Physical findings
   a. Pallor
   b. Tachycardia
   c. Blood pressure variable
   d. Edema
   e. Ascites
   f. Variable hepatosplenomegaly
3. Laboratory findings
   a. Anemia
   b. Increased reticulocyte count
   c. Positive maternal Kleihauer-Betke test

    d. Radiographic evidence of cardiomegaly, edema, ascites, and pleural effusions

  4. Initial management—*avoid high-output congestive heart failure*
    a. Respiratory support
    b. Vascular access (umbilical)
    c. Measure hematocrit
    d. If symptomatic, perform *partial exchange transfusion* by administering 50–80 mL/kg of O-negative packed red blood cells while removing an identical volume of whole blood. Try to achieve a hematocrit of 40–50%.
    e. If asymptomatic, provide supportive care.

  5. Stabilization
    a. Restrict fluids (60 mL/kg/d)
    b. Maintain urine output
    c. Avoid fluid overload
    d. Cardiac evaluation; consider echocardiogram

VI. Outcome

A. Perinatal mortality 1 per 1000 pregnancies
B. Death rate approaches 100% for volumes >200 mL
C. Variable neurologic outcomes among survivors

Suggested Reading

Zak LK, Donn SM: Feto-maternal hemorrhage. In Donn SM, Faix RG (eds): Neonatal Emergencies. Mt. Kisco, NY, Futura Publishing, 1991, pp 423–430.

Chapter 68

Phototherapy

Cyril Engmann, MBBS, and Robert E. Schumacher, M.D.

I. Definition

Use of light to chemically alter cutaneous bilirubin in the management of hyperbilirubinemia. This has been the standard of care for four decades.

II. Mechanisms of Action

A. Incompletely understood

B. Bilirubin absorbs light (450–460 nm) resulting in photo-oxidation and photo-isomerization.

C. Labile and stable photo-isomers are generated.

1. The important stable photo-isomer is lumirubin.
2. Lumirubin is polar, water soluble.
3. Lumirubin formation is the rate-limiting step in elimination of bilirubin by phototherapy.
4. Lumirubin is excreted through the biliary tract (without need for conjugation) and subsequently eliminated in stool and urine.

III. Efficacy Factors

A. Light dosage/irradiance depends on power of light and distance from the infant (standard phototherapy lamps should be positioned within 15–20 cm from the patient).

B. Spectral emission (blue-green region of visible spectrum most effective)

C. Surface area illuminated (conventional phototherapy involves exposing maximal areas of skin to irradiance of 7–10 $\mu W/cm^2/nm$)

D. Initial bilirubin load

E. Rate of bilirubin production

IV. Indications

A. Establish etiology first—exact algorithm used depends on the infant (e.g., preterm vs. term)

1. History
2. Physical examination
3. Laboratory studies
   a. Blood typing/antibody test

      b. CBC, differential, platelets

      c. RBC morphology

      d. Sepsis should be ruled out

B. After diagnostic studies are completed, phototherapy is indicated when serum bilirubin is sufficiently high, or in the absence of treatment, predicted to be so high that incremental changes place infant at risk for neurologic sequelae. Theoretically, this value is different for each infant. Practicality dictates the need for guidelines.

C. In *healthy term* newborns consider phototherapy at bilirubin values (mg/dL) of > 12 at age 25–48 hours, > 15 at 48–72 hours, and > 17 at age > 72 hours.

D. Other considerations/guidelines

    1. Phototherapy may be considered at lower bilirubin levels that involve individual clinical judgment, especially so in sick newborns.

    2. Phototherapy is indicated at bilirubin levels that are about 5 mg/dL less than exchange transfusion levels.

    3. Intensive phototherapy (number of lights, distance from infant, special lights) may be indicated when making plans for exchange transfusion. Consider a fiber-optic unit under the infant, combined with overhead unit. Intensive therapy should lower values 1–2 mg/dL within 4–6 hours. The key factor in using multiple phototherapy sources is to irradiate more of the infant's body surface area.

    4. "Prophylactic" phototherapy may be indicated for extensive bruising (especially in a small baby), the diagnosis of hemolytic disease, or in extremely low birthweight infants.

V.   Techniques

A. Several different light sources available

    1. Fluorescent (several types, including "special blue"; irradiance is currently thought more important)

    2. Quartz halogen

    3. Fiber-optic blankets generate little heat and can be placed nearer the infant. They provide up to 50 μW/cm^2/nm. They have been shown to be less effective than conventional therapy but more effective than no therapy.

B. Minimum irradiance required—a standard phototherapy unit with 8 new daylight lamps operating under optimal conditions provides minimally effective levels of phototherapy (5 μW/cm^2/nm). Measure energy output.

C. Infant care
   1. Shield the eyes (animal data suggest retinal degeneration may occur after several days of continuous use).
   2. Monitor temperature closely.
   3. Follow fluid balance carefully; many jaundiced term infants are also dehydrated. Phototherapy may increase transepidermal water losses. It may be necessary to compensate with an increase by 25% above estimated fluid needs without phototherapy. Overhydrating is not of proven benefit.
   4. Determine serum bilirubin concentration every 8–12 hours. Be cognizant of the range of laboratory error in comparing values.
   5. Avoid phototherapy in infants with cholestatic jaundice (conjugated bilirubin $\geq$ 2.0 mg/dL); there is the risk of bronze baby syndrome.
   6. In most instances, phototherapy can be interrupted for nursing and parent visits.

VI. Termination of Therapy
   A. Generally discontinued when serum bilirubin value not likely to rise to a dangerous level
   B. Rebound phenomena in infants $\geq$ 1800 g has been cast into doubt by recent literature.
   C. For healthy term infant, stable values of $\leq$ 14–15 mg/dL are usually appropriate.
   D. Obtain bilirubin measurements as needed after phototherapy.

VII. Prevention of Neurologic Sequelae
   A. Gestational age
   B. Postnatal age
   C. Birthweight
   D. Etiology of hyperbilirubinemia
   E. Overall patient condition

VIII. Potential/Theoretical Risks and Complications
   A. Impaired maternal–infant bonding (consider fiber-optic unit)
   B. Retinal damage
   C. Diarrhea
   D. Dehydration
   E. Hyperthermia
   F. Isomerization/oxidation of drugs, other compounds, or cellular structures
   G. Apnea (from eye shields occluding nares)

H. Thrombocytopenia
I. Hyperpigmentation (especially black babies)
J. Bronze baby syndrome
K. Patent ductus arteriosus
L. Riboflavin, calcium, other deficiencies
M. Blue hue produced by blue lamps has been associated with nausea and dizziness in caregivers as well as impairing assessment of skin color (jaundice).

Suggested Reading

American Academy of Pediatrics: Practice parameter: Management of hyperbilirubinemia in the healthy term infant. Pediatrics 94:558–565, 1994.

Dennery PA, Seidman DS, Stevenson DK: Neonatal hyperbilirubinemia. N Engl J Med 344:581–590, 2001.

Halamek LP Stevenson DK: Neonatal jaundice and liver disease. In Fanaroff AA, Martin RJ (eds): Neonatal-Perinatal Medicine, 7th ed. St. Louis, Mosby-Year Book, 2002, pp 1327–1332.

Maisels MJ (ed): Neonatal Jaundice. Clinics in Perinatology, vol. 7. Philadelphia, W.B. Saunders, 1990.

Tan KL: Phototherapy for neonatal jaundice. Clin Perinatol 18:423–439, 1991.

Chapter 69

Exchange Transfusion

Steven M. Donn, M.D., and Suzanne H. Butch, M.A., M.T. (ASCP), S.B.B.

I. Indications

A. Correction of anemia

B. Removal of sensitized red blood cells

C. Reduction of serum bilirubin

D. Severe sepsis

E. Immune thrombocytopenia caused by maternal autoantibodies

F. Removal of drugs, toxins, metabolites, or other undesirable substances

G. Miscellaneous—some centers have advocated exchange transfusion for the treatment of disorders such as RDS and DIC. Efficacy remains equivocal.

II. Exchange Transfusions

Consider for the following situations:

A. Fetomaternal incompatibility such as Rh (D, E, C, c) or Kell or other antibodies + sensitized mother + positive cord blood antibody test:

1. Initial hemoglobin < 12 mg/dL. (For severe anemia and/or hydrops, first exchange should be a partial exchange with packed red blood cells.)

2. Cord blood bilirubin > 5 mg/dL

3. Bilirubin > 10 mg/dL by 12 hours of age

4. Bilirubin > 20 mg/dL at any age (lower level if associated clinical conditions warrant)

5. Clinical evidence of kernicterus (at *any* bilirubin level)

B. ABO incompatibility with positive antibody test or eluate (*see* II, A, 4 and 5 above).

C. Hyperbilirubinemia other than II. A and B. The level at which exchange needs to be initiated is influenced by the interaction of several factors:

1. Low total protein (theoretical albumin-binding capacity is total protein × 3.7. This approximates how much indirect bilirubin can be bound by circulating albumin.)

2. pH (acidosis increases albumin-bilirubin dissociation)

3. Presence of substances that compete for binding sites on the albumin molecule (free fatty acids in lipid emulsion,

furosemide, benzoic acid, diazepam, some cyclosporins, sul-
fonamides)
4. Asphyxia neonatorum—this lowers the "exchange level" by
rendering the brain more susceptible to kernicterus.
5. VLBW infants—when bilirubin level (mg/dL) = BW (g)/100,
evaluate and determine exchange necessity. Weigh risk-to-
benefit in VLBW. Some centers do not exchange until bilirubin
is ≥ 10 mg/dL regardless of infant's birthweight.
D. Metabolic-toxic: certain conditions can be palliated by repetitive
exchange transfusions (e.g., hyperammonemia secondary to urea
cycle defects, drug overdose).

III. Blood Request

A. Whole blood < 24 hours old is not generally available. "Whole
blood equivalent," prepared from red blood cells and fresh frozen
plasma, is most frequently used. The red blood cells should be:
1. Freshest available (< 7–10 days old)
2. Leukocyte-reduced or CMV seronegative
3. Tested and found to lack hemoglobin S (SickleDex negative)
4. Irradiated
5. Crossmatched—when fetomaternal incompatibility is suspected, compatibility testing should be performed using maternal blood.
B. When preparing blood *before* delivery for the infant of a sensitized
mother, O-negative red blood cells that are negative for the antigens against which the mother has antibodies will be resuspended
in AB fresh frozen plasma. Specify the approximate HCT desired
(48–52%).
C. The blood products should be prepared well in advance of the delivery and be available, if needed, in the delivery or stabilization
room.
D. Before beginning, make sure enough blood is present for a total exchange. A double volume exchange is generally performed. Using a
blood volume of 85 mL per kg of body weight times 2, calculate the
volume to be removed and replaced. One unit of reconstituted whole
blood may be adequate in many cases. Weigh the unit(s). Subtract
the weight of the empty plastic bag(s) (35 g). Total the weight of the
units. Divide the weight by 1.06 to get the approximate volume.
E. Consider checking the K^+, pH, and HCT of the exchange unit.
F. It may also be necessary to use O-negative packed red blood cells
acutely, either as a push transfusion or partial exchange transfusion if the baby is unstable and severely anemic.

G. The blood should be mixed periodically during the exchange as the blood will settle in the container and the desired HCT will not be maintained.

IV. Technique

A. Neonatologist supervision is mandatory. Obtain informed consent from parents.

B. Place a UVC after aspirating gastric contents; if infant already has a UAC, this is acceptable. However, an umbilical artery catheter should *not* be placed solely for the purposes of performing an exchange transfusion. (Use 5-F or 8-F catheter from commercially available exchange tray for vein, *never* for artery.)

C. Simultaneous arterial-venous two-line exchange may be preferable in some infants—consult with neonatologist.

D. Make sure enough blood is present for total exchange. *Weigh each unit before beginning the exchange.* Subtract the weight of the empty plastic bag (35 g). The final weight should be within 6% of the stated volume of blood.

E. Blood should be crossmatched. When fetomaternal incompatibility is suspected, compatibility testing should be performed using maternal blood. When preparing blood *before* delivery for the infant of an Rh-sensitized mother, request O-negative red blood cells resuspended in AB+ fresh frozen plasma to an HCT of about 50%. It may also be necessary to use O-negative packed red blood cells acutely, either as a push transfusion or partial exchange transfusion if the baby is unstable and severely anemic. These components should be prepared well in advance of the delivery and be available, if needed, in the delivery or stabilization room.

F. Whole blood or its equivalent is used. Aim for a single donor.

G. *Use a blood warmer* for all exchange transfusions.

H. UVC insertion should equal the distance from umbilicus to xiphoid process. Alternatively, a "low" position, with the catheter inserted 4–6 cm is acceptable for performance of the exchange transfusion, provided that hypertonic solutions are avoided. A free-flow return of blood suggests that the tip of the UVC is not in the portal system.

I. Pre-exchange studies:
1. Obtain written informed consent from a parent.
2. Bilirubin (total and direct)
3. HCT, reticulocyte count
4. Check CVP (normal, 5–8 cm H_2O)
5. HCT of the donor unit: if blood > 24 hours old, consider

checking K^+, pH on donor unit, especially in VLBW or as-phyxiated infants.

J. Exchange is carried out in 10 mL increments (5 mL if < 1 kg) for the first 50–100 mL, then may increase to 20 mL in larger infants, 10 mL in small. Blood should be infused slowly, *but steadily*. All aliquots must be carefully and accurately recorded. Allow about ½ hour per volume exchanged (e.g., approximately 1–2 min per cycle).

K. 10% calcium gluconate is given *slowly* through stopcock following each 100 mL exchanged. Watch for bradycardia. Dose is 1 mL (100 mg)/100 mL blood exchanged.

L. Monitor vital signs closely throughout procedure, especially for arrhythmias, hypotension, and temperature change.

M. Post-exchange studies:
1. Recheck CVP.
2. Consider removal of catheter.
3. Check HCT and platelet counts serially.
4. Check bilirubin serially.
5. Document procedure note on chart; communicate with parents.
6. Check serum calcium and electrolytes 6–12 hours post-exchange.

N. Miscellaneous
1. Discuss with neonatologist whether to "prime" with albumin prior to exchange.
2. Complications (incidence is 3.6%) include:
   a. Infection (may treat with antibiotics if umbilical cord is old or looks like a source of potential bacteremia); transfusion-acquired viral infections
   b. Thrombosis
   c. Blood loss/anemia
   d. Hepatic necrosis/hepatitis
   e. Usual complications of umbilical catheters
   f. Arrhythmias
   g. Fluid overload
   h. Hypoglycemia
   i. Hypocalcemia
   j. Hyperkalemia
   k. Necrotizing enterocolitis
   l. Thrombocytopenia
   m. Hypernatremia
   n. Acidosis
   o. Death (0.5%)

3. Consult with neonatologist regarding reinstitution of feeds. If stable, consider feeds 4–6 hours after exchange.
4. Certain pharmacologic agents are removed by exchange transfusion. Consider "reloading" infant following exchange, especially for antibiotics, anticonvulsants, and methylxanthines (Table 44).

TABLE 44
Drug Loss during Exchange Transfusion

	Percent Loss	
Drug	One Volume	Two Volume
Amikacin	7.1	13.8
Ampicillin	7.7	14.7
Carbamazepine	3.7	7.2
Carbenicillin	5.6	10.9
Colistin	18.7	33.9
Diazepam	2.3	4.5
Digoxin*	1.2	2.4
Furosemide	4.9	9.5
Gentamicin	5.2	10.1
Kanamycin	5.6	10.9
Methicillin	10.1	19.1
Oxacillin	19.6	35.4
Penicillin G (crystalline)	6.0	11.6
Penicillin G (procaine)	2.4	4.8
Phenobarbital	6.4	12.3
Phenytoin	3.1	6.2
Theophylline*	17.8	32.4
Tobramycin	10.3	19.6
Vancomycin	5.7	11.0

*Whole blood volume used in calculation.
From Lackner TE: Drug replacement following exchange transfusion. J Pediatr 100: 811–814, 1982, with permission.

Suggested Reading

Ahlfors CE: Criteria for exchange transfusion in jaundiced newborns. Pediatrics 93:488–494, 1994.

Cashore WJ, Stern L: The management of hyperbilirubinemia. Clin Perinatol 11:339–357, 1984.

Keenan WJ, Novak, KK, Sutherland JM, et al: Morbidity and mortality associated with exchange transfusion. Pediatrics 75:417–421, 1985.

Section XI. RENAL PROBLEMS

Chapter 70

Hematuria

Mohammad A. Attar, M.D.

I. Definition

Excretion of red blood cells into urine causing dipstick positive for blood with documentation of > 3–5 RBC/HPF on microscopic exam (urine dipstick reacts with hemoglobin)

II. Etiologies

- **A.** Hypoxia
- **B.** Generalized hemorrhagic disease
- **C.** Renal venous or arterial thrombosis
- **D.** Obstructive uropathy
- **E.** Cortical or medullary necrosis
- **F.** Infection
- **G.** Congenital malformations (such as renal cystic diseases)
- **H.** Blood dyscrasias
- **I.** Renal stones
- **J.** Drugs/nephrotoxins
- **K.** Trauma (especially after suprapubic tap)
- **L.** Congenital neoplasms

III. False Positives

- **A.** Positive urine dipstick but no RBCs
  1. Myoglobinuria—secondary to rhabdomyolysis resulting from prolonged seizures, steroid use, severe ischemic injury, or myopathies
  2. Hemoglobinuria—secondary to erythroblastosis fetalis and other hemolytic diseases
- **B.** Red or orange urine but negative dipstick for blood
  1. Urate crystals (seen as orange/red discoloration in diaper)
  2. Rifampin

IV. Diagnosis

- **A.** Examine freshly voided urine (dipstick and microscopic)
  1. RBC casts—diagnostic of glomerular disease
  2. WBC casts—suggestive of pyelonephritis
  3. WBCs—suggestive of infection

    4. Leukocyte esterase—suggestive of infection
    5. Nitrites—suggestive of infection
B. Other diagnostic modalities may be utilized based on history, physical exam, and urinalysis, and include:
    1. Urine culture (catheterized is preferable)
    2. Renal ultrasound with Doppler flow of renal vessels (to rule out structural causes such as stones, nephrocalcinosis, cysts, obstruction)
    3. Renal radionuclide scan (to assess renal function and/or structure)
    4. Urine calcium-to-creatinine ratio (to rule out hypercalciuria)
    5. VCUG (uncommon, to rule our vesicoureteral reflux)
    6. IVP (rarely, to assess renal function and/or structure; perform with caution in newborns)
    7. Cystoscopy (rarely)
    8. Arteriography (rarely)

Suggested Reading

Brem AS: Neonatal hematuria and proteinuria. Clin Perinatol 8:321–332, 1981.

Chapter 71

Renal Failure

Mohammad A. Attar, M.D., and William E. Smoyer, M.D.

I. Definition

Impaired renal function characterized by the inability to adequately regulate salt and water balance and/or eliminate waste products. Usually characterized by elevated serum creatinine.

II. Etiologies

A. Prerenal (most common)

  1. Hypotension

   a. Hemorrhage

   b. Septic shock

   c. Dehydration

  2. Renal hypoperfusion

   a. Hypoxia/asphyxia

   b. Congestive heart failure

   c. Patent ductus arteriosus

   d. NSAIDs (indomethacin; reduces glomerular filtration rate [GFR])

   e. ACE inhibitors (enalaprilat; reduces GFR)

B. Intrarenal (less common)

  1. Ischemia (resulting in proximal tubular cell death or acute tubular necrosis; more severe injury can result in glomerular cell death or acute cortical necrosis)

   a. Shock

   b. Hemorrhage

   c. Dehydration

   d. Sepsis

   e. Hypoxia

  2. Renal anomalies

   a. Renal agenesis

   b. Renal dysplasia

   c. Polycystic kidneys

  3. Vascular

   a. Renal arterial thrombosis (risk increased by UAC)

   b. Renal venous thrombosis (risk increased by UVC)

  4. Interstitial (uncommon)

       a. Allergic drug reaction (e.g., penicillin or NSAIDs)

       b. Drug toxicity (e.g., aminoglycosides)

    5. Hyperuricemia (rare; seen in setting of high WBC with release of intracellular uric acid)

    6. Drugs that reduce intrarenal blood flow (e.g., indomethacin)

C. Postrenal (less common)

    1. Urinary tract obstruction (anatomical)

       a. Posterior urethral valves (most common)

       b. Urethral trauma/atresia

       c. Imperforate prepuce

       d. Urethral diverticulum

       e. Megacystis-megaureter syndrome

       f. Ureteropelvic obstruction (UPJ; would need to be bilateral to induce renal failure)

       g. Ureterovesical obstruction (UVJ; would need to be bilateral to induce renal failure)

    2. Urinary tract obstruction (functional)—neurogenic bladder

III. Clinical and Laboratory Findings

A. Fluids and electrolytes

    1. Serum sodium—usually decreased

    2. Serum potassium—usually normal, but increases with severe renal failure

    3. Serum calcium—frequently decreased (especially if subacute or chronic)

    4. Serum phosphorus—frequently increased (especially if subacute or chronic)

    5. Serum bicarbonate—usually decreased (as part of an increased anion gap metabolic acidosis)

B. Oliguria (< 0.5 mL/kg/h) or anuria—most common in prerenal causes of acute renal failure

C. Polyuria (> 4 mL/kg/h)—most common in renal dysplasia or obstructive uropathy

D. Increased BUN and creatinine are diagnostic of all forms of renal failure, but a markedly increased BUN:creatinine ratio is suggestive of prerenal acute renal failure.

E. Abnormal urinary indices (only helpful in oliguric acute renal failure and if the baby has not had diuretics)

    1. Prerenal

       a. Urine osmolality—usually > 400 mOsm/L

       b. Urinalysis—usually normal, but with increased specific gravity

    c. Urine sodium—usually < 20 mEq/L

    d. Urine-to-plasma urea ratio—usually > 20

    e. Fractional excretion of sodium (FE_{Na})—usually < 1.0%

  2. Intrarenal

    a. Urine osmolality—usually < 400 mOsm/L

    b. Urinalysis—may see hematuria, proteinuria, pyuria, or casts

    c. Urine sodium—usually > 20 mEq/L

    d. Urine to plasma urea ratio—usually < 10

    e. FE_{Na}—usually > 2.0%

IV. Diagnosis

A. History (asphyxia, hemorrhage, UAC, congenital heart disease, drugs)

B. Physical examination (edema vs. volume depletion, abdominal mass, Potter facies, preauricular skin tag or pit, two-vessel umbilical cord, sacral dimple)

C. Serum/urine laboratory studies

  1. Serum electrolytes, BUN, creatinine, calcium, phosphorus, magnesium, albumin

  2. Consider urine sodium (if oliguric and not on diuretics)

D. Renal ultrasound

E. Renal radionuclide scan (uncommonly used)

F. Renal biopsy (rarely used)

V. Treatment

A. Correct underlying cause if possible.

B. Consider placement of a Foley catheter.

C. Correct hypovolemia if present; replace blood/fluid losses.

D. Consider fluid challenge (10–20 mL/kg over 1 hr) if intravascular volume depletion suspected.

E. Consider diuretics (if oliguric and not volume depleted)—furosemide 1–2 mg/kg/dose IV over 30 min (to prevent ototoxicity).

F. Consider vasopressors (dopamine and/or dobutamine) for persistent hypotension and consider echocardiogram to assess cardiac function.

G. Treat hyperkalemia aggressively, if present.

H. Correct metabolic acidosis—$NaHCO_3$, 1–3 mEq/kg/d IV or PO divided three times a day. For severe acidosis, consider THAM.

I. Fluid management

  1. Meticulously monitor intake of all fluids and electrolytes, and renal and nonrenal output.

2. If normovolemic, restrict fluids to insensible losses plus urine output.
   a. Insensible loss (mL/kg/hr):
      Term (days 1–3):   0.7–1.0
      Preterm: 2.0–2.5
      Phototherapy (open warmer): add 15–20 mL/kg/d
   b. Replace urine output milliliter for milliliter with electrolytes matched to urinary electrolytes (usually 0.2–0.45% NaCl).
   c. Replace all other output milliliter for milliliter based on fluid composition.
   d. Strict intake and output measurements and daily weights
   e. Attempt to provide 100 kcal/kg/d.
   f. Consider use of radiant warmer to augment insensible losses.
   g. Monitor electrolytes frequently, watching especially for potential hyperkalemia or hyponatremia.
J. Adjust drug doses as indicated for the degree of renal failure, and dose only by trough levels where possible.
K. Treat hypertension if present.

VI. Renal Replacement Therapy Options in Newborns
A. Peritoneal dialysis (most common; *see* Chapter 72)
B. Continuous renal replacement therapy (CRRT) (less common)
   1. Continuous arteriovenous (CAVH) and venovenous (CVVH) hemofiltration
      a. Blood passes through a hemofilter, plasma ultrafiltrate is removed, and a portion of the ultrafiltrate volume is replaced with a physiologic replacement fluid.
      b. Main advantages—precise control of fluid removal; better tolerated by hemodynamically unstable patients than peritoneal or hemodialysis.
   2. Continuous arteriovenous (CAVHD) and venovenous (CVVHD) hemodialysis
      a. Blood passes through a hemofilter and is continuously dialyzed across the semipermeable filter membrane by countercurrent flow of a physiologic dialysis solution, and a portion of the combined ultrafiltrate and dialysate is removed from the body.
      b. Main advantages—precise control of fluid removal; better tolerated by hemodynamically unstable patients than peritoneal or hemodialysis; possibly less filter clotting than with CAVH or CVVH.

C. Hemodialysis
1. Purpose—removal of free water and removal of free solutes.
2. Performed in intermittent periods of treatment, usually 3–4 hours, 3–4 times weekly.
3. Rapid countercurrent dialysis flow quickly removes fluids and solutes from the patient's blood.
4. Fastest way to clear solute from the body; therefore, more effective for neonatal hyperammonemia than either peritoneal dialysis or any type of CRRT.

VII. Prognosis
A. Outcome is dependent on the underlying cause of the renal failure.
B. Most newborns and infants who receive the appropriate treatment have an excellent prognosis.
C. Outcome in infants with congenital urinary tract obstruction depends on the degree of renal dysplasia.
D. Infants with the intrinsic acute renal failure have a poorer prognosis than other groups.

Suggested Reading

Engle WD: Acute renal failure. In Donn SM, Faix RG (eds): Neonatal Emergencies. Mt. Kisco, NY, Futura Publishing, 1991, pp 409–420.

Karlowicz MG, Adelman RD: Acute renal failure in the neonate. Clin Perinatol 19:139–158, 1992.

Mathew OP, Jones AS, James E, et al: Neonatal renal failure: Usefulness of diagnostic indices. Pediatrics 65:57–60, 1980.

Shaffer SE, Norman ME: Renal function and renal failure in the newborn. Clin Perinatol 16:199–218, 1989.

Vogt BA, Davis ID, Avner ED: The kidney. In Klaus MH, Fanaroff AA (eds): Care of the High Risk Neonate, 5th ed. Philadelphia, W.B. Saunders, 2001, pp 425–446.

Chapter 72

Neonatal Peritoneal Dialysis

Mohammad A. Attar, M.D., and William E. Smoyer, M.D.

I. Indications
A. Refractory severe or symptomatic uremia
B. Refractory hyperkalemia
C. Refractory severe fluid overload
D. Refractory metabolic acidosis
E. Refractory severe or symptomatic hypocalcemia
F. Hyperammonemia
   1. Dialysis usually required if ammonia >200 μg/mL
   2. Preferred initial management is acute hemodialysis, as it results in much faster reduction in plasma ammonia levels.

II. Comments
A. Peritoneum is freely permeable to electrolytes such as urea, glucose, and ammonia.
B. Peritoneum is semipermeable to proteins.
C. Peritoneal dialysis is unlikely to cause dysequilibrium syndrome because it corrects electrolyte disturbances relatively slowly.
D. Peritonitis (chemical or bacterial) is *not* a contraindication.
E. Peritoneal dialysis itself is not painful; sedation and analgesia are not indicated except for catheter insertion (morphine may be used).
F. Relative contraindications include NEC, ventriculoperitoneal shunt, and bleeding diathesis.
G. Informed consent must be obtained.

III. Procedure
A. Consult nephrology if dialysis is indicated.
B. Order dialysis solution and manual peritoneal dialysis setup per recommendations of nephrologist.
C. Warm dialysis solution to 37°C.
D. Cycles should last approximately 1 hour:
   1. 5–10 min for dialysis solution to fill
   2. 40–50 min for dialysis solution to dwell
   3. 5–10 min for dialysate solution to drain
E. Start with cycle volumes of 10 mL/kg (based on dry weight) and

gradually (over weeks) increase the cycle volume to a maximum of 40–50 mL/kg unless patient develops abdominal distention, respiratory distress, or catheter leakage at the exit site.

F. Laboratory studies
  1. Calcium and electrolytes every 6 hr initially
  2. Electrolytes, BUN, creatinine, total protein, albumin, calcium, phosphorus every 24 hr.

G. Weigh patient every 12 hr.

H. Since there can be significant losses of albumin, 1.0 g/kg of 25% albumin should be given for serum albumin < 2.8 g/dL. This may be required frequently. Albumin should be given over 4–6 hours.

I. Because peritoneal dialysis removes fluid by using glucose as an osmotic agent to draw fluid across the peritoneal membrane, higher concentrations of glucose (range is usually 1.5–4.25%) will result in greater amounts of fluid removal.

J. Since dialysis solution does not usually contain either potassium or phosphorus, these must sometimes be supplemented. This can be easily done by adding KCl and/or K_3PO_4 to the dialysis solution at doses of 2–4 mEq/L.

K. Although dialysis solution can be made with either bicarbonate or lactate as the source of base, only bicarbonate should be used to manage patients with severe metabolic acidosis or liver failure.

L. The length of dialysis depends on the patient's indications and clinical course.

IV. Complications

A. Perforation of viscus
B. Perforation of bladder
C. Peritonitis
D. Sepsis
E. Hypocalcemia
F. Hypovolemia (especially with 4.25% glucose solution)
G. Hyperglycemia (may require an insulin drip)

Suggested Reading

Engle WD: Acute renal failure. In Donn SM, Faix RG (eds): Neonatal Emergencies. Mt. Kisco, NY, Futura Publishing, 1991, pp 409–420.

Vogt BA, Davis ID, Avner ED: The kidney. In Klaus MH, Faranoff, AA (eds): Care of the High Risk Neonate, 5th ed. Philadelphia, W.B. Saunders, 2001, pp 425–446.

Section XII.   METABOLIC DISEASE

Chapter 73

Metabolic Disease

Steven M. Donn, M.D., and Charles R. Neal, Jr., M.D., Ph.D.

I. **Metabolic Defects Causing Catastrophic Illness**
   - **A.** Amino acids
   - **B.** Organic acids
   - **C.** Fatty acids
   - **D.** Carbohydrates
   - **E.** Urea cycle
   - **F.** Mitochondrial
   - **G.** Lysosomal

II. **Signs of Metabolic Disease**
   - **A.** Gastrointestinal
     1. Poor feeding
     2. Vomiting
     3. Diarrhea
   - **B.** Respiratory
     1. Apnea
     2. Tachypnea, respiratory distress
   - **C.** Hepatic
     1. Hepatomegaly
     2. Jaundice
   - **D.** Neurologic
     1. Lethargy, coma
     2. Poor suck, abnormal reflexes
     3. Abnormal tone
     4. Seizures
   - **E.** Hematologic
     1. Thrombocytopenia
     2. Neutropenia
   - **F.** Metabolic
     1. Acidosis
     2. Ketosis
   - **G.** Dysmorphic features
   - **H.** Abnormal odors
     1. Glutaric aciduria II—acrid, sweaty feet
     2. Isovaleric acidemia—sweaty feet

3. Maple syrup urine disease
4. 3-Methylcrotonyl-CoA carboxylase deficiency—cat urine
5. PKU—musty or barny
6. Trimethylaminuria—fishy
7. Tyrosinemia—musty or boiled cabbage

III. Laboratory Work-up
A. Routine studies
1. CBC, differential, platelets
2. Serum electrolytes; calculate anion gap
3. Blood glucose
4. ABG
5. Plasma ammonia, lactate, pyruvate
6. U/A (include ketones, reducing substances)

B. Specialized studies
1. Urine
   a. Amino acids
   b. Organic acids
2. Plasma
   a. Amino acids
   b. Carnitine

IV. Active Management
A. General supportive care
1. Assisted ventilation (especially for hyperammonemia)
2. Correct dehydration
3. Acid–base balance
4. Antibiotics

B. Removal of toxic metabolites (e.g., NH_3)
1. Exchange transfusion
2. Peritoneal dialysis
3. Hemodialysis (most effective)

C. Nutritional
1. Stop protein initially
2. Provide 125–150 kcal/kg/d
3. Gradually reintroduce protein at 0.5 g/kg/d and advance slowly

D. Therapy (usually defect-specific)
1. Obtain metabolic/genetics consult ASAP
2. Arginine (essential amino acid when urea cycle defect present) 750 mg/kg/d IV
3. Sodium benzoate—conjugates with glycine to form hippuric acid

4. Phenylacetate—conjugates with glutamine to form phenyl-
   acetylglutamine
5. Carnitine (organic acidemias)
6. Pharmacologic vitamin doses

V. Practical Hints

A. Infants are usually clinically normal at birth and deteriorate after
sufficient protein challenge.

B. Classic presenting "triad":
   1. Vomiting
   2. Seizures
   3. Stupor or coma

C. Diagnosis generally requires some degree of suspicion, awareness,
and anticipation.

D. Outcome is related to rapidity of reversal of coma. Do not delay in
initiating therapy. Encourage prompt transfer. Preserve specimens,
especially urine.

E. Preservation of umbilical vessels for either exchange transfusion
or hemodialysis is crucial. Inexperienced individuals should not
attempt catheterization.

F. Pay careful attention to family history, especially early, unexplained neonatal deaths. Most disorders are autosomal recessive in
inheritance.

G. Make every effort to obtain postmortem examination of nonsur-
vivors. Coordinate any special studies with metabolic experts.

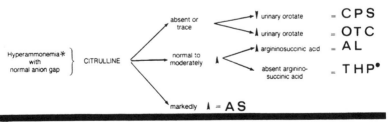

* Hyperammonemia + acidosis + ▲ anion gap = ORGANIC ACIDEMIA
● THP, normal plasma arginine

Figure 9. Algorithmic approach to neonatal hyperammonemia. CPS = carbamyl-
phosphate synthetase deficiency; OTC = ornithine transcarbamylase deficiency;
AL = argininosuccinate lyase deficiency; THP = transient hyperammonemia of
prematurity; AS = arginine succinate synthetase deficiency. (From Donn SM,
Banagale RC: Neonatal hyperammonemia. Pediatr Rev 5:206, 1984, with permission.)

H. The algorithm shown in Figure 9 is useful in differential diagnosis of neonatal hyperammonemia and urea cycle defects.

Suggested Reading

Donn SM, Banagale RC: Neonatal hyperammonemia. Pediatr Rev 5:203, 1984.

Muenzer J: Catastrophic metabolic disease in the newborn. In Donn SM, Faix RG (eds): Neonatal Emergencies. Mt. Kisco, NY, Futura Publishing, 1991.

Section XIII. SURGICAL ISSUES

Chapter 74

Neonatal Pain and Sedation

Charles R. Neal, Jr., M.D., Ph.D., and Wendy Kenyon, R.N.

I. **Definitions**
   A. Pain—an unpleasant sensory and emotional experience associated with actual or potential tissue damage or described in terms of such damage (International Association of the Study of Pain)
   B. Nociception—the activity of the nervous system, that may lead to the perception of pain
   C. Analgesia—a state of being where one is theoretically unable to feel pain, conscious or not
   D. Analgesics—medications that reduce or eliminate pain
      1. Opium—a narcotic drug obtained from the unripe seed pods of the opium poppy (*Papaver somniferum*)
      2. Opioid—generally, a term to cover all natural and synthetic opiates with an emphasis on modern pharmacologic pain-killing formulas that have a chemical structure substantially related to morphine, heroin (natural), or methadone (synthetic)
      3. Narcotic—any drug that produces analgesia, narcosis (state of stupor or sleep), addiction or physical dependence, or euphoria
   E. Sedation—an altered state of consciousness
   F. Tolerance—decreasing effectiveness of a drug after repeated administration, requiring an increase in the dose to maintain the same clinical effect
   G. Addiction—a psychological dependence to a drug that leads to a pattern of compulsive drug use characterized by a continued craving for any drug for uses other than indicated

II. **Neuroanatomy and Neurophysiology**
   A. Pain transmission—the neural pain pathway extends from the sensory receptors in the skin to the cerebral cortex.
      1. Pain perception begins with activation of cutaneous nociceptors with afferent axons that reach the dorsal horn of the spinal cord via parasympathetic, sympathetic, and splanchnic nerves.
      2. The signal is then received by nociceptive-specific neurons within the substantia gelatinosa of the dorsal horn and is either amplified or reduced by descending input from several forebrain and brainstem nuclei.

3. Ensuing output of the dorsal horn is next transmitted via the spinothalamic tract to the thalamus, and then relayed to the cerebral cortex where the pain sensation is discriminated and localized (perceived).

B. Theoretical framework: the "gate control" theory of pain

1. Melzack and Wall (1965) were the first to propose that pain perception is an integrated process, that involves coordinated input from many brain centers. This concept differed markedly from other theories, which recognized only one specific brain area for pain perception.

2. Neurons within the substantia gelatinosa extend the length of the spinal cord and act as a gate-control system in that they modulate transmission of impulses from the periphery to central brain structures.

   a. Large and small diameter fibers transmit nociceptive information via impulses centrally.

   b. Central brain structures then either facilitate or inhibit the propagation of painful perception.

   c. Synapses within the substantia gelatinosa maintain a presynaptic "gate" that modulates the transmission of nociceptive impulses.

   d. This presynaptic gate is open in its resting state.

3. Large-diameter fibers are activated first in pain.

   a. Impulses from large fibers activate central pain centers, bringing about the perception of a noxious stimulus as painful.

   b. Negative feedback from descending cortical and limbic systems close the presynaptic gate of large-diameter fibers after repeated stimulation.

4. Small-diameter fibers are modulated by a central positive feedback system, which serves to propagate impulses.

C. Embryology

1. Synaptic development

   a. Synapses, which directly link incoming sensory fibers with receptive interneurons in the dorsal horn of the spinal cord, first appear during the 6th week of gestation.

   b. Differentiation of dorsal horn neurons begins at 13 weeks of gestation.

   c. The region of the dorsal horn associated with pain transmission, substantia gelatinosa, reaches maturity by 30 weeks of gestation.

2. Cutaneous receptor development

    a. Essential for pain perception, the nociceptive nerve endings in the skin of the newborn equal or exceed the number found in the adult skin.

    b. The first cutaneous sensory receptors appear in the periorbital area of the fetus by 7 weeks of gestation.

    c. By 15 weeks of gestation, cutaneous sensory receptors are present on the trunk, arms, legs, the palms of the hands, the soles of the feet, and the face.

    d. Cutaneous sensory receptors are present on all surfaces by 20 weeks of gestation.

3. Myelination

    a. Paucity of myelination is a common rationale for the argument that conduction of pain impulses in the newborn is minimal. However, much pain transmission in the newborn is via *unmyelinated* fibers.

    b. There are two categories of nociceptors involved in transmission of noxious stimuli:

       i. High threshold nociceptors are mechanoreceptors that respond only to pressure.

         (a) Their axons are myelinated, and conduction velocity is about 25 m/sec (A-delta velocity range).

         (b) These fibers are the primary response to injury.

       ii. *Polymodal nociceptors* respond to pressure and heat or chemical irritation.

         (a) Their axons are unmyelinated, and conduction velocity is about 2 m/sec (C-delta velocity range).

         (b) These fibers are the secondary response to pain.

         (c) Although lack of myelination may decrease the conduction velocity of an impulse, the newborn's shorter interneuronal distance often offsets the slower conduction velocity.

         (d) Myelination of the pain pathways terminating in the thalamus and brainstem are complete by 30 weeks of gestation. The pain fibers in the posterior limb of the corona radiata and the internal capsule are myelinated completely by 37 weeks.

4. Cerebral cortex development

    a. Development of the cortex begins at 8 weeks of gestation, and by 20 weeks, the fetus has 10 billion neurons.

    b. Maturation of the cerebral cortex is complex, and includes several processes such as neuronal migration and cell death. This maturation continues throughout the remainder of fetal development and postnatally, as does refinement of pain perception and an integrated pain response.

    5. Pain-related neurochemical ontogeny
        a. Excitatory
            i. Substance P, calcitonin-gene-related peptide, and somatostatin are expressed in the dorsal horn of the spinal cord by 8–10 weeks of gestation.
            ii. Vasoactive intestinal polypeptide neuropeptide Y and glutamate appear at 12–16 weeks of gestation.
        b. Inhibitory
            i. Dopamine and norepinephrine are expressed at 34–36 weeks of gestation.
            ii. Serotonin appears postnatally.

III.   Assessment

  A. Ongoing assessment is critical in the premature and term newborn because infants are unable to verbally express pain.

  B. Signs of pain
    1. Physiologic
        a. Early signs include tachycardia, hypertension, tachypnea, and increased intracranial pressure.
        b. Late signs include bradycardia, hypotension, hypoxia, and apnea.
        c. Preterm infants have less autonomic stability than more mature infants, and may present with late signs of pain much more quickly than term infants.
    2. Behavioral
        a. State instability, grimace, brow bulge, flailing, and prolonged crying are common painful behaviors.
        b. It is important to remember that, although preterm infants have much less facial response to pain than term infants, they still do feel and perceive pain.

IV.   Pain and Sedation Management

Newborns in the NICU are subject to innumerable daily noxious stimuli. The goal in optimizing long-term neurodevelopmental outcome of these infants begins with decreasing nociceptive activity, eliminating pain, and minimizing stress.

  A. Pharmacologic intervention for pain management
    1. Method of drug delivery
        a. Continuous infusions should be provided if a constant

painful stimulus is present (e.g., ECMO, mechanical ventilation, multiple chest tubes, fractures).

   b. Bolus dosing should be provided prior to all painful procedures (e.g., lumbar puncture, central catheter placement,
chest tube insertion).

2. Opiates are uniformly effective analgesic drugs, with variable
sedative effects.

   a. Opioid alkaloids share similar structures, and all have broad
functional physiologic effects.

   b. Opiates act throughout the peripheral and central nervous
systems, but their strongest analgesic effects are within the
dorsal horn of the spinal cord.

     i. Via presynaptic inhibition, they decrease substance P re-
lease, slowing pain transmission at the synaptic level.

     ii. Opiates also function by reducing cutaneous receptor
fields, via inhibition of transmission along C fibers.

     iii. In order for opioids to have an effect, a painful stimulus
must be present.

   c. Common opiates used in the NICU setting

     i. Morphine is a highly addictive narcotic analgesic drug
used in the form of its hydrochloride, sulfate, and acetate
salts.

       (a) When given intravenously, it has an immediate on-
set of action.

       (b) Its analgesic and sedative effects peak at about 20
minutes.

       (c) Duration of action is approximately 2–4 hours, but
may be longer in preterm infants.

       (d) Dosing

         (i) Begin bolus dosing at 0.05 mg/kg/dose, every
2–6 hr. If the infant requires conscious sedation
for longer than 72 hr, dosing should be increased to 0.1 mg/kg/dose.

         (ii) Continuous infusions may be helpful for new-
borns requiring prolonged opiate treatment
(e.g., prolonged intubation, critically ill), or
those that are difficult to monitor (e.g., elective
paralysis).

          (aa) Infusions should be started at 10 µg/kg/h.

          (bb) A bolus dose should be administered be-
fore beginning a continuous infusion.

      (e) Side effects include respiratory depression, mild abdominal ileus with feeding intolerance, urinary retention, and hypotension (uncommon in preterm infants when opiate used alone).

    ii. Fentanyl is a synthetic opiate that is 80–100 times as potent as morphine.

       (a) When given intravenously, it has an immediate onset of action.

       (b) Its analgesic and sedative effects peak at about 5 minutes, making it ideal for use with emergent procedures, especially in infants receiving morphine.

       (c) Duration of action is approximately 30–60 minutes, but may be longer in preterm infants.

       (d) Dosing

         (i) Begin bolus dosing at 1–5 µg/kg/dose, every 1–2 hr.

         (ii) Continuous infusions may be helpful for infants requiring prolonged opiate treatment (e.g., prolonged intubation, critically ill), or those that are difficult to monitor (e.g., elective paralysis).

           (aa) Infusion should be started at 1–3 µg/kg/h.

           (bb) A bolus dose should be administered before beginning a continuous infusion.

           (cc) Tolerance can develop more rapidly with fentanyl compared to morphine, requiring more diligent monitoring of analgesia to provide adequate dosing.

       (e) Side effects potentially can be similar to those of morphine, as with any opiate, but most common is chest wall rigidity.

  3. Opiate antagonists are very effective for reversing sedative and respiratory side effects of opioid drugs.

    a. Narcan (naloxone) can be given intravenously, intramuscularly or subcutaneously, at 1–4 µg/kg/dose.

    b. Naltrexone is not used in the NICU setting.

    c. An opiate antagonist should *never* be given to an infant to reverse opiate-induced apnea or respiratory depression if there is a history of chronic opiate exposure, *in utero* or postnatally.

B. Pharmacologic management for sedation

  1. Method of drug delivery

    a. Continuous infusions of sedatives should be provided only if absolutely necessary.

    b. PRN administration of sedatives may be administered in addition to opiates to maximize conscious sedation in intubated infants.

2. Sedatives provide no analgesia, but may be used in combination with an analgesic for enhanced conscious sedation.

   a. Benzodiazepines act on gamma-aminobutyric acid (GABA) receptors, which are distributed throughout the central nervous system. All benzodiazepines induce hypnosis, sedation, and amnesia through their actions.

      i. Midazolam (Versed) is a short-acting sedative.

         (a) Its active metabolite, 1-hydroxy-midazolam, can accumulate, leading to prolonged sedation.

         (b) Intubated preterm and term infants requiring midazolam are rare, but if necessary, continuous intravenous infusions should be initiated at a rate of 0.03 mg/kg/h in infants < 32 weeks and 0.06 mg/kg/h in infants > 32 weeks.

            (i) Intravenous loading doses should not be used in newborns; rather, the infusion may be run more rapidly for the first several hours to establish therapeutic plasma levels.

            (ii) The rate of infusion should be carefully and frequently reassessed, particularly after the first 24 hours to insure administration of the lowest possible effective dose and reduce the potential for drug accumulation.

         (c) Hypotension may be observed in patients who are critically ill and in preterm and term infants, particularly those receiving an opiate and/or when midazolam is administered rapidly.

            (i) Because of an increased risk of apnea, extreme caution is advised when sedating preterm and former preterm patients who are not intubated.

            (ii) It is important to bear in mind that midazolam may potentially lower the seizure threshold in some patients, so it should not be given to infants at risk for seizures.

      ii. Diazepam (Valium) is a longer acting sedative.

         (a) Seldom used for sedation in the NICU setting

         (b) Begin dosing at 0.05 mg/kg/dose every 2–4 hr. Up to 0.3 mg/kg/dose may be given if necessary.

         (c) Side effects include respiratory depression and hypotension.

        iii. Lorazepam (Ativan) is a long-acting sedative, with a half-life of 10–20 hours.

          (a) It has no active metabolites.

          (b) Begin dosing at 0.1 mg/kg/dose every 4–6 hr. Up to 0.4 mg/kg/dose may be given, but this is rarely necessary.

          (c) Side effects are not common.

            (i) Hypotension may be observed in critically ill patients and in preterm and term infants, particularly those also receiving an opiate.

            (ii) A gasping syndrome has been described for the metabolic acidosis and shock seen with lorazepam use as a result of benzyl alcohol overdose from its preservative. This side effect is highly unlikely in the doses used in the NICU setting.

        iv. Flumazenil is a benzodiazepine antagonist.

          (a) May be used in the NICU to reverse respiratory depression, especially if you do not wish to intubate an infant

          (b) Dose for reversal is 8–15 μg/kg/dose.

   b. Phenobarbital provides excellent sedation.

     i. It has a half-life of up to 100–200 hours in preterm and sick term infants.

     ii. It is an excellent sedative for use in infants with neonatal abstinence syndrome.

     iii. Begin with a loading dose of 20 mg/kg, followed by maintenance dosing of 3–5 mg/kg/d.

   c. Chloral hydrate is a sedative-hypnotic.

     i. It has a half-life of about 8–60 hr.

     ii. It is excellent for use in infants requiring mild sedation, as for an MRI.

     iii. Dosing is 50–75 mg/kg/dose, PO or PR.

V.   Local Anesthetic Agents

A. EMLA (eutectic mixture of local anesthetics) is a mixture of prilocaine and lidocaine.

   1. Apply topically 30–60 minutes prior to any minor procedure.

   2. Duration of anesthesia is about 1 hr.

B. Lidocaine, 0.5% solution

   1. A subcutaneous injection into the region is as effective as EMLA, but more painful.

   2. Onset of action is almost immediate.

VI. Nonpharmacologic Interventions for Pain

A. Non-nutritive sucking

1. Provide a pacifier to calm an infant prior to any painful or stressful procedure.
2. Can be a plain pacifier, or one dipped in sucrose

B. Sucrose as an analgesic agent

1. Sweet taste elicits endogenous opioid release.
2. Indicated for relief of minor procedural pain
3. Administered to anterior part of tongue
   a. Give via pacifier, syringe, or gloved finger.
   b. Should be administered 2 minutes prior to procedure.
4. Dosage guidelines
   a. Administer in 0.05–0.1-mL increments as needed and as tolerated.
   b. Preterm infants
      i. For those weighing < 1000 g, give 0.05–0.1 mL.
      ii. For those weighing 1000–2000 g, give 0.05–0.2 mL.
      iii. For those weighing > 1000 g, give 0.05–0.5 mL.
   c. Term infants
      i. Give 0.05–0.5 mL.
      ii. Up to 2 mL may be given to term infants following a painful procedure.
      iii. There are no known side effects to this therapy.

C. Swaddling, containment, or facilitated tucking

D. Music therapy

E. Therapeutic touch/infant massage

Suggested Reading

Anand KJ: International Evidence-Based Group for Neonatal Pain: Consensus statement for the prevention and management of pain in the newborn. Arch Pediatr Adolesc Med 155:173–180, 2001.

Anand KJ: Effects of perinatal pain and stress. Prog Brain Res 122:117–129, 2000.

Anand KJ, Barton BA, McIntosh N, et al: Analgesia and sedation in preterm neonates who require ventilatory support: Results from the NOPAIN trial. Arch Pediatr Adolesc Med 153:331–338, 1999.

Anand KJ, Carr DB: The neuroanatomy, neurophysiology and neurochemistry of pain, stress and analgesia in newborns and children. Pediatr Clin North Am 36:795–822, 1989.

Anand KJ, Hickey PR: Pain and its effect on the human neonate and fetus. N Engl J Med 317:1321–1329, 1987.

Bell SG: The national pain management guideline: Implications for neonatal intensive care. Agency for Health Care Policy and Research. Neonatal Netw 13:9–17, 1994.

Chiswick ML: Assessment of pain in neonates. Lancet 355:6–8, 2000.

Deshpande J, Tobias J: The Pediatric Pain Handbook. St. Louis, Mosby, 1996.

Melzack R, Wall P: Pain mechanisms: A new theory. Science 150:971–979, 1965.

Chapter 75

Neonatal Anesthesia Considerations

Shobha Malviya, M.D., and Lori Q. Riegger, M.D.

I. Challenges

The high-risk newborn confronts the anesthesiologist with unique challenges that include:

A. Obvious difficulties related to smaller size: vascular access, airway management, and thermoregulation

B. Differences in pharmacokinetics of anesthetic and other drugs

C. Unique aspects of developmental physiology, such as the risk of post anesthetic apnea in preterm and former preterm infants.

D. Higher anesthesia-related morbidity and mortality in newborns compared with older children and adults.

II. Fasting Schedule

The minimal acceptable period between oral intake and sedation, anesthesia, and surgery at University of Michigan's C.S. Mott Children's Hospital is presented in Table 45.

TABLE 45
Fasting Schedule for Pediatric Anesthesia at
C.S. Mott Children's Hospital

Clear Liquids	Breast Milk	Solid Food (Including Cow's Milk and Formula)
2 hours	4 hours	6 hours

III. Pharmacology of Anesthetic Drugs in Newborns

Response to therapeutic agents differs significantly in newborns compared with older children and adults.

A. Volatile anesthetics

1. Newborns experience a higher incidence of cardiovascular instability and hemodynamic compromise during induction of anesthesia via the inhaled route because of rapid equilibration, rapid myocardial uptake, and increased sensitivity of the myocardium. Of all volatile anesthetic agents, sevoflurane provides the most stable hemodynamic conditions during induction and maintenance of anesthesia.

2. The immature autonomic nervous system in newborns predisposes

them to greater depression of baroreceptor responses when exposed to volatile anesthetics, particularly halothane.

3. Minimum alveolar concentration (MAC) of a volatile anesthetic agent that produces immobility in 50% of subjects exposed to a noxious stimulus is lower in preterm and term newborns than in infants 1–6 months of age. In the case of sevoflurane, however, the MAC remains stable in the neonatal period through 6 months of age.

4. Despite these differences, volatile anesthetics should not be withheld from newborns but should be used judiciously with close monitoring of blood pressure and heart rate.

B. Intravenous anesthetics

1. Requirement for intravenous induction agents sodium thiopental and ketamine is increased in newborns and young infants. However, the half-life of thiopental is very prolonged in preterm and term newborns and may result in delayed emergence or a risk for postanesthetic apnea.

2. Elimination half-life of morphine is significantly prolonged in newborns compared with older children and adults (13.9 vs. 2 hr, respectively). Furthermore, newborns have been shown to have decreased clearance, higher serum concentrations, and greater penetration of morphine in the brain. Newborns have also been shown to have decreased requirements of fentanyl when used as a sole anesthetic compared with older children and adults. In the unstable newborn, however, the use of high doses of opioids (fentanyl 10–30 μg/kg) for maintenance of anesthesia provides hemodynamic stability, ablates neuroendocrine stress responses, and improves surgical outcomes.

C. Muscle relaxants

1. Although newborns may be more sensitive to muscle relaxants, they require the same dose per m^2 of body surface area as adults because of the larger volume of distribution of most muscle relaxants in newborns.

2. Newborns eliminate muscle relaxants more slowly because of the larger volume of distribution and reduced glomerular filtration. Adequate reversal of muscle relaxants is therefore essential in newborns prior to extubation.

IV. Airway Management

A. Even during short procedures, ventilation should be assisted because anesthetics cause significant airway depression in newborns.

B. A laryngeal mask airway (LMA) is an alternative to an endotracheal tube.

1. The end of the LMA sits in the posterior pharynx just above the epiglottis. A correctly placed LMA avoids airway obstruction from the tongue and pharyngeal soft tissue, but because it sits above the larynx, the airway is not protected from aspiration or laryngospasm.
2. Ventilation of a newborn with an LMA must be gently assisted because of the high incidence of hypercapnia with their use. However, aggressive ventilation may lead to gastric distension/aspiration.
3. The LMA is a useful device in patients who are difficult to intubate and is included in the American Society of Anesthesiologists Difficult Airway Algorithm.

C. Endotracheal intubation is used for the majority of neonatal anesthetics. Most intubations are performed under general anesthesia to avoid increases in intracranial pressure associated with intubations of awake infants.

V. Postanesthetic Apnea

A. Former preterm infants recovering from even relatively minor surgical procedures under anesthesia are at increased risk of postanesthetic apnea.

B. Several studies that attempted to define the upper postconceptual age (PCA) at risk for apnea failed to establish a consistent policy because of small sample sizes and inconsistencies in monitoring anesthetic practices. Using a combined analysis of the existing data, Coté et al. reported that the risk of apnea was < 5% at 48 weeks' PCA and < 1% at 54–56 weeks' PCA.

C. The risk of apnea has been found to be inversely proportional to PCA and gestational age. Associated risk factors include anemia and a history of ongoing apnea in the immediate preoperative period.

D. Regional anesthesia techniques, such as spinal or epidural anesthesia, decrease the risk of apnea after surgery but do not eliminate it.

E. For these reasons, it is the policy of our institution to monitor ECG, respiratory rate and oxygen saturation in all former preterm infants less than 50 weeks' PCA for a minimum of 12 apnea-free hours after anesthesia, regardless of the extent of the surgical procedure. The use of prophylactic caffeine reduces the incidence of apnea after anesthesia, but does not eliminate the need for monitoring.

VI. Anesthetic Considerations Related to Specific Procedures

A. Tracheoesophageal fistula

1. The risk of aspiration must be minimized by aspirating any secretions in the upper esophageal pouch prior to rapid sequence induction of general anesthesia using an intravenous induction agent, such as thiopental, or ketamine and succinylcholine.

2. Bronchoscopy may be required in some infants to identify the fistula and seal it with a balloon-tipped catheter to avoid gastric distention with positive pressure ventilation. Alternatively, needle aspiration gastrostomy may be performed for decompression of the stomach.

3. Monitoring should include measuring arterial blood pressure invasively particularly in the unstable newborn.

4. Maintenance of anesthesia may be achieved by judicious use of a volatile anesthetic in combination with an opioid anesthetic, such as fentanyl, depending on whether the infant will be ventilated postoperatively.

5. Brief episodes of desaturation and blood pressure instability from compression of the lungs, trachea, and large blood vessels should be expected during the repair and may have to be tolerated to allow completion of the procedure.

B. Congenital diaphragmatic hernia

1. The severity of the malformation depends on the extent of herniation of abdominal contents into the thoracic cavity. Minor herniations may be asymptomatic at birth, while the most severe present with respiratory distress, hypoxemia, and episodes of life-threatening pulmonary hypertension with right-to-left shunting from a severely hypoplastic lung.

2. Immediate surgery is not needed. In fact, stabilization of the patient and treatment of pulmonary hypertension before surgery have improved outcomes.

3. In addition to routine monitoring, most patients require an arterial line and central line for monitoring. Measurement of preductal and postductal oxygen saturations is helpful to assess the degree of right-to-left shunting.

4. All but the most stable patients are intubated and ventilated before surgery. Anesthesia in these cases usually consists of an analgesic such as fentanyl, an amnestic, and varying amounts of volatile anesthetics depending on patient stability.

5. Care must be taken when ventilating these patients because of

the risk of contralateral pneumothorax, which must be recognized and treated immediately.

6. In the most severe cases, the procedure may need to be performed while the patient is breathing nitric oxide or on ECMO.

C. Patent ductus arteriosus ligation

1. Anesthesia usually consists of an opioid analgesic (generally fentanyl) and an amnestic, such as midazolam or lorazepam.

2. During the procedure, compression of the left lung is unavoidable. Therefore, periods of desaturation often must be tolerated to finish the ligation, but the response to bradycardia should be reinflation of the lung to improve gas exchange.

3. During the procedure, a thin stethoscope is often placed on the right side of the chest to monitor breath sounds from the lung not compressed by the surgery and to confirm that the PDA murmur disappears once the duct is ligated.

4. Hypotension is frequent during the ligation and should be treated with 10–15 mL/kg 5% albumin. Dopamine (5–10 μg/kg/min) may also be required.

5. Before closing the incision, the surgeon is encouraged to perform multilevel intercostal nerve blocks to provide postoperative analgesia.

D. Omphalocele

1. Paralytic ileus in the majority of patients places them at risk for aspiration. A nasogastric tube should be suctioned prior to a rapid sequence induction using thiopental or ketamine with succinylcholine.

2. Anesthetic maintenance may be achieved with opioids and inhalational agents.

3. Evaporative fluid loss (10–20 mL/kg/h) and heat loss should be expected because of the exposed gut. Volume should be replaced with 5% albumin and crystalloid. The room should be warmed and convection heating used to keep the baby warm.

4. Closing a minor defect or tenting a larger defect should be uneventful. Closure of a large defect, however, may lead to hemodynamic and respiratory compromise. Additionally, because of pressure on the liver and kidneys, function of these organs may be impaired. Clearance of drugs may be diminished and/or oliguria or anuria may occur. Dopamine may be required, and in some cases the surgeons may need to change their plan to a less aggressive one.

Suggested Reading

Anand KJ, Brown MJ, Causon RC, et al: Can the human newborn mount an endocrine and metabolic response to surgery? J Pediatr Surg 20:41–48, 1985.

Bikhazi GB, Davis PJ: Anesthesia for newborns and premature infants. In Motoyama EK, Davis PJ (eds): Smith's Anesthesia for Infants and Children. St. Louis, Mosby, 1996, pp 445–474.

Coté CJ, Zaslavsky A, Downes JJ, et al: Postoperative apnea in former preterm infants after inguinal herniorrhaphy: A combined analysis. Anesthesiology 82:809–822, 1995.

Crone RK, Sorensen GK, Orr RJ: Anaesthesia for the newborn. Can J Anaesth 38:R105–R125, 1991.

Lerman J, Sikich N, Kleinman S, Yentis S: The pharmacology of sevoflurane in infants and children. Anesthesiology 80:814–824, 1994.

Lönnqvist PA: Management of the newborn: Anesthetic considerations and postoperative management. In Bissonnette B, Dalens B (eds): Pediatric Anesthesia: Principles and Practice. New York, McGraw-Hill, 2002, pp 995–1030.

Lönnqvist PA: Successful use of laryngeal mask airway in low-weight ex-premature infants undergoing cryotherapy for retinopathy of the premature. Anesthesiology 83:422–424, 1995.

Malviya S, Swartz J, Lerman J: Are all preterm infants younger than 60 weeks postconceptual age at risk for postanesthetic apnea? Anesthesiology 78:1076–1081, 1993.

Morray JP, Geiduschek JM, Ramamoorthy C, et al: Anesthesia-related cardiac arrest in children: Initial findings of the Pediatric Perioperative Cardiac Arrest (POCA) Registry. Anesthesiology 93:6–14, 2000.

Chapter 76

Surgical Emergencies

Ronald B. Hirschl, M.D., and Steven M. Donn, M.D.

In addition to congenital diaphragmatic hernia (*see* Chapter 77), a number of other neonatal surgical emergencies may be encountered in the delivery room or other locations.

I. **Esophageal Atresia (EA) with or without Tracheoesophageal Fistula (TEF)**
   A. Incidence
      1. Approximately 1/4500 live births
      2. Usually sporadic, although familial or sibling cases reported
      3. Often associated with multiple anomalies
   B. Anatomic types (combinations of EA and TEF)
      1. Esophageal atresia and distal TEF (87%)
      2. Isolated esophageal atresia (7%)
      3. H-type TEF only (4%)
      4. Esophageal atresia and proximal TEF (1%)
      5. Esophageal atresia and proximal and distal TEF (1%)
   C. VATER (VACTERL) association
      1. *V*ertebral
      2. *A*nal (imperforate anus)
      3. *C*ardiac
      4. *T*racheo-
      5. *E*sophageal
      6. *R*enal
      7. *L*imb (radial) dysplasia
   D. Clinical manifestations
      1. Polyhydramnios with esophageal atresia
      2. Copious secretions, coughing, choking
      3. Intermittent cyanosis
      4. Abdominal distention with TEF
      5. Recurrent gastroesophageal reflux (GE) and aspiration
   E. Diagnosis
      1. Requires high clinical suspicion
      2. Esophageal atresia
         a. Inability to pass orogastric tube

      b. Plain radiography with simultaneous injection of 10 mL air into proximal pouch, *or*

      c. "Pouch-o-gram" to rule out proximal pouch fistula (contrast study; be careful to avoid contrast aspiration)

   3. H-type fistula—bronchoscopy/esophagoscopy

F. Preoperative management

   1. Position patient upright at 30° angle.

   2. Suction catheter (Replogle) to upper pouch.

   3. Frequent airway suctioning

   4. Respiratory support as needed (avoid intubation if possible)

   5. Antibiotics

   6. Echocardiogram to evaluate for CHD and to identify side of aortic arch

   7. Renal sonography if indicated

G. Surgical management

   1. Esophageal atresia with distal TEF

      a. Preoperative management

         i. Cardiac echocardiogram

         ii. Proximal pouch continuous suction

         iii. Head of bed elevated 30°

      b. Delay in primary repair should be considered under the following circumstances:

         i. Life-threatening anomalies

         ii. Weight < 1.5 kg

         iii. Significant respiratory compromise

      c. Operation

         i. Posterolateral thoracotomy on side opposite aortic arch

         ii. Fistula ligation

         iii. Esophagoesophagostomy

      d. Delayed primary repair (days to weeks) under the following circumstances:

         i. Prematurity

         ii. Pneumonia

         iii. Life-threatening anomaly, typically cardiac

         iv. Clinical deterioration prior to repair

            (a) Preliminary decompressive and feeding gastrostomy

            (b) Proximal pouch suction (Replogle)

      e. TEF and RDS

         i. Infants with TEF and RDS and severely compromised pulmonary compliance may be difficult to ventilate. Delivered gas will take path of least resistance, through

TEF and into stomach or gastrostomy tube, limiting pulmonary gas exchange.

   ii. Management

     (a) Place gastrostomy tube to underwater seal.

     (b) High-frequency jet ventilation

     (c) Insertion of Fogarty balloon catheter to occlude fistula

     (d) Consider early fistula ligation.

2. Pure esophageal atresia

  a. Preoperative management (3–12 weeks)

    i. Gastrostomy tube placement

    ii. Proximal pouch continuous suction (Replogle)

    iii. Daily dilation of proximal pouch

    iv. Weekly assessment of proximal and distal pouch growth under fluoroscopy starting at 3 weeks post-gastrostomy tube placement

    v. Preoperative proximal pouch contrast study

  b. Intraoperative management

    i. Esophagoesophagostomy preferred

     (a) Stomach may be mobilized into chest if necessary.

     (b) Incision of muscularis (myotomy) may increase length.

    ii. Cervical esophagostomy

     (a) Proximal pouch brought out on left neck

     (b) G-tube, sham oral feeds

     (c) Will require eventual esophageal replacement with stomach, colon, small bowel

3. Isolated *H* or *N* type TEF intraoperative management

  a. Bronchoscopy with placement of Fogarty balloon catheter through the fistula

  b. Fistula ligation, usually via cervical approach

H. Postoperative care

1. Assisted ventilatory management as required. *Reintubation and endotracheal tube manipulation should be performed with extreme care.*

2. Frequent suctioning of posterior pharynx, *proximal to esophageal anastomosis only*

3. Parenteral nutrition

4. Gastrostomy or NG/OG feeding after return of GI function

5. Antibiotics

6. Maintain chest tube until barium study rules out leak (7 days).

7. Oral feedings initiated and chest tube removed after leak is ruled out
8. Evaluate VACTERL with spine films, sacral sonography (rule out tethered cord), abdominal sonography, echocardiography
9. Maintain head of bed at 45° angle, neck flexed slightly. *Do not extend head because it places tension on the esophageal anastomosis.*

I. Prognosis
  1. Success and survival factors
     a. Severe pulmonary dysfunction with preoperative ventilator dependence
     b. Associated major anomalies
  2. No major or life-threatening anomalies, *not* ventilator dependent = 93%
  3. Severe associated anomalies, preoperative ventilator dependence = 31% survival

J. Complications
  1. Anastomotic
     a. Disruption (2–3%)
        i. Mediastinitis
        ii. Requires operation—repair can sometimes be performed; most frequently requires formation of cervical esophagostomy and gastrostomy tube placement.
        iii. If esophagostomy performed, may reconstruct esophagus with stomach, colon, small bowel at > 6 months of age
     b. Small anastomotic leak (15%)
        i. Maintain NPO, parenteral nutrition
        ii. Leave chest tube in place
        iii. Most will resolve
     c. Recurrent TEF
        i. Requires operation
        ii. Bronchoscopy with placement of catheter across fistula
        iii. Ligation of fistula with pericardial patch reinforcement of closure
  2. Esophageal strictures (15%)
     a. Usually observed at 2–6 weeks
     b. Require repeated dilation
     c. May result from GE reflux
     d. Rarely require resection
  3. Respiratory
     a. Tracheomalacia
        i. Respiratory stridor

    ii. Bark with cough
   b. Bronchospastic airways
   c. Symptoms may result from GE reflux
  4. GE reflux (70%)
   a. Recurrent pneumonia
   b. Increasing respiratory dysfunction/"asthma"
   c. Vomiting
   d. Failure to thrive
   e. Esophageal strictures
   f. May require fundoplication (20%)

II. The Acute Abdomen

 A. General clinical manifestations
  1. Bilious vomiting
  2. Abdominal distention (increased with distal bowel obstruction)
  3. Lethargy
  4. Irritability
  5. Failure to tolerate feedings
  6. Failure to pass meconium
 B. Additional physical findings
  1. Tenderness
  2. Discoloration, edema, or erythema of abdominal wall
 C. Other nonspecific indicators of abdominal disease
  1. Septic appearance
  2. Apnea, bradycardia
  3. Thrombocytopenia
  4. Temperature instability
  5. Abnormal leukocyte count
 D. Gastrointestinal obstruction
  1. Gastric web
  2. Acute gastric volvulus
  3. Pyloric stenosis or atresia
  4. Duodenal obstruction
   a. Complete
     i. Atresia with gap
    ii. Web
    iii. Annular pancreas
   b. Incomplete
     i. Diaphragm with perforation
    ii. Stenosis
    iii. Prepyloric vein
  5. Malrotation

      a. Ladd's bands
      b. Volvulus
   6. Jejunal or ileal atresia
   7. Meconium ileus
   8. Colonic atresia (rare)
   9. Hirschsprung's disease
  10. Imperforate anus
  11. Incarcerated inguinal hernia
  12. Intussusception

E. Acute visceral perforation
   1. Manifestations
      a. Free intraperitoneal air
      b. Localized abscess (unusual)
      c. Abdominal distention
      d. Abdominal wall discoloration or erythema
      e. Generalized peritonitis
      f. Generalized sepsis
   2. Etiologies
      a. Complication of other condition
         i. Atresia
        ii. Meconium ileus
       iii. Malrotation
      b. NEC
      c. Iatrogenic perforation
      d. Spontaneous perforation

F. Evaluation
   1. Physical examination
   2. Laboratory
      a. CBC, differential, platelets
      b. Serum electrolytes, BUN, creatinine, glucose, bicarbonate
      c. Coagulation studies (with bleeding or profound sepsis)
      d. Blood gases
   3. Radiographic studies
      a. Plain radiographs of chest, abdomen—free air, dilated/fixed bowel loops, portal venous air
      b. Cross-table lateral and/or left lateral decubitus views of abdomen—free air
      c. Upper/lower gastrointestinal contrast studies if indicated (no barium if perforation suspected)

G. Acute management
   1. NPO, NG/OG decompression
   2. Establish vascular access.

3. Basic resuscitative measures (fluid, blood)
4. Support hemodynamic status.
5. Respiratory support as necessary
6. Monitor urinary output.
7. Antibiotics
8. Immediate surgical consultation

III. Abdominal Wall Defects

A. Gastroschisis

1. Anomaly consists of a 2–3 cm full-thickness defect with herniation of variable amount of uncovered intestine, stomach, fallopian tubes, ovaries, or testes. Liver is normally positioned. Defect is almost always to the right and adjacent to the umbilical cord.
2. Features
   a. Normal umbilical cord
   b. No sac or remnant of peritoneum
   c. Bowel is thick, edematous, and matted.
   d. Intestine shorter than normal, nonrotated
3. Incidence: 1/3000–1/8000 live births
4. Associated anomalies are rare except for bowel atresia (10%).

B. Omphalocele/hernia of the umbilical cord

1. Anomaly consists of a defect of the abdominal wall fascia with herniation of varying amounts of abdominal viscera (including liver) into a translucent sac composed of amnion and peritoneum. Hernia of the umbilical cord if < 4 cm; omphalocele if ≥ 4 cm.
2. Features
   a. Umbilical cord is attached to sac.
   b. Sac is always present; may be ruptured.
   c. Size of defect and sac determine degree of herniation.
   d. Intestine is generally nonrotated, but otherwise normal.
3. Incidence: 1/6000–1/10,000 live births
4. Associated anomalies frequent (50–60%)
   a. Cardiac
   b. Neurologic
   c. Genitourinary
   d. Skeletal
   e. Chromosomal
   f. Beckwith-Wiedemann syndrome
   g. Other gastrointestinal
      i. Malrotation
      ii. Meckel's diverticulum

      iii. Intestinal atresia

      iv. Diaphragmatic hernia

C. Acute management

  1. Place 10-F gastric sump catheter and aspirate stomach.

  2. Wrap herniated viscera with warm saline-soaked gauze and place legs/abdomen in plastic bag (bowel bag) to prevent fluid and heat loss.

  3. For gastroschisis, support intestine on top of abdomen to avoid loops hanging over edge of defect, which may compromise venous drainage and induce bowel edema.

  4. Consider placement of spring-loaded preformed silo if available.

  5. Secure vascular access.

  6. Support hemodynamic status; large volumes of fluid may be necessary (2–4 times basal requirements) if viscera are exposed.

  7. Respiratory support as needed

  8. Broad-spectrum antibiotics

  9. Rule out coexisting anomalies.

D. Other defects

  1. Exstrophy of the bladder

    a. Incidence: 1/10,000–1/50,000 live births

    b. Rare associated anomalies

  2. Cloacal exstrophy

    a. Incidence: 1/400,000 live births

    b. Includes multiple anomalies

      i. Omphalocele

      ii. Genital deformities

      iii. Musculoskeletal

      iv. Anorectal

      v. Neural tube

      vi. Chromosomal

    c. Gender reassignment may be necessary. Many issues discussed in Chapter 84, Ambiguous Genitalia, are pertinent and should be reviewed vis-a-vis the psychosocial emergency of this situation.

Suggested Reading

Coran AG: Esophageal atresia and tracheoesophageal fistula. In Donn SM, Faix RG (eds): Neonatal Emergencies. Mt. Kisco, NY, Futura Publishing 1991, pp 515–528.

Donn SM, Zak LK, Bozynski ME, et al: Use of high-frequency jet ventilation in the management of congenital tracheoesophageal fistula associated with respiratory distress syndrome. J Pediatr Surg 25:1219–1221, 1990.

Hirschl RB: Intestinal obstruction in the neonate. In Burg FD, Gershon A, Polin RA, Ingelfinger JR (eds): Current Pediatric Therapy, 14th ed. St. Louis, Mosby, 1996, pp 213–217.

Polley TZ: The acute abdomen. In Donn SM, Faix RG (eds): Neonatal Emergencies. Mt. Kisco, NY, Futura Publishing, 1991, pp 529–550.

Wesley JR: Abdominal wall defects. In Donn SM, Faix RG (eds): Neonatal Emergencies. Mt. Kisco, NY, Futura Publishing, 1991, pp 551–568.

Chapter 77

Congenital Diaphragmatic Hernia

*Ronald B. Hirschl, M.D., Oliver S. Soldes, M.D.,
and Robert E. Schumacher, M.D.*

I. Description

Congenital diaphragmatic hernia (CDH) is a defect in the diaphragm that allows the abdominal viscera to migrate into the chest. Diaphragmatic hernias occur in three locations: posterolateral (Bochdalek), retrosternal (Morgagni), and at the esophageal hiatus. The term CDH is generally used to refer to Bochdalek hernias. Bochdalek CDH should be suspected in infants with severe respiratory distress shortly after birth.

II. Epidemiology

A. The incidence of CDH is estimated to be 1 in 2200–5000 live births.

B. Mortality rates are generally high nationally (37%). Early survival has increased to as much as $\pm$ 80% with the use of lung-protective ventilation strategies, ECMO, and delayed repair at selected centers.

C. The etiology of CDH unknown. Females are affected twice as often as males. Most cases occur sporadically. CDH may be associated with other anomalies (up to 39%), most commonly congenital heart defects. Congenital heart disease and prematurity significantly increase the risk of mortality.

III. Embryology and Anatomy

A. Failure of closure of the pleuroperitoneal canals results in CDH. Visceral herniation into the chest produces pulmonary hypoplasia.

B. Bochdalek hernias account for 85–90% of neonatal CDH and are associated with respiratory failure. The left diaphragm is most often involved (80–90% of posterolateral CDH).

C. The ipsilateral lung and sometimes the contralateral lungs are hypoplastic. The number of bronchial divisions and alveoli is reduced. The pulmonary vessels have a significantly increased muscle mass and vasoreactivity.

IV. Pathophysiology

A. Pulmonary hypoplasia and persistent pulmonary hypertension of the newborn (PPHN) result in hypercarbia, hypoxia, and acidosis.

B. The pulmonary vasoreactivity causes episodic exacerbations of existing pulmonary hypertension and worsening right-to-left shunting, diminished cardiac output, hypoxia, and acidosis.

C. Newborns with CDH have small, immature lungs with limited gas exchange resulting in hypoventilation. A surfactant deficiency may exist, but replacement therapy has not proven beneficial.

V. Presentation and Diagnosis

A. Early diagnosis is critical for a successful outcome. Antenatal diagnosis is now common, allowing a planned delivery at a center equipped to manage these patients (e.g., an ECMO center).

B. Classically, infants with Bochdalek CDH present with acute respiratory distress shortly after birth. However, they can present with a wide range of severity, from asymptomatic to profound respiratory failure. Other physical findings include:

1. Diminished breath sounds on the affected side
2. A scaphoid or flat abdomen
3. Displaced heart sounds and point of maximum intensity (PMI) of cardiac pulsations
4. Bowel sounds in the chest

C. The diagnosis is usually established radiographically. Findings include:

1. A bowel gas pattern in the thorax on the affected side
2. The NG/OG tube may be above the diaphragm.
3. Displacement of the heart away from the affected side
4. Opacification of the hemithorax with displacement of the heart is a less frequent mode of presentation.
5. CDH may mimic other conditions such as an intrathoracic stomach, pleural effusion, congenital lobar hyperinflation, diaphragmatic eventration, or congenital cystic adenomatoid malformation of the lung.
6. Umbilical venous catheter may be displaced toward the affected side with a left-sided CDH.

D. Infants with Morgagni and hiatal hernia usually present after the immediate newborn period with gastrointestinal signs.

VI. Management

A. The focus of clinical management has shifted from emergent surgical repair to medical stabilization, followed by delayed primary repair of the CDH.

B. Initial steps to take after diagnosis:

1. Minimize bag-mask ventilation to reduce gaseous distention of

the bowel. Intubate the infant if assisted ventilation is needed. Place an orogastric or nasogastric tube to decompress the intestine.

2. Place arterial and central venous catheters for monitoring and medication administration. Pre- and postductal pulse oximeters (right arm and left leg) are desirable to assess the degree of shunting.

3. Urine output should be checked frequently as one index of organ perfusion.

4. An oxygen-enriched environment should be provided and blood gas values and evidence of PPHN checked frequently.

5. A neutral thermal environment should be provided to help minimize oxygen requirements. Stimulation should be minimized to avoid precipitating episodic worsening of pulmonary hypertension.

6. Intravenous fluids providing 10% glucose should be given pre- and postoperatively at a maintenance rate. Meticulous attention to fluid and electrolyte balance is essential.

7. Be aware of the high risk for pneumothorax in the contralateral lung. Chest tubes are placed therapeutically for pneumothorax and should be connected to suction.

C. Ventilator management should be directed toward minimizing barotrauma while maintaining reasonable gas exchange parameters (pH > 7.2, preductal saturation $\geq 90\%$, $PaO_2 > 50$ mmHg). A strategy of permissive hypercapnia, spontaneous respiration, and elective surgical repair has been used with variable success.

D. Pressors are frequently required to support the blood pressure and perfusion. Dopamine is usually the first-line agent. Dobutamine may be added if increased support is required.

E. Anemia should be avoided, and blood transfusions may be necessary to maintain an adequate oxygen delivery carrying capacity, particularly in infants on ECMO and postoperatively.

F. The timing of repair of CDH may be subdivided into three categories: **immediate** operation (< 24 hours), **delayed** operation (24–72 hr), and **very delayed** operation (> 72 hr). The effect of survival of a delayed approach has not been definitively demonstrated. It is known that there is no detrimental effect of delayed repair. There is a trend toward improved survival, reduced ECMO utilization, and reduced morbidity with a very delayed approach. In general, surgical correction should be undertaken when a child is physiologically stable and ventilator support has been weaned as much as possible.

G. Third space fluid and electrolyte losses into the chest and abdomen increase intraoperative and postoperative fluid requirements. Be prepared to administer fluids judiciously to the infant with CDH to maintain ventricular filling pressures during and after operation.

H. Postoperative management

1. Inotropic therapy should be instituted early, possibly routinely.
2. The degree of ductal shunting is followed by monitoring pre- and postductal SaO_2.
3. Chest tubes may or may not be used. If a chest tube is placed on the ipsilateral side, it should be left connected to water seal, not suction. Expect a pneumothorax or hydropneumothorax on chest x-rays in the immediate postoperative period. The hypoplastic lung will not fill the entire hemithorax after reduction and repair of the CDH. Contralateral chest tubes are not necessary unless a pneumothorax exists.

I. Treatment of PPHN consists of efforts to ensure adequate ventilation and to maximize pulmonary blood flow. Deliberate hyperventilation or systemic alkalinization is discouraged because of associated lung injury and other adverse effects upon cardiopulmonary physiology. High-frequency oscillatory ventilation may be a useful adjunct in selected cases.

J. Pharmacologic therapy for PPHN with intravenous vasodilating agents (e.g., tolazoline, prostanoids) in infants with CDH has had only modest success and is now infrequently used. Inhaled nitric oxide (NO) may lower pulmonary vascular resistance and improve oxygenation. However, NO has failed to improve survival or reduce the need for ECMO in patients with CDH.

K. Surfactant may be deficient in patients with CDH. However, limited clinical data have failed to demonstrate the efficacy of surfactant replacement therapy in infants with CDH.

L. Long-term problems in children with CDH include symptomatic gastroesophageal reflux, feeding difficulties, adhesive bowel obstruction, scoliosis, pectus excavatum, and recurrent diaphragmatic hernia.

M. Innovative approaches

1. The use ECMO is one therapeutic regimen that has altered the mortality rate in infants with CDH.
2. Fetal tracheal occlusion in high-risk fetuses with CDH may produce lung growth and possibly improved survival. Repair of the CDH *in utero* does not improve outcome.
3. Lobar lung transplantation has been tried.

Suggested Reading

Boloker J, Bateman DA, Wung JT, Stolar CJ: Congenital diaphragmatic hernia in 120 infants treated consecutively with permissive hypercapnia/spontaneous respiration/elective repair. J Pediatr Surg 37:357–366, 2002.

Greenholz SK: Congenital diaphragmatic hernia: An overview. Semin Pediatr Surg 5:216–223, 1996.

Hirschl RB: Innovative therapies in the management of newborns with congenital diaphragmatic hernia. Semin Pediatr Surg 5:256–265, 1996.

Nakayama DK: Congenital diaphragmatic hernia. In Nakayama DK, Bose CL, Chescheir NC, et al (eds): Critical Care of the Surgical Newborn. Armonk, NY, Futura Publishing, 1997, pp 173–201.

The Neonatal Inhaled Nitric Oxide Study Group (NINOS): Inhaled nitric oxide and hypoxic respiratory failure in infants with congenital diaphragmatic hernia. Pediatrics 99:838–845, 1997.

Chapter 78

Meconium Aspiration Syndrome

Robert E. Schumacher, M.D., and Steven M. Donn, M.D.

I.   Pathophysiology

A. The passage of meconium *in utero* may occur as a result of hypoxic stimulation of peristalsis followed by hypoxic relaxation of the anal sphincter. Passage of meconium may also be a normal physiologic event associated with increased fetal maturity and increasing concentrations of the hormone motilin.

B. Intrauterine meconium aspiration may occur when hypoxia and acidosis stimulate deep gasping and relaxation of the glottic sphincter. Animal models of chronic uterine ischemia and oligohydramnios demonstrate "aspiration" of amniotic fluid with normal fetal breathing movements. Further, meconium in the pharynx can be aspirated at birth with the onset of respirations.

C. Among all infants with meconium-stained liquor, infants with evidence of intrauterine asphyxia are at the greatest risk of developing meconium aspiration syndrome (MAS).

D. If not removed from the airways, meconium can produce problems secondary to air trapping and atelectasis. This results in a mixture of overdistention (high lung volumes) and atelectasis (low lung volumes). Air leaks can occur. Following aspiration, inflammation and pneumonitis can ensue. MAS may be associated with persistent pulmonary hypertension, especially in asphyxiated infants.

II.   Diagnosis

A. History of meconium-stained amniotic fluid

B. Presence of meconium in the trachea

C. Subsequent respiratory distress

D. Chest radiograph (hyperinflation and patchy or fluffy infiltrates)

III.   Associations

A. Signs of postmaturity or dysmaturity (e.g., thin cord, muscle and fat wasting, peeling skin, SGA)

B. Meconium staining of skin, nails, and umbilical cord

C. Other systemic consequences of asphyxia (e.g., acute tubular necrosis, hypoxic-ischemic encephalopathy, transient myocardial ischemia)

IV. Differential Diagnosis

A. Transient tachypnea of the newborn after tracheal suctioning of meconium

B. Congenital respiratory or cardiac malformation with coincident meconium staining

C. Bacterial sepsis or pneumonia (increased incidence in MAS)

V. Management

The presence of meconium in the amniotic fluid should increase suspicion of fetal distress and lead to closer fetal monitoring. The individual responsible for the infant should not simultaneously be responsible for the mother's care, because airway management and possibly resuscitation of an asphyxiated infant may be needed.

A. Preventive airway management at delivery

1. Thorough obstetric suctioning of the infant's mouth and pharynx before shoulders are delivered with DeLee mucus trap attached to suction, 10–12-F catheter suction, or bulb syringe. However, this practice has been recently questioned.

2. Guidelines for delivery room management of the infant

   a. An individual skilled in management of the infant airway should be immediately available at deliveries in which there is meconium-stained amniotic fluid.

   b. If the infant appears vigorous (strong respiratory efforts, good muscle tone, and heart rate > 100 bpm), endotracheal suctioning is not routinely indicated.

   c. If the infant is not vigorous, laryngoscopy and intubation should be done, and the mouth and trachea should be suctioned prior to the institution of positive pressure.

   e. If meconium is still retrievable after multiple passes, consider leaving the endotracheal tube in for continued airway management.

3. Endotracheal suction pointers

   a. Use largest size ETT, usually 3.5- or 4-mm internal diameter in term infant.

   b. Withdraw ETT with continuous application of suction (maximum suction: -100 cm H_2O). Suction tubing may be attached to ETT connector by a commercially available adapter; alternatively, modified ETTs with an integrated suction adapter are available commercially. ***Do not*** apply direct mouth suction to ETT as was done in the past.

   c. *Resist* the temptation to begin immediate ventilation prior to suctioning of the profoundly asphyxiated infant who is meconium stained. However, do not delay positive pressure ventilation of the depressed infant once the airway has been cleared. If meconium is recovered, continue to check the heart rate. With significant bradycardia, positive pressure may be administered without repeating the procedure.

   f. Laryngoscopy and intubation may cause reflex bradycardia. This usually responds to ventilation and oxygen.

4. Some delivery room personnel and parents may voice concerns about "needless" intubation of a seemingly "normal" infant. These concerns can generally be allayed by an explanation beforehand of the reasons for the procedure and the serious consequences of MAS.

B. Subsequent management

1. If respiratory distress (e.g., tachypnea, retractions, grunting, cyanosis) follows aspiration of meconium from the trachea, admit infant to a level II or level III nursery for continuous nursing observation with cardiorespiratory and noninvasive oxygen monitoring. Handling should be minimized, because it tends to produce episodes of desaturation.

2. Except in the mildest cases, a blood gas study and a chest radiograph should be ordered (early film is most useful to rule out other diagnoses, e.g., air leaks, rather than making a positive diagnosis of MAS).

3. Supply generous oxygen supplementation: keep PaO_2 or $TCPO_2$ 60–70 mmHg or $SaO_2 > 95\%$. However, beware of false sense of security when need for O_2 or $PaCO_2$ is rising!

4. Consider obtaining arterial access if $FiO_2 \geq 0.4$, because arterial punctures cause significant desaturation episodes.

5. Institute positive pressure ventilation for rising $PaCO_2$ (> 50 mmHg) or need for high FiO_2 (e.g., ≥ 0.6) to maintain oxygenation.

6. Ventilator strategy—initially, deal with high expiratory resistance and often normal compliance, (e.g., tendency to air-trap). This includes short inspiratory time and an adequate expiratory time to produce selective ventilation of low resistance lung units. If pneumonitis develops (lower compliance), strategy may change to include higher PEEP.

7. Artificial surfactant as a bolus therapy has been studied and probably may prevent the need for ECMO. Artificial surfactant as a lavage is under investigation. Both procedures are still unapproved for clinical practice.

8. Consider sedation or pharmacologic paralysis if infant is

worsening his or her own condition by agitation. Higher pressures or rates may be necessary after paralysis.

9. Consider drawing blood culture and instituting broad-spectrum antibiotics (e.g., ampicillin and gentamicin).

10. If practicing in a level II setting, have a low threshold for transfer to a level III unit. Warning signs include dusky spells with handling, rising $PaCO_2$, and rising O_2 need ($FiO_2 \geq 0.5$).

Suggested Reading

Halliday HL: Endotracheal intubation at birth for preventing morbidity and mortality in vigorous, meconium-stained infants born at term. Cochrane Database of Systematic Reviews [Computer File] (2):CD000500, 2000.

Niermeyer S, Kattwinkel J, Van Reempts P, et al: International guidelines for neonatal resuscitation: An excerpt from the guidelines 2000 for cardiopulmonary resuscitation and emergency cardiovascular care. International Consensus on Science. Contributors and Reviewers for the Neonatal Resuscitation Guidelines. Pediatrics 106:E29, 2000.

Wiswell TE, Gannon CM, Jacob J, et al: Delivery room management of the apparently vigorous meconium-stained neonate: Results of the multi-center, international collaborative trial. Pediatrics 105:1–7, 2000.

Wiswell TE: Handling the meconium-stained infant. Semin Neonatol 6:225–231, 2001.

Persistent Pulmonary Hypertension of the Newborn

Robert E. Schumacher, M.D., and Steven M. Donn, M.D.

I. Definition

Persistent pulmonary hypertension of the newborn (PPHN) is a condition in which there is high pulmonary vascular resistance and variable right-to-left shunting through a patent foramen ovale or ductus arteriosus, resulting in arterial hypoxemia.

II. Normal Pulmonary Vascular Development

A. Most alveoli develop after birth; thus the newborn's intra-acinar blood vessels also develop after birth. The newborn has a decreased cross-sectional area available for pulmonary blood flow, and vascular resistance is high.

B. The newborn's pulmonary vascular smooth muscle development does not fully extend to the level of the alveolus, but when smooth muscle is present there is often medial thickening relative to that seen in the adult. Increased muscular development occurs near term; hence, PPHN is not as common in the preterm infant.

C. At term, pulmonary vascular resistance is relatively high. When measured at birth, the term newborn's pulmonary artery pressure is at approximately systemic levels.

D. At or near term, the pulmonary vasculature is sensitive to a number of stimuli, including oxygen, carbon dioxide, and pH. Hypoxia, hypercarbia, and acidosis may trigger vasoconstriction and increased pulmonary vascular resistance. This can interfere with the normal transition from intrauterine to extrauterine circulation.

III. Pathogenesis: Three Basic Mechanisms with Some Overlap

A. Normal pulmonary vascular morphology with myocardial dysfunction or increased reactivity of the vasculature to vasoconstrictive stimuli

   1. Associated with asphyxia

      a. Hypoxia or acidosis may lead to pulmonary vasoconstriction and increased pulmonary vascular resistance.

      b. Left ventricular myocardial dysfunction from asphyxia may cause pulmonary venous hypertension and subsequent pulmonary arterial hypertension with right-to-left ductal shunting. When cardiac function improves, so does the PPHN.

2. Meconium aspiration syndrome

   a. An appropriate response to alveolar hypoxia is vasoconstriction. This can present a major diagnostic problem in differentiating the relative contributions of severe pulmonary disease vs. PPHN to ongoing hypoxemia.

   b. Some infants with MAS also may have anatomic pulmonary vascular changes (see below).

3. Sepsis and pneumonia

   Release of vasoactive substances by bacteria (particularly group B streptococci) and possibly by granulocytes increases pulmonary vascular resistance.

4. Thrombus or microthrombus formation with release of vasoactive substances

B. Anatomically abnormal pulmonary vasculature

1. An abnormal extension of the vascular smooth muscle, so that it is thickened and reaches more distal vessels in the pulmonary vascular tree, resulting in increased resistance

   a. Idiopathic PPHN (chronic hypoxia *in utero?*)

   b. Meconium aspiration syndrome (some cases)

   c. Premature closure (*in utero*) of the ductus arteriosus

2. Decreased cross-sectional area of the pulmonary vascular bed secondary to abnormally small lungs *along with* marked thickening and abnormal distal extension of the pulmonary vascular smooth muscle

   a. Congenital diaphragmatic hernia

   b. Congenital cystic adenomatoid malformation

   c. Pulmonary hypoplasia—primary, or secondary to oligohydramnios

C. Structural congenital heart disease (CHD)—this is usually considered a separate category.

1. Anomalous pulmonary venous return

2. Myopathic left ventricular disease

3. Left ventricular outflow obstruction

4. Any structural abnormality resulting in obligate right-to-left shunting

5. Ebstein's anomaly

IV. Diagnosis

The differential diagnosis of hypoxemia in the full-term infant includes primary pulmonary disease, cyanotic CHD, and PPHN. Pulmonary disease and PPHN can often coexist. Determining which is the primary problem is frequently difficult but is of paramount importance.

A. Baseline data, similar to that obtained for any sick newborn, may be useful:

1. History—maternal fever or possible infection, meconium staining, postdatism, IUGR, maternal aspirin ingestion
2. Physical examination—no specific physical findings confirm the diagnosis of PPHN, but many will suggest other specific diagnoses that, early on, may mimic PPHN (e.g., the hypoxemic infant with decreased breath sounds unilaterally from a tension pneumothorax).
3. Chest radiograph—no specific findings confirm the diagnosis of PPHN; it is most useful for suggesting or excluding other diagnoses.
4. *Arterial* blood gas—low PaO_2 in the face of high FiO_2. Abnormal $PaCO_2$ and pH should be corrected before attributing hypoxia to possible PPHN.

B. Hyperoxia test

1. Place the infant in 1.0 FiO_2.
2. With pulmonary disease, the PaO_2 *should* increase. The PaO_2 *may* increase if PPHN is present but usually does not. If cyanotic heart disease is present, the PaO_2 *usually* does not increase.

C. Simultaneous pre- and postductal arterial blood gases

1. Obtain an ABG from the right radial artery (preductal) and umbilical artery catheter or posterior tibial artery (postductal) *simultaneously.*
2. A higher PaO_2 in right radial sample (20 mmHg difference) indicates some degree of right-to-left ductal shunting. If both values are high (> 100 mmHg), there is little or no shunting, and PPHN is unlikely *at that time,* despite a difference of ≥ 20 mmHg. If both values are low but essentially equal, the primary site of shunting may be via the foramen ovale and PPHN is *not* ruled out. This scenario is very common. A large difference when present is diagnostic of right-to-left ductal shunting.
3. The use of double site transcutaneous PO_2 or pulse oximetry values is helpful, especially if the gold standard blood gas values are not available.

D. Hyperoxia-hyperventilation test

Hypoxemia and acidosis cause pulmonary vasoconstriction. Alkalosis and increased blood oxygen can decrease pulmonary vascular resistance. By increasing minute ventilation, $PaCO_2$ falls and pH rises. This, often coupled with sodium bicarbonate infusion, markedly increases pH and may result in a dramatic rise in PaO_2. One must differentiate between an increase in PaO_2 secondary to increased mean airway pressure from that secondary to alkalosis. A dramatic increase along with extreme lability of the PaO_2 is more suggestive of PPHN.

   E. Cardiology consultation (echocardiography)
1. Rule out anatomic congenital heart disease.
2. Evaluate myocardial function.
3. May allow direct visualization of shunting using Doppler techniques, although the interpretation of this is semiquantitative.

V.   Treatment
   A. Prenatal
1. High-risk pregnancies (e.g., congenital diaphragmatic hernia, prolonged oligohydramnios) should be delivered at a tertiary center.
2. Identification and adequate management of other at-risk pregnancies, such as postdatism, maternal chorioamnionitis, and meconium-stained infants, are crucial.

   B. Postnatal—prevention is always the first step.
1. *Adequate resuscitation*
2. Avoid hypothermia, hypovolemia.
3. Avoid hypercarbia, acidosis, and hypoxia. Oxygen is an excellent pulmonary vasodilator.
4. Treat suspected sepsis, seizures, and electrolyte imbalances or other problems promptly.

   C. Make the diagnosis carefully by ruling out other clinically similar problems.

   D. General supportive measures
1. Use appropriate ventilatory modality and strategy.
2. Support systemic blood pressure (see below).
3. Maximize oxygen carrying capacity (e.g., maintain hematocrit $\geq 40\%$).
4. Treatment of underlying disorder
   a. Surfactant replacement, if deficient
   b. Antimicrobials, if indicated
   c. Alleviate mechanical problems (e.g., pneumothorax, pleural effusion, ascites)

   E. Mechanical ventilation
1. First ensure adequate *normal* ventilation and treat underlying pulmonary disease if present (e.g., drain pneumothorax, treat pneumonia, position ETT correctly).

2. If the diagnosis of PPHN is made, two diametrically opposite general ventilatory approaches exist; controlled studies on relative efficacies are lacking.

   a. *Alkalosis/hyperventilation* consists of achieving alkalosis by increased ventilation (decreased $PaCO_2$) and bicarbonate infusion. This leads to decreased pulmonary vascular resistance and markedly increased PaO_2. The use of muscle relaxants is common. Support is weaned *very* slowly.

   b. *Conservative ventilation* consists of the least necessary ventilation to achieve normal to slightly elevated $PaCO_2$ and PaO_2 of 45–70 mmHg. Use of muscle relaxants and sedatives is discouraged. Much lower pH is also tolerated.

   c. A modified approach that attempts to achieve reasonable blood gases using moderate ventilatory support is also acceptable.

3. With either approach, realize that these infants are *extremely labile* and that small changes in ventilatory support and FiO_2 are the rule. A transition phase is reached after 3–5 days when ventilatory support can be weaned more quickly.

F. Pharmacologic therapy

1. Ensure adequate cardiac output and blood pressure. Right-to-left shunting is dependent on the differential resistances between the pulmonary and the systemic circulations; thus, avoiding systemic hypotension is important. A CVP line may be helpful.

   a. Volume administration

   b. Cardiotonic drugs, including dopamine, dobutamine, and epinephrine

2. Sodium bicarbonate may be given initially as periodic boluses or as an infusion (≤ 1.0 mEq/hr) to help increase pH. Be careful of sodium and fluid overload.

3. Nitric oxide (NO; administered via inhalation in concentrations reported from 5 to 80 parts per million (*see* page 283)

G. Other therapy

1. High-frequency ventilation (*see* page 269)

2. Infants failing to respond to the above measures may be considered for extracorporeal membrane oxygenation (ECMO) (*see* page 286)

3. Follow-up—infants are generally at risk for problems.

   a. PPHN and focal seizures are associated with neonatal stroke.

   b. PPHN is associated with progressive hearing loss; serial follow-up is recommended.

Suggested Reading

Walsh MC, Stork EK: Persistent pulmonary hypertension of the newborn: Rational therapy based on pathophysiology. Clin Perinatol 28:609–627, 2001.

Chapter 80

Infant of Diabetic Mother

William M. Bellas, D.O., and Robert E. Schumacher, M.D.

I. **Incidence**

Diabetes mellitus is the most common medical complication of pregnancy, affecting 2–3% of pregnancies. Approximately 100,000 infant(s) of diabetic mothers (IDMs) are born in the United States each year, comprising 5% of all neonatal admissions. Insulin-dependent diabetes complicates 0.5% of all pregnancies. Better maternal control of glucose alters the incidence of nearly every IDM outcome. Point estimates of incidence vary tremendously. Familiarity with outcomes-associated local practice can guide care providers' behavior.

II. **Classification**

For the neonatal care provider, the most useful method for classifying the pregnant woman is to define the onset of carbohydrate intolerance (pregestational vs. gestational) and the requirement for exogenous insulin (insulin-dependent diabetes vs. non–insulin-dependent diabetes). A global estimate of "control" by the obstetric team should also prove helpful.

III. **Pathophysiology**

The developing embryo/fetus is exposed to an abnormal metabolic milieu. The impact on cellular growth and differentiation depends on when during gestation the onset of diabetes occurs.

    A. Pedersen hypothesis: maternal hyperglycemia causes high concentrations on glucose to cross the placenta. This stimulates the fetal pancreas to produce excessive insulin. Fetal insulin functions as a growth factor and may interfere with corticosteroid-stimulated pulmonary maturation.

    B. Altered metabolic fuels: maternal hyperglycemia, hyperketonemia, arachidonic acid deficiency, myoinositol deficiency, sorbitol accumulation, and free oxygen radicals may all contribute to diabetes-associated embryopathies.

IV. **Clinical Presentation**

    A. General: the classic appearance is usually that of a large ruddy, edematous, and flexed infant with round facies. Infrequently, a small-appearing newborn will subsequently be identified as an IDM. This scenario may suggest signs of a chronic *in utero* insult (e.g., placental insufficiency).

B. Macrosomia: incidence is reported in textbooks to be as high as 20–50%, but recent cohorts/series in the 1980s and 1990s show 14–28% with disproportionate (high ponderal index) macrosomia. Maternal HbA_{1C} does not accurately predict the occurrence of macrosomia. There is an increased risk for shoulder dystocia and resultant birth injuries, including fracture of the humerus or clavicle, cephalohematoma, subdural hemorrhage, Erb's palsy, and injury to abdominal viscera. Point estimates of risk of trauma in IDMs are approximately 1%.

C. Hypoglycemia: defined as serum glucose < 35 mg/dL in term newborns and < 25 mg/dL in preterm newborns. However, there are inherent problems with using this definition in clinical practice. First, blood glucose values do not measure glucose or "energy" delivery. Second, glucose screening tests are not as accurate as once thought. Consequently, there may be a large discrepancy between serum and whole blood glucose values. Depending on definition, hypoglycemia occurs in 2–40% of infants whose mothers required insulin. Good metabolic control lowers the risk. Serum glucose is usually lowest at 1–3 hours of age; it may present as lethargy, hypotonia, sweating, seizures, poor feeding, apnea, or jitters. However, severe hypoglycemia (< 10 mg/dL) frequently occurs without apparent signs.

D. Hypocalcemia: classic literature reports a high incidence (50%) of asymptomatic hypocalcemia, occasionally with hypomagnesemia (see below), secondary to suppressed fetal parathyroid function related to severity of maternal diabetes. Serum calcium reaches its nadir at 24–72 hours of age. Recent studies, controlled for gestational age and concurrent illness, show a lower incidence (5–18%) sometimes not significantly increased from controls.

E. Hypomagnesemia: this is a direct result of maternal magnesium deficiency, understood to be related to maternal diabetes severity and nephropathic losses of magnesium. Low serum levels of magnesium in the newborn alter calcium metabolism by way of the calcium-sensitive, magnesium-dependent adenylate cyclase system.

F. Respiratory distress syndrome (RDS): in the past, the incidence of RDS was increased in IDMs. Recent data suggest this is no longer true. Elective premature delivery by cesarean section without labor increases the risk of RDS. In animal models, hyperinsulinemia interferes with enzymes necessary for surfactant synthesis. The value of some amniotic fluid fetal lung maturity testing in IDMs, particularly the L/S ratio, has been questioned. Current data suggest that other tests, especially the presence of PG, accurately predict maturity.

G. Cardiomegaly: intraventricular septal thickening and increased left ventricular mass are common (28–50%), but symptomatic hypertrophic obstructive cardiomyopathy is now rare. Although hyperinsulinism seems related to hypertrophy, good metabolic control does not decrease the risk. It is usually a self-limited process and resolves without medical intervention.

H. Hyperbilirubinemia: the incidence varies in relation to maternal glucose control. The probable etiology is related to a secondary increase in RBC production mediated by the hyperinsulinemic state and subsequent hemolysis.

I. Polycythemia/hyperviscosity: recent studies report no greater risk than controls; however, it was previously reported in up to 13%. The etiology is still unclear; increased erythropoiesis and decreased RBC deformability probably play a role. Recent studies are looking at the effects of insulin growth factor and its role in erythroid progenitor cell stimulation. Thrombophilia, particularly renal vein thrombosis, may result.

J. Congenital malformations: these occur in pregestational diabetics as a result of the disordered metabolic milieu during organogenesis and account for the greatest proportion of morbidity and mortality. In many series, gestational diabetics do not have an increased risk. Increased risk can be mitigated by good metabolic control prior to conception. Studies have correlated HbA_{1C} levels $\geq 8\%$ with increasing malformation rates as high as 24%. Most common malformations include heart defects, neural tube and sacrococcygeal defects, renal anomalies, and small left colon syndrome. Many can be identified by ultrasound.

V. Management Guidelines

A. Delivery room: be aware of the increased incidence of preterm delivery (25%) and cesarean section. It is imperative to be fully prepared for cardiopulmonary resuscitation at birth because of the high risk of macrosomia and birth trauma. Make a rapid assessment for common congenital anomalies (e.g., cyanosis, neural tube defects, abdominal masses).

B. Fluids and electrolytes
  1. Hypoglycemia
    a. To prevent hypoglycemia, early and frequent feedings

(every 2–3 hr) with either formula or breast milk are recommended, while monitoring for signs of hypoglycemia by capillary glucose before feeding. If using standard formula (6.9 g CHO/100 mL), 7 mL/kg/hr is required to deliver 8 mg/kg/min of carbohydrate load. Observe closely for feeding intolerance (small left colon syndrome). If at additional risk, it may be prudent to begin an immediate IV infusion of $D_{10}W$ at 7–8 mg/kg/min (100–115 mL/kg/day) for poorly controlled, non–insulin-treated mother.

b. Bedside capillary glucose testing should be performed frequently. Reagent test strips often overestimate the incidence of hypoglycemia, particularly with concurrent polycythemia. Laboratory confirmation of reagent readings < 40 mg/dL should be obtained.

c. Treat initial symptomatic hypoglycemia (serum glucose < 40 mg/dL) with a 5 mL/kg IV bolus of $D_{10}W$ given over 20 min (500 mg/kg glucose). Repeat this therapy if low capillary glucose (CG) < 40 mg/dL after each mini-bolus. Once CG is ≥ 40 mg/dL immediately after mini-bolus therapy, IV therapy should be adjusted to 5 mL/kg/hr while checking CG every 30 min. After two successive CG ≥ 40 mg/dL, change frequency monitoring to every 2–4 hr.

  i. Subsequent CG ≥ 40 mg/dL
    (a) If able to oral/OG feed: attempt feeding at 2–3 hr intervals with CG before feeding. After two subsequent CG ≥ 40 mg/dL, begin weaning IV 20% every feed.
    (b) If unable to oral/OG feed: continue IV dextrose therapy and obtain CG every 3 hr or with signs.

  ii. Subsequent CG < 40 mg/dL with or without signs of hypoglycemia
    (a) Signs present: mini-bolus 5 mL/kg $D_{10}W$ IV and increase maintenance IV by 2 mg/kg/min. Reassess CG immediately after bolus.
    (b) Signs absent: increase infusion rate by 2 mg/kg/min (1.2 mL/kg/hr). Reassess CG.

d. After achieving stable euglycemia, IV glucose can typically be weaned over 24–48 hr in decrements of 20% of the original infusion every feed as oral intake is increased and CG remains > 40 mg/dL. IDMs often feed poorly.

2. Hypocalcemia: metabolically unstable, ill, or premature IDMs (insulin and non–insulin-treated) should have serum calcium

determined between 24 and 48 hr or if symptomatic. If not responsive to exogenous calcium, measure serum magnesium.

C. Respiratory distress: if showing signs, obtain chest radiograph and
arterial blood gas. Look for evidence of RDS, pneumothorax, or
cardiomegaly.

D. Cardiomegaly, hypotension, or poor perfusion: assure normoglycemia, obtain four-limb blood pressures, chest radiograph, arterial blood gas, and echocardiography if evidence of CHD. Symptomatic hypertrophic cardiomyopathy is managed with increased
preload and avoidance of vasopressors and digoxin. The role of
propranolol and calcium channel blockers is controversial.

E. Hyperbilirubinemia: measure serum bilirubin as clinically warranted (jaundice).

F. Polycythemia/hyperviscosity. With clinical signs, hematocrit
should be obtained. If polycythemic, consider partial exchange
transfusion (*see* Polycythemia, page 321).

G. Vascular access: peripheral IV lines may be difficult to start in
macrosomic IDMs. In the presence of definite hypoglycemia, use
the umbilical vein for rapid treatment. If a UAC is indicated, insert a
low (tip at L3–L4) line to avoid high concentrations of glucose in
the pancreatic circulation. Glucagon (0.025–0.1 mg/kg/dose every
20–30 min) can be given IM while access is being achieved. Caution should be used with administration secondary to its promotion
of hyperglycemia and secondary pancreatic secretion of insulin.

Suggested Reading

ACOG technical bulletin. Diabetes and pregnancy. Int J Gynaecol Obstet
48:331–339, 1995.

Cordero L, Treuer SH, Landon MB, Gabbe SG: Management of infants of
diabetic mothers. Arch Pediatr Adolesc Med 152:249–254, 1998.

Cowett RM: Hypoglycemia and hyperglycemia in the newborn. In Polin
RA, Fox WW (eds): Fetal and Neonatal Physiology. Philadelphia, W.B.
Saunders, 1998, p 596.

Hunter DJ, Burrows RF, Mohide PT, Whyte RK: Influence of maternal
insulin-dependent diabetes mellitus on neonatal morbidity. Can Med-
Assoc J 149:47–52, 1993.

Langer O, Levy J, Brustman L, et al: Glycemic control in gestational diabetes mellitus—how tight is tight enough: Small for gestational age versus large for gestational age? Am J Obstet Gynecol 161:646–653, 1989.

Mace S, Hirschfield SS, Riggs T, et al: Echocardiographic abnormalities in
infants of diabetic mothers. J Pediatr 95:1013–1019, 1979.

Miller E, Hare JW, Cloherty JP, et al: Elevated maternal hemoglobin A_{1c} in early pregnancy and major congenital anomalies in infants of diabetic mothers. N Engl J Med 304:1331–1334, 1988.
Noguchi A, Eren M, Tsang RC: Parathyroid hormone in hypocalcemia and normocalcemic infants of diabetic mothers. J Pediatr 97:112–114, 1980.
Tyrala EE: The infant of the diabetic mother. Obstet Gynecol Clin North Am 23:221–241, 1996.

Chapter 81

Small for Gestational Age Infant

Cyril Engmann, MBBS, and Mohammad A. Attar, M.D.

I. Definition

A. Less than the third percentile for gestational age

B. More than two standard deviations below the mean for gestational age, using norms based on an appropriate reference population

1. Usher and McLean, in 1969, established sea level reference curves for an urban, heterogeneous, North American population.
2. The Lubchenco curves (derived from a population in Denver). If used at sea level, the classification of small for gestational age (SGA) is approximated by a weight less than the 10th percentile because of lower birthweights at higher altitudes.

C. Based on the above definitions, however, some infants will be constitutionally small and should be distinguished from those with intrauterine growth restriction (IUGR) (previously referred to as *intrauterine growth retardation*). IUGR is a pathologic condition.

D. It is critical to have accurate assessment of the gestational age in order to make the classification of SGA.

E. A distinction is made between symmetric and asymmetric growth restriction.

1. Symmetric—head circumference, height, and weight are *all* proportionately reduced for gestational age. Symmetric SGA results from extrinsic conditions or decreased growth potential, both occurring early in pregnancy. It results in a reduction in the total number of cells. This limits the potential for "catch-up" growth.
2. Asymmetric—fetal weight or weight and length are reduced out of proportion to head circumference. There is relative sparing of brain growth. This occurs later in pregnancy and results in a normal number of cells that are hypoplastic, but that retain the potential for "catch-up" growth.

II. Etiologic Factors

A. Maternal

1. Reduced uteroplacental perfusion (leading cause of IUGR in the USA). Examples: hypertension (chronic, acute, or pregnancy induced), chronic vascular disease, advanced diabetes, autoimmune disease.

2. Multiple gestation—separate growth norms should be used for multifetal gestation.
3. Socioeconomic factors, e.g., young and advanced maternal age, lower socioeconomic status
4. Drugs (tobacco, cocaine, ethanol, opiates, others)
5. Hypoxemia (e.g., altitude, maternal heart disease, chronic pulmonary insufficiency)
6. Uterine anomalies
7. Severe malnutrition—the greatest effect on fetal growth is in the third trimester.

B. Fetal
1. Chromosomal abnormality
2. Congenital anomalies
3. Congenital infection
4. Dysmorphic syndromes

C. Placental—fetal growth is determined mostly by innate growth potential during the first and second trimesters. Placental factors assume the predominant role for fetal growth in the third trimester.
1. Anatomic abnormality (e.g., circumvallate insertion of the umbilical cord, hemangiomas, multiple infarcts)
2. Microscopic (e.g., villitis, either secondary to infection or idiopathic)
3. Implantation site (e.g., old uterine scar)

C. Racial and ethnic populations—these may systematically differ from reference norms based on other populations; it may be necessary to generate population-specific growth curves based on healthy, uncomplicated births.

D. Statistical definition of SGA makes it unavoidable that some normal infants will be so classified.

III. Diagnosis

A. Determine gestational age (LMP, second trimester fetal ultrasound, physical examination).

B. Clinical history and examinations (serial maternal weight and fundal height determination)

C. Ultrasonography is most commonly used in morphometric analysis of fetal growth. Serial measures of the following used in combination have a high degree of accuracy.
1. *Biparietal diameter* (head sparing in asymmetric IUGR makes this less sensitive)
2. *Abdominal circumference* at the level of the umbilical vein (the liver is the first organ to manifest effects of growth restriction)

3. Ratio of *head circumference to abdominal circumference*
4. *Femur length* provides early reproducible measure of fetal length.

IV. Neonatal Assessment

A. Reduced birthweight for gestational age

B. Use of the ponderal index:
(birthweight in g) $\times$ 100 $\div$ (length in cm)^3

C. Use of Dubowitz or Ballard scoring system to estimate gestational age (accurate to within 2 weeks in infants weighing more than 999 g and at 30–42 hours of age.) However, if infant has significant IUGR, these systems will underestimate the true gestational age, because the physical factors that make the baby small, such as decreased breast tissue, will cost points on the score.

V. Problems that Occur with Increased Frequency in the IUGR Infant

A. Asphyxia (IUGR infants tolerate the stress of labor poorly)

B. Meconium aspiration (post-term IUGR infants are at particular risk)

C. Hypoglycemia (diminished glycogen stores and capacity for gluconeogenesis)

D. Polycythemia/hyperviscosity (fetal hypoxia and increased erythropoietin levels may induce excessive RBC production)

E. Poor thermoregulation (diminished subcutaneous adipose tissue resulting in poor insulation)

F. Thrombocytopenia

G. Anemia

H. Congenital anomalies

I. Immunologic dysfunction

J. Transplacental effects of drugs used to treat associated or underlying maternal disease

K. Poor postnatal weight gain

L. Inguinal hernias

M. Pulmonary hemorrhage (rare)

N. Delayed ossification (increased fontanel size)

O. Normal variant—apparent "cardiomegaly"

VI. Management

A. Determine etiology
1. Detailed maternal history
2. Placental examination
3. Thorough neonatal examination
4. Indicated laboratory studies

    B. Laboratory studies
       1. Strongly recommended
         a. Serum glucose monitoring
         b. CBC and platelet count—central HCT if peripheral HCT $> 65\%$
       2. For infants suspected of having congenital infection (e.g., symptomatic, hepatosplenomegaly, anemic, microcephalic, etc.), obtain appropriate cultures and serologic studies (*see* Chapter 38).
       3. For infants with dysmorphic features, consider karyotype, genetics and dysmorphology consultation.
    C. Anticipate need for support.
       1. Glucose
       2. Temperature control
       3. May have greatly increased caloric needs for growth
       4. Consider hydration or partial exchange transfusion for polycythemia/hyperviscosity.

VII. Outcome

    A. Perinatal mortality among SGA infants is 5–20 times higher than for appropriately grown infants.
    B. Depends on the etiology of the growth restriction as well as asymmetrical versus symmetrical (poorer outcome)
    C. Many of the reported handicaps may be secondary to adverse perinatal events (asphyxia, polycythemia) or underlying fetal anomalies or infections.
    D. The infant may or may not experience catch-up growth; recent studies suggest most catch-up occurs in the first year of life.
    E. Epidemiologic evidence suggests that insulin resistance, diabetes, obesity, and cardiovascular disease are more common in adults who were IUGR at birth. Mechanisms for this are not yet clearly established.
    F. Outcome is widely variable but generally good.

Suggested Reading

Anderson MS, Hay WW: Intrauterine growth restriction and the small-for-gestational-age (SGA) infant. In Avery GB, Fletcher MA, MacDonald MG (eds): Neonatology: Pathophysiology and Management of the Newborn, 5th ed. Philadelphia, J.B. Lippincott, 1999, p 411.

Doctor BA, O'Riordan MA, Kirchner HL, et al: Perinatal correlates and neonatal outcome of small for gestational age infants born at term gestation. Am J Obstet Gynecol 183:652–659, 2001.

Hay WW, Thureen PJ, Anderson MS: Intrauterine growth restriction. Neo-Reviews 2:e129, 2001.

Kliegman RM: Intrauterine growth retardation: Determinants of aberrant fetal growth. In Fanaroff AA, Martin RJ (eds): Neonatal-Perinatal Medicine, 6th ed. St. Louis, Mosby, 1997, pp 221–240.

Lubchenco LO, Hansman C, Dressler M, Boyd E: Intrauterine growth as estimated from liveborn birth-weight data at 24 to 42 weeks gestation. Pediatrics 32:793, 1963.

Usher R, McLean F: Intrauterine growth of live born Caucasian infants at sea level: Standards obtained from measurements in 7 dimensions of infants born between 25 and 44 weeks of gestation. J Pediatr 74:901–910, 1969.

Chapter 82

Very Low Birthweight Infant Management

Mary E.A. Bozynski, M.D., M.S., and Jennifer L. Grow, M.D.

I. **Unique Neurologic Responses of the VLBW (< 1500 g) Infant**
   A. Inability to regulate autonomic responses to environmental stresses
      1. Hypoxemia in response to handling, "routine" care procedures, noise, light
      2. Inability to tolerate cold stresses, with resultant hypoxemia, hypoglycemia, and acidemia
   B. Possible adverse neurodevelopmental consequences of extrauterine (intensive care nursery) environment
   C. Some suggested modifications to the environment
      1. Low ambient lighting
      2. Low ambient noise (e.g., no radios, quiet conversation; exercise care with room and incubator doors)
      3. Careful scheduling of procedures and handling in consultation with bedside nurse
      4. "Quiet time" 24 hours a day
      5. Identification of VLBW infant protocol by a notice on the incubator
      6. Developmental program based on infant's "readiness"
   D. Some studies suggest that by reducing environmental stressors, the severity of medical complications such as BPD and IVH may be reduced, thus improving neurodevelopmental outcomes. This should begin at delivery and especially in the treatment room where light and noise levels are often overlooked.

II. **Skin Problems of the VLBW Infant**
   A. Immaturity of the skin
      1. High ratio of surface area to body mass
      2. Highly permeable, both directions
         a. High insensible water losses
         b. Absorption of iodine from antiseptics leading to hypothyroidism
      3. Fragile in response to chemical (e.g., antiseptic solutions) or physical (e.g., adhesive tape) trauma
   B. Suggested interventions
      1. Avoid open-bed warmers except in the acutely unstable infant.

2. Cover ELBW infant under an open-bed warmer with a transparent plastic heat shield or plastic-wrap blanket (ELBW = < 1000 g).
3. Use double-walled incubator or cover infant with heat shield or plastic wrap.
4. Add extra humidity to incubator.
5. Use elasticized sleeves in all incubator portholes.
6. Minimize use of adhesive tapes and tincture of benzoin.
7. If possible, use cotton cling wrap (or other nonadhesive tape) or decrease tape adhesiveness by touching with a cotton ball when wrapping around an extremity.
8. Use iodine-containing solutions sparingly and promptly clean skin with water.
9. Be alert to risk of hidden iodine burn to back after umbilical catheterization.

III. Renal Problems of the VLBW Infant

A. Immature kidneys
1. Poor ability to conserve water
2. Poor ability to conserve sodium

B. Suggested interventions
1. Attempt to minimize insensible water losses by measures outlined in II,B above and by adequate ventilator humidification.
2. Carefully monitor hydration status
   a. Daily weight
   b. Serial heart rate and blood pressure measurements
   c. Frequent serum Na, K, glucose, and HCT determination
   d. Serial clinical examination of hydration status
   e. Beware of relying on urine output and specific gravity (high obligatory losses, *see* III,A above).
3. Watch for hyperglycemia and glycosuria as IV fluid intake increases; be prepared to decrease glucose content of IV fluids.
4. Accept some weight loss—it is normal!

IV. Educating Parents of the VLBW Infant

A. Gradually prepare parents in advance for common possible medical complications.
1. Cerebral hemorrhages or ischemic lesions
2. Early onset respiratory distress
3. Later onset chronic lung disease
4. Apnea
5. Feeding difficulties

      6. Patent ductus arteriosus
      7. Suspected sepsis
  B. Psychosocial issues
      1. Parental expectations for their infant at 1 month, 6 months,
         2 years, and after
      2. Expected discharge to home around time of original due date
      3. Availability of parent support groups, social services, hospital
         chaplains

Suggested Reading

Als H, Lawhon G, Brown E, et al: Individualized behavioral and environ-
    mental care for the very low birth weight preterm infant at high risk for
    bronchopulmonary dysplasia: Neonatal intensive care unit and develop-
    mental outcome. Pediatrics 78:1123–1132, 1986.

Als H, Lawhon G, Duffy F, et al: Individualized developmental care for the
    very low-birth-weight preterm infant: Medical and neurofunctional ef-
    fects. JAMA 272:853–858, 1994.

Long JG, Lucey JF, Philip AGS: Noise and hypoxemia in the intensive care
    nursery. Pediatrics 65:143–145, 1980.

Long JG, Philip AGS, Lucey JF: Excessive handling as a cause of hypoxemia.
    Pediatrics 65:203–207, 1980.

Widerstrom A, Mowder B, Sandall S: At-Risk and Handicapped Newborns
    and Infants: Development, Assessment, and Intervention. Englewood
    Cliffs, NJ, Prentice-Hall, 1991.

Chapter 83

Hydrops Fetalis

Steven M. Donn, M.D.

I. **Definition**

Soft tissue edema and fluid accumulation in serous cavities of the fetus. Usually divided into **immune hydrops** if it results from feto-maternal blood group incompatibility (isoimmunization), and **non-immune hydrops** if from other causes.

II. **Associations**

The following is a partial list of the many associations.

A. Cardiovascular—approximately 26% of cases
   1. Anatomic cardiac malformations—left heart hypoplasia, A-V canal defect, right heart hypoplasia, cardiomyopathy, multiple other defects
   2. Tachyarrhythmias (SVT) and bradyarrhythmias (congenital heart block)
   3. High-output cardiac failure secondary to vascular malformations—sacrococcygeal teratoma, fetal or placental angioma, arteriovenous malformation

B. Chromosomal abnormalities—approximately 10% of cases
   1. 45, X
   2. Trisomy 21
   3. Multiple other trisomies, aneuploidies, deletions, and duplications

C. Thoracic abnormalities—approximately 9% of cases
   1. Cystadenomatoid malformation of the lung
   2. Chondrodysplasia
   3. Congenital diaphragmatic hernia
   4. Pulmonary sequestration, chylothorax
   5. Osteogenesis imperfecta
   6. Asphyxiating thoracic dystrophy

D. Twin–twin transfusion—approximately 8% of cases
   1. Donor—may become anemic
   2. Recipient—at risk for vascular accidents secondary to poly-cythemia

E. Anemia—approximately 6% of cases
   1. Hemolytic anemias

      a. Alloimmune—e.g., Rh sensitization, α-thalassemia
      b. RBC enzyme deficiencies
   2. Other anemias
      a. Fetomaternal transfusion
      b. Parvovirus B19 infection
F. Infection—approximately 4% of cases
   1. Cytomegalovirus
   2. Bacterial agents
   3. Toxoplasmosis
   4. Syphilis
   5. Others (e.g., parvovirus)
G. Other—each accounting for ≤ 3% of cases, including urinary tract malformation, cystic hygroma, impaired fetal movement, peritonitis, hepatic causes, genetic metabolic diseases, nephrotic syndrome, miscellaneous
H. Idiopathic—approximately 15–20% of cases in more recent series

III. Pathophysiology

Although this is often not clear, several patterns are evident, which usually coexist.

A. Increased systemic venous pressure—this includes many of the anatomic heart lesions and rhythm disturbances, thoracic lesions, and high output congestive heart failure.

B. Anemia—severity of the hydrops is not well correlated with the degree of anemia present, but is undoubtedly a major factor in many cases.

C. Hypoalbuminemia—often occurs concomitantly with anemia, but even without anemia is an important condition.

D. Unknown—mechanism is unclear in many cases of hydrops fetalis.

IV. Management

A. Prenatal
   1. If the condition is discovered prenatally, extensive investigations regarding etiology are warranted. These include:
      a. Maternal and family health histories
      b. Maternal blood type and antibody studies
      c. Glucose tolerance test
      d. Kleihauer-Betke test
      e. Syphilis serology, CMV, toxoplasmosis, and parvovirus titers
      f. Fetal ultrasound with echocardiography

g. Amniocentesis or cordocentesis for karyotype and fetal hematologic studies

h. Consider hemoglobin electrophoresis for thalassemia and RBC enzyme studies.

2. Frequent assessments of fetal well being are crucial because emergent delivery may become necessary.

3. Fetal intrauterine transfusions may be beneficial in instances of hemolytic or nonhemolytic anemias.

4. Once hydrops develops it rarely resolves spontaneously *in utero*.

B. Postnatal

1. Management depends greatly on etiology.

2. In prenatally diagnosed cases of hydrops, delivery should take place at a hospital that has not only neonatology, but pediatric cardiology and pediatric surgery personnel available. Resuscitation is often much more extensive than with other sick newborns. *Immediate* intubation and establishment of vascular access is required.

3. If the heart rate or color fails to improve and poor chest movement is noted, evacuation of fluid from serous cavities, especially the pleural spaces and the peritoneum, may be required. Thoracostomy tubes are recommended rather than needle thoracentesis.

4. If severe anemia is present, an isovolemic partial exchange transfusion with whole blood or packed red blood cells should be done immediately. Avoid giving large volume boluses, because the total body water is increased and intravascular volume may be normal or increased. A number of tubes of blood (including several red, lavender, and green top tubes) for laboratory work-up should be obtained before beginning the transfusion.

5. Laboratory studies may include:

   a. CBC with differential and platelets; reticulocyte count

   b. Blood type, direct antibody test

   c. Syphilis serology

   d. Bilirubin, total and direct

   e. Total serum protein, albumin

   f. Karyotype

   g. Liver enzymes

   h. BUN, serum creatinine

   i. TORCH, IgM-specific antibodies

   j. Cultures (bacterial, viral)

   k. Save blood for:

      i. RBC enzymes

      ii. Hgb electrophoresis

   l. Urine metabolic screen

6. Other diagnostic studies to consider:
   a. Echocardiography, ECG
   b. Radiographs: chest, abdomen, long bones, skull
   c. Placental pathology
   d. Genetics consultation
   e. Diagnostic thoracentesis, paracentesis
7. Management will vary based on etiology and active clinical problems. Major problems generally include respiratory and fluid management.
   a. High peak inspiratory pressure or PEEP may be necessary.
   b. Fluid administration should be conservative, and measures to maintain perfusion and mobilize edema are usually required.
   c. Remember to base drug and fluid doses on estimated dry weight or surface area. The volume of distribution in these infants may be highly variable. Thus, follow drug levels whenever possible.

V.   Outcome

A. Reports on outcome vary widely, ranging from 50% to 98% mortality. Higher mortality is seen in cases with underlying lethal conditions. The best prognosis is usually seen in idiopathic cases.

B. Many of the causes of hydrops are currently untreatable.

C. The main factors affecting outcome in any infant will be etiology of the hydrops, condition prior to delivery, and the effectiveness of the resuscitation.

Suggested Reading

Davis CL: Diagnosis and management of nonimmune hydrops fetalis. J Reprod Med 27:594–600, 1982.

Davis CL: Hydrops fetalis. In Donn SM, Faix RG (eds): Neonatal Emergencies. Mt. Kisco, NY, Futura Publishing, 1991, pp 461–473.

Machin GA: Hydrops revisited: Literature review of 1,414 cases published in the 1980s. Am J Med Genet 34:366–390, 1989.

Phibbs RA: Hydrops fetalis and other causes of neonatal edema and ascites. In Polin RA, Fox WW (eds): Fetal and Neonatal Physiology, 2nd ed. Philadelphia, W.B. Saunders, 1998, pp 1730–1736.

Chapter 84

Ambiguous Genitalia

Mohammad A. Attar, M.D., and Jennifer L. Grow, M.D.

I. **General**

A. Consider a newborn as having ambiguous genitalia if experienced examiners have doubts as to the correct anatomic sex assignment.

B. Characteristics of sexual development

1. Genetic sex—determined at fertilization

2. Gonadal sex—determined by genetic sex

3. Phenotypic sex—regulated by the differentiation of gonads during the first half of fetal life

4. Psychological sex—acquired postnatally; influenced by hormones and society

C. Reasons for the need for early recognition and diagnosis of ambiguous genitalia

1. Designation of the correct sex for child-rearing

2. Diagnosis of congenital adrenal hyperplasia (CAH) before the onset of adrenal crisis

3. Identification of individuals at risk for gonadal tumors

4. Provision of genetic counseling and the option for prenatal diagnosis with future pregnancies

5. Institution of early corrective measures to promote normal body image and gender identity

D. Impression of ambiguity depends on many factors

1. Penile or clitoral length—penile length measured with a ruler placed on the pubic symphysis; penis is maximally stretched for measurement; length is from base to tip of glans (not foreskin)

2. Appearance of labia (rugated or smooth)

3. Number of orifices identified

4. Presence or absence (and location) of palpable gonads

5. Presence or absence of median raphe

D. Genitalia need not be overtly "ambiguous"; an intersex problem is likely if either of the following two situations exists:

1. Two or more abnormalities of the external genitalia are present

a. Phallus size

b. Urethral meatus (location)

c. Labioscrotal folds (fusion)

d. Gonad(s) (location or size)

2. Any one of the following abnormalities is present:
   a. With male-appearing genitalia
      i. Micropenis
      ii. Hypospadias (more severe; e.g., separation of scrotal sacs; undescended testes)
      iii. Impalpable gonads
      iv. Small gonads
      v. Inguinal mass (uterus or tube)
   b. With female-appearing genitalia
      i. Clitoromegaly/clitoral hypertrophy
      ii. Posterior labial fusion
      iii. Palpable gonads
      iv. Inguinal hernia or mass
      v. Shortened vulva with single opening

II. Diagnostic Evaluation of the Infant with Ambiguous Genitalia

A. History and physical exam; inquire about:
   1. Maternal drug exposures
   2. Family history of previously affected siblings, neonatal deaths, infertility in maternal aunts
B. Obtain buccal smear for rapid screening of X and Y chromatin.
C. Send peripheral blood at 6–48 hours for:
   1. Karyotype (may take 2–3 weeks for completion; bone marrow aspirate results are more rapid)
   2. Serum hormone levels (e.g., testosterone, 17-OH progesterone, 11-deoxycortisol, 17-OH pregnenolone, estradiol, LD, FSH)
D. Daily electrolytes (Na, K) to assess for aldosterone deficiency in CAH
E. Radiologic studies to identify internal reproductive structures
   1. Abdominal and pelvic ultrasound
   2. Retrograde urography, CT scan
F. Obtain pediatric endocrinology, genetics, and pediatric urology or surgery consultations

III. Differential Diagnosis

A. True hermaphroditism—discrepancy between external genitalia and internal gonadal structures; both testis and ovary are present in the same individual.
B. Female pseudohermaphroditism—masculinization of the female infant. Etiologies include:
   1. CAH—most common, especially 21-hydroxylase deficiency

2. Exposure of fetus to maternal androgenic hormones *in utero* (maternal virilizing tumor, maternal CAH, maternal ingestion of exogenous androgenic drugs)

C. Male pseudohermaphroditism—inadequate virilization of male infants
   1. Disorder of testicular differentiation or development (XX male syndrome, mixed gonadal dysgenesis, persistent müllerian duct syndrome)
   2. Defect in testosterone synthesis (CAH, other enzyme deficiencies); association of micropenis and hypoglycemia suggests panhypopituitarism
   3. Defect in testosterone metabolism (5α-reductase deficiency)
   4. Defects in testosterone action (incomplete androgen insensitivity or testicular feminization)

D. Chromosome abnormalities—do not usually lead to ambiguous genitalia. However, mixed gonadal dysgenesis (presence of a normal or partially differentiated testis and an undifferentiated or streak gonad) is usually associated with 45, X/46, XY mosaicism and ambiguity of the external genitalia.

IV. Management

A. Inability to determine sex assignment is a psychosocial emergency!
   1. *Do not* make guesses as to what the genetic sex probably is. Ultimately, structure determines functional sexual identity regardless of gonadal or chromosomal sex; sex assignment is not made until chromosomes and müllerian duct status is known.
   2. Inform parents: "Your baby's genitalia have not developed completely. Further tests and exams by experts are needed in order to determine which sex your baby was intended to be reared."
   3. *Do not* circumcise!

B. If CAH is strongly suspected in a newborn with ambiguous genitalia, treatment with cortisol, Florinef, and salt replacement should be started immediately. Continue to monitor electrolytes daily.

C. Considerations beyond the immediate neonatal period:
   1. Surgical procedures (depending on the sex of rearing) such as clitorectomy, dilation of the introits, definitive angioplasty, hypostasis repair, orchiopexy, removal of heterologous or dysgenetic gonads)
   2. Hormone replacement therapy
   3. Long-term psychological counseling should be available for the parents and child.

Suggested Reading

American Academy of Pediatrics Committee on Genetics: Evaluation of the newborn with developmental anomalies of the external genitalia. Pediatrics 106:138–142, 2000.

Bacon GE, Spencer ML, Hopwood NJ, Kelch RP: A Practical Approach to Pediatric Endocrinology, 3rd ed. Chicago, Year Book, 1990.

Danish RK, Dahms WT: Abnormalities of sexual differentiation. In Fanaroff AA, Martin RJ (eds): Neonatal-Perinatal Medicine: Diseases of the Fetus and Infant, 7th ed. St. Louis, Mosby, 2001, pp 1416–1467.

Zajac JD, Warne GL: Disorders of sexual development. Baillieres Clin Endocrinol Metab 9:555–579, 1995.

Chapter 85

Retinopathy of Prematurity

Charles R. Neal, Jr., M.D., Ph.D., and Cyril Engmann, MBBS

I. Definition

Retinopathy of prematurity (ROP) is best defined as a vasculoproliferative disorder that is known to occur almost exclusively in premature infants.

II. Incidence

Data from the cryotherapy trial (1986–1987):

A. The study included 4009 infants who weighed < 1251 g at birth (Table 46).

Table 46
Incidence of ROP

Birthweight (g)	ROP Present %
< 1251	66
1000–1250	47
750–1000	78
< 750	90

B. Moderately severe and severe ROP made up smaller proportions of the cases.

    1. Almost all ROP-related vision loss was associated with the severe degree.

    2. Extrapolating the data from this study to the country's population of premature births indicates that about 420 infants per year experience vision loss from ROP.

C. Improved survival of extremely low birthweight infants after the era of surfactant administration has not been associated with an increase in the incidence of ROP in this population.

III. Pathophysiology

A. Retinopathy of prematurity results from an injury to the developing retinal capillary bed.

    1. Development of moderate or severe disease tends to occur at the same postconceptional age, thought to be 34–36 weeks.

      a. Median age for stage 1 ROP is 34.3 weeks.

      b. Median age for stage 2 ROP is 35.4 weeks.

      c. Median age for stage 3 ROP is 36.6 weeks.

      d. Median age for *plus disease* is 36.3 weeks.

      e. Median age for threshold ROP is 36.9 weeks.

   2. It does not occur necessarily at the same chronologic age.

B. New vessel growth regresses about 80% of the time, with the other 20% progressing to neovascularization, scar formation, hemorrhage, or retinal detachment.

C. With regression, the excessive vessels involute and remodel into a nearly normal pattern.

IV. Risk Factors

A. Prematurity is the greatest risk factor for ROP.

   1. Only those infants whose retinal vessels have not completed their migration from the optic disc to the ora serrata develop ROP.

   2. There are case reports of ROP in full-term infants whose injury to the developing retinal vessels could have occurred antenatally.

B. Hyperoxia is a widely accepted risk factor.

   1. No safe level of arterial PaO_2 can be identified.

      a. Continuous oxygen saturation monitoring cannot eliminate ROP.

      b. Some infants develop ROP even without the administration of supplemental oxygen.

      c. ROP has also been reported in infants with cyanotic congenital heart disease, where PaO_2 levels are known to be lower.

   2. AAP guidelines recommend oxygen tension monitoring if supplemental oxygen is required beyond an emergency period for newborns delivered before 36 weeks of gestation.

      a. Attempts should be made to maintain PaO_2 in the range of 50–80 mmHg.

      b. These same guidelines also acknowledge that, in some situations, it may be prudent to maintain PaO_2 levels > 100 mmHg, especially if attempts to decrease the inspired oxygen concentration dramatically reduce the PaO_2 to very low levels.

   3. The concomitantly increased risk of ROP may not be avoidable during such periods.

      a. The infant's medical record needs to reflect this justification.

      b. Under these circumstances, it is important that the associated risks and benefits of increased O_2 requirements are discussed with the parents.

C. Other potential risk factors

   1. Hypoxia, *in utero* ischemia, hypercarbia, and hypocarbia

   2. Degree of illness

      a. Increased ROP incidence is observed concomitantly with IVH, PDA, sepsis, and development of BPD.

      b. Need for exchange and replacement transfusions correlates with an increased incidence of ROP.

      c. Prolonged length of stay in the hospital, an indicator of the severity of illness, also positively correlates with ROP.

   3. Use of prostaglandins

   4. Vitamin E deficiency

   5. Prolonged exposure to bright light

   6. Lactic acidosis

   7. Prenatal factors, both maternal and fetal, are positively correlated with ROP incidence.

      a. Fetal factors include congenital anomalies, such as anencephaly and trisomy 18.

      b. Maternal factors include preeclampsia, maternal diabetes, third trimester bleeding, and heavy smoking.

   8. Genetic predisposition

V. Description of ROP Using the International Classification of ROP (ICROP)

A. Location of the disease:

Zone I	Extends from the optic disc to twice the distance from the disc to the center of the macula.
Zone II	Extends from the edge of zone I to the nasal ora serrata and to the area near the temporal anatomic equator.
Zone III	The residual crescent of retina anterior to zone II. This is the last zone to be vascularized and is most frequently involved in ROP.

B. Severity of the disease:

Stage 1	Demarcation line: a thin white demarcation line separates the vascular from the avascular retina.
Stage 2	Ridge: a clear ridge that elevates above the retina is observed at the demarcation.
Stage 3	Ridge with proliferation: the ridge is now noted to have extraretinal fibrovascular proliferation.
Stage 4	Subtotal retinal detachment
Stage 5	Total retinal detachment

C. Extent of the disease is measured around the retina in clock hours (1–12).

D. Special designation for the accelerated inflammation with poor prognosis: plus disease.

VI. Ophthalmologic ROP Screening Examination of Premature Infants

A. AAP recommendations (2001)

1. Who meets criteria for ROP exam?
   a. All infants < 28 weeks' gestational age or with birthweights < 1500 g, regardless of oxygen exposure
   b. Selected premature infants with birthweights between 1500 and 2000 g and an unstable clinical course or premature infants who are believed to be at high risk by the attending neonatologist
   c. ROP examinations are very important and *should never be taken lightly.*
      i. Hypertension, reflex bradycardia, and apneic events can be caused by mydriatic eye drops.
      ii. Similar untoward effects often occur during these very difficult eye examinations.
   d. Infants selected to have ROP screening should have at least two examinations, unless on initial exam the retina is unequivocally shown to be fully vascularized bilaterally.
2. Who performs the examination?
   a. A person experienced in pediatric ophthalmology and indirect ophthalmoscopy should do the exams.
   b. The examiner should have sufficient regular experience and knowledge in the examination of preterm infants for ROP to identify the location and sequential retinal changes in the disorder.
3. When should the first examination occur?
   a. The first examination should generally be performed between 4 and 6 weeks of chronologic (postnatal) age.
      i. Alternatively, the AAP also suggests within the 31st to 33rd week of postconceptional or postmenstrual age, whichever is later.
      ii. This age is determined as gestational age at birth plus chronologic age.
   b. It is best if the first examination is performed prior to discharge.
   c. Timing of the initial screening examination may be adjusted

appropriately on the basis of other reliable data, such as local incidence and onset of ROP, preference of ophthalmologic specialist, and presence of other recognizable risk factors.

B. Examination findings and prognosis

1. The location and sequential retinal changes, if any, should be recorded using ICROP nomenclature.
2. The object of the examination is to provide timely recognition of disease that could be amenable to therapy, and to provide prognosis.

   a. If the first examination shows that retinal vessels are in zone 3, serious ROP or visual sequelae rarely develop and prognosis is good.

   b. If there is stage 1 or 2 disease in zone II, subsequent examinations are needed.

      i. Exams are scheduled at 2-week intervals.

      ii. Rapid progression of the disease is a serious prognostic sign and more frequent exams are needed.

   c. If the infant has stage 3 disease or stage 2 in zone II with plus disease, weekly examinations are advised.

   d. If the ROP reaches "threshold" severity, the risk of poor retinal outcome increases to about 50%.

      i. Threshold severity is defined as more than 5.5 continuous clock hours or 8 total clock hours of stage 3 with plus disease in zone II or zone I.

      ii. Ophthalmic surgery should be arranged for this condition.

   e. ROP with vessels ending in zone I is unusual. These infants are more likely to develop rapidly progressive ROP (Rush disease).

VII. Complications of ROP

A. Varying degrees of visual impairment, including retinal detachment and blindness in worst cases

B. Later complications include glaucoma, strabismus, cataracts, and amblyopia.

VIII. Prevention of ROP

A. All factors being equal, the reality is that the only way to prevent ROP from occurring is to prevent premature deliveries.

B. Factors that may help decrease the incidence of ROP

1. Control of oxygen administration
2. Decreased hospitalization-associated morbidities
3. Vitamin E replacement therapy

a. Vitamin E is a theoretical treatment with no proven effectiveness.
b. Significant morbidity has been reported with prolonged high doses.
4. Reduction of the ambient light
a. A controversial subject
b. The contribution of this factor to ROP remains under significant investigation, with mostly equivocal results in follow-up studies.

IX. Treatment

A. Cryotherapy
1. Works by freezing the avascular retina, preventing further abnormal vessel proliferation
2. Complications include scarring of the retina, cell destruction, and possible retinal detachments.
3. At 10-year follow-up exams, *eyes that had received cryotherapy were much less likely than control eyes to be blind.* Follow-up results show long-term value from cryotherapy in preserving visual acuity in eyes with threshold ROP.

B. Laser therapy
1. Argon or iodide laser therapy is used to perform photocoagulation of the avascular periphery of the retina. It is less invasive and less traumatic to the eye than cryotherapy, requiring no anesthetics.
2. Complications include scarring, choroidal hemorrhage, and pain.

C. Investigational oxygen therapy
1. The theory is that neovascularization of ROP is a response to tissue ischemia and hypoxia that follows the injury and loss of newly growing retinal vessels.
2. Trials of gradually weaning infants from high oxygen over several days are being conducted.

Suggested Reading

American Academy of Pediatrics, Section on Ophthalmology: Screening examination of premature infants for retinopathy of prematurity. Pediatrics 108:809, 2002.
American Academy of Pediatrics/American College of Obstetricians and Gynecologists: Guidelines for Perinatal Care, 3rd ed. Elk Grove Village, IL, AAP, 1992, pp 197–203.

Banach MJ, Berinstein DM: Laser therapy for retinopathy of prematurity. Curr Opin Ophthalmol 12:164–170, 2001.

Committee for the Classification of Retinopathy of Prematurity: The international classification of retinopathy of prematurity. Arch Ophthalmol 102:1130–1134, 1984.

Cryotherapy for Retinopathy of Prematurity Cooperative Group: Multicenter trial of cryotherapy for retinopathy of prematurity: One-year outcome—structure and function. Arch Ophthalmol 108:1408–1416, 1990.

Cryotherapy for Retinopathy of Prematurity Cooperative Group: Multicenter trial of cryotherapy for retinopathy of prematurity. Ophthalmological outcomes at 10 years. Arch Ophthalmol 119:1110–1118, 2001.

Hunsucker K: Laser surgery for retinopathy of prematurity. Neonatal Netw 14:21–26, 1995.

Isenberg S (ed): The Eye in Infancy, 2nd ed. St. Louis, Mosby, 1994, pp 437–470.

Palmer EA, Flynn J, Hardy R, et al: Incidence and early course of retinopathy of prematurity: The Cryotherapy for Retinopathy of Prematurity Cooperative Group. Ophthalmology 11:1628–1640, 1991.

The STOP-ROP Multicenter Study Group: Supplemental therapeutic oxygen for prethreshold retinopathy of prematurity (STOP-ROP): A randomized, controlled trial. I: Primary outcomes. Pediatrics 105:295–310, 2000.

Chapter 86

Congenital Epidermolysis Bullosa and Related Disorders

John D.E. Barks, M.D., B. Jane Scheff, R.N., and Eileen G. Wright, R.N.

I. Definition

A. A group of heterogeneous skin diseases that are characterized by the formation of blisters in response to minor trauma or heat

B. The diseases can be classified by the location of formation of the blisters (intraepidermal, junctional, or subepidermal), mode of transmission, or the presence or absence of scarring.

C. Over 25 different types have been identified.

D. Differential diagnosis includes several congenital ichthyoses with extensive desquamation but no true bullae, e.g., harlequin ichthyosis, collodion baby, epidermolytic hyperkeratosis, and congenital ichthyosiform erythroderma.

II. Diagnosis

A. Family history and clinical examination

B. Skin biopsy is the cornerstone.

C. Immunofluorescence and microscopy are helpful in identifying the cleavage plane.

D. Electron microscopy is helpful in distinguishing between various types.

III. Treatment

Similar principles apply to both bullous and nonbullous disorders.

A. Thermoregulation—when using a radiant warmer, use as low a temperature setting as the situation allows; heat may exacerbate epidermolysis bullosa (EB) and lead to increased insensible fluid losses. Yet, wet dressings and exfoliation may exaggerate heat loss.

B. Skin care—the overall goals are to minimize trauma to skin and the risk of infection. Gentle handling is critical.

1. Avoid tape, adhesives, identification bracelets. UAC and UVC are usually sutured in. CR monitor leads are secured with Coban or other material that sticks to itself but not the infant's skin.

2. Bedding and clothing—Affected infants should lay on sheepskin. Dress in soft, loose-fitting clothing and diapers. Place loose mittens on hands.

3. Bath—daily or less often depending on topical therapy used
   a. Soak dressings to remove, using sterile water.
   b. Pat dry; avoid friction.
   c. Treatment of blisters is determined on an individual basis. They may be left intact or decompressed using sterile technique.
4. Dressing changes
   a. Sterile application of an antibacterial ointment as recommended by Dermatology, Plastic Surgery, or Burn Service (bacitracin, silver sulfadiazine, or nystatin are commonly used).
   b. An alternative topical therapy is silver-impregnated gauze dressing (e.g., Acticoat), often used in burn patients, soaked in warmed sterile water at the time of application, periodically moistened with sterile water from a spray bottle.
   c. Use fine mesh gauze to separate digits.
   d. Wrap affected areas with soft, lint-free gauze.
5. Minimize contractures
   a. Maintain extremities in the flexed position.
   b. Gentle range of motion exercises
   c. Request physical therapy consultation.
C. Maintain comfort
   1. Administer analgesics prior to bath, dressing changes, and range of motion exercises.
   2. Swabbing mouth with mixture of viscous lidocaine and Mylanta may relieve the discomfort associated with feedings in patients with facial or oral lesions.
D. Fluids, electrolytes, and nutrition
   1. Potential for high insensible water losses, especially in recessive forms of the disease, and some ichthyoses, similar to a burn. This may require higher than usual maintenance fluids, as well as periodic fluid boluses while assessing basal fluid needs.
   2. TPN may be required until full enteral feeds are established.
   3. Gentle oral feeding is necessary. Special nontraumatic nipples may be used to avoid oropharyngeal trauma. Avoid NG tubes if possible; however, if needed, use one designed to be left in place long term (e.g., Corpak polyurethane tubes can be left in for 30 days).
   4. In recessive forms, a nutritionist should be consulted early to optimize caloric intake.
E. Close attention to possible sepsis and prompt treatment with antibiotics is required in all variants of the disease.

F. If airway protection and assisted ventilation are required, ETT can be secured to nonadhesive cloth tape strap tied around the head.

G. Red cell transfusions may be required in junctional EB (JEB).

H. Specific pharmacotherapy may be indicated in some conditions, e.g., phenytoin may reduce blister formation in recessive dystrophic EB and JEB; retinoic acid may attenuate harlequin ichthyosis. Dermatology consultation is required.

I. Genetic consultation and counseling for the parents is advised.

Suggested Reading

Drolet BA, Esterly NB: The skin. In Fanaroff AA, Martin RJ (eds): Neonatal-Perinatal Medicine, 7th ed. St. Louis, Mosby, 2002, pp 1537–1567.

Denyer J: Management of severe blistering disorders. Semin Neonatol 5:321–324, 2000.

Fine JD: National Epidermolysis Bullosa Registry, University of North Carolina, Chapel Hill, NC. Available at http://www.med.unc.edu/derm/nebr_site/index.htm

Frieden IJ, Howard R: Vesicles, pustules, bullae, erosions and ulcerations. In Eichenfeld LF, Frieden IJ, Esterley NB (eds): Textbook of Neonatal Dermatology. Philadelphia, W.B. Saunders, 2001, pp 137–178.

Paller AS: Disorders of cornification (icthyosis). In Eichenfeld LF, Frieden IJ, Esterley NB (eds): Textbook of Neonatal Dermatology. Philadelphia, W.B. Saunders, 2001, pp 276–293.

Section XV. TRANSPORT AND OUTREACH

Chapter 87

Neonatal Transports

Steven M. Donn, M.D., and Molly R. Gates, M.S., R.N.C.

I. Levels of Acceptance

Referrals to tertiary care centers may arise from:

A. Community (level I or II hospitals within or beyond a designated geographic region)

B. Level III NICUs for provision of specialized services (e.g., pediatric surgery, ECMO, high-frequency ventilation, hemodialysis)

C. Need for specialized diagnostic studies (metabolic, neurologic, cardiology)

D. Limited availability of beds in other NICUs

E. Maternal transports to the obstetrical service of mothers whose infants may require NICU services

II. General Considerations

Transports should generally be accepted unless there are extenuating circumstances.

A. Consider care requirements of existing patients. Will addition of another critically ill baby adversely impact the care of existing patients?

B. Check the delivery rooms for pending or imminent high-risk deliveries.

C. Does the capability for back-transport or transfer to a less acute unit exist for stable infants in the NICU?

D. Project patient moves over the next few days. It is almost impossible to delineate guidelines for every situation that might occur.

E. Communication between all members of the health care team is essential to facilitate acceptance of a patient or, alternatively, refusal, without undue delay to the referring physician.

III. Logistics of Neonatal Transports: The University of Michigan Model

A. Requests

1. All requests for neonatal transports are made to the Neonatology Service at all times of the day.

2. The call is taken by the transport physician or the charge nurse, if the physician is occupied.

      3. The physician receiving the call communicates the request to the charge nurse to assure bed and staffing availability.

B. Basic information

    1. The physician responding to the call obtains and records identifying information on an Infant Referral Form, including:

      a. Name and phone number of referring physician and hospital

      b. Infant's name and birth date

      c. Infant's clinical history and present condition

    2. Appropriate consultative advice may be offered. The referring physician should be asked whether parents have been informed of transfer and to notify the UM service immediately if the infant expires.

    3. The referring physician should be informed immediately of any delays in transport team departure or anticipated arrival.

    4. The UM Hospital Admissions Office is notified by the NICU clerk about the pending transfer, and a registration card and hospital chart are prepared.

    5. Although it is necessary to obtain basic clinical data, it is also important to consider the current position and stress on the referring physician. Keep questions brief; try not to have the physician repeat the entire history and course to multiple people. Consider whether the information you are collecting is needed immediately for decision-making and interim management or if it could be deferred until the transport team arrives.

C. Physician responsibilities for initiating transport

    1. Notify Respiratory Therapy (they will contact Dispatch to arrange for vehicle). Unless otherwise requested, the vehicles will be prepared as quickly as possible. It is expected that all nonelective transports will depart within 30 minutes of acceptance.

    2. Notify the charge nurse who arranges for nursing coverage.

    3. The neonatology fellow or neonatal nurse practitioner (NNP) determines the composition of the team, based on the severity or the patient's problems. In general, the team will consist of a physician or NNP, neonatal staff or EMS nurse, and respiratory therapist (many centers have successfully used an all-nurse or nurse–respiratory therapist team that maintains physician contact by telephone or radio during the transport).

D. Transport

    1. The physician (or designated nurse) has the overall responsibility for the transport and all personnel, including the ambulance attendants. Judgment should be exercised regarding safety, speed, and route. Drivers should not be requested to drive faster

than their comfort level allows. Likewise, drivers should not drive faster than the crew can tolerate.

2. Before departure, air and oxygen tank levels must be checked. Distance and special needs may require provision of additional oxygen supply.
3. Team members must be familiar with all ambulance or aircraft equipment (e.g., electrical connections, oxygen sources, suction, lights). All equipment should be secured so that with sudden stops no potentially dangerous items (e.g., tanks, monitors) are loosened.
4. Vehicles are equipped with radio communications to Dispatch. This may be used to give arrival times to hospitals, to request assistance (e.g., police escort), or to alert the NICU to unusual circumstances.
5. Only individuals specifically oriented to aircraft transport may fly.

E. Conduct at a referring hospital
  1. General principles
    a. The transport team represents the tertiary center.
    b. Do not underestimate the value of positive public relations.
    c. Transport provides a valuable opportunity for education and exchange of ideas.
  2. The reason for sending a team to the originating hospital is to stabilize the infant and make him/her fit for transport. The extent of procedures to be done may depend on the time and distance involved (e.g., an infant from a nearby hospital may not require an umbilical artery catheter immediately, enabling deferral of the procedure until admission to the NICU). All necessary diagnostic and therapeutic procedures should be done with the approval of the referring physician, to whom the team acts as consultants. Technically, care of the infant is transferred at the time the transport team assumes his/her care.
  3. The physician on the transport team is responsible for obtaining complete maternal and neonatal histories, all laboratory data, and radiographs (consider having copies made of significant findings). Document the amount of blood drawn for studies.
  4. The transport physician and nurse must talk with the parents, provide printed materials about the NICU, and obtain written consent for transport, admission, and treatment. Give the parents an opportunity to see *and touch* the infant. If possible, leave a photograph of the infant for the mother (obtain permission first).

    5. Notify the NICU before leaving the referring hospital. Advise the charge nurse of the estimated time of arrival, need for equipment (e.g., ventilator settings, infusion pumps), and medications (e.g., pressor drips), as well as the patient's general condition.

F. Costs

    1. Insurance benefits vary among carriers.

    2. Questions should be addressed to the UM Business Office.

G. Return trip

    1. Excessive speed is seldom, if ever, warranted if the infant is properly stabilized.

    2. The ambulance must be stopped if invasive procedures (e.g., intubation) become necessary.

    3. Remember that the transport vehicle serves as an extension of the NICU and appropriate observation, charting, and care should be provided.

H. After the trip

    1. Physician and nurse write appropriate transport notes.

    2. Transport evaluation forms are to be completed and returned to the nursing office for review. All identified problems will be referred to the appropriate discipline for correction.

    3. The referring physician should be notified of the infant's status within 24 hours.

    4. Parents should be notified that the infant arrived safely.

I. Back transport

    1. The possibility of back transfer, following resolution of acute illness, should be discussed with each family *early* in the infant's course.

    2. Suitable candidates should be sent with the least necessary staff and equipment.

    3. Complete medical and nursing summaries must accompany the infant. Also, if available, comments related to management of subsequent pregnancies should be included.

    4. Arrangements for back transfer

       a. Consult family; determine private physician.

       b. Contact private physician for approval.

       c. Contact receiving hospital nursery for approval.

       d. Consult nursing to arrange specific details (staffing, vehicle, equipment).

J. Refusal of service

    1. The neonatal transport team generally cannot respond to requests to attend deliveries in outside hospitals. However, under extenuating circumstances, exceptions are made. Efforts should

be directed at maternal transport (whenever possible) and neonatal resuscitation.

2. The neonatal transport team is not equipped or staffed to transport older infants or children. Requests to do so should be channeled to the appropriate service.

3. The following circumstances (or combination) may make an immediate response to a request impossible or inadvisable:
   a. Transport team has already been dispatched elsewhere.
   b. Excessive distance involved
   c. Inclement weather
   d. No available beds

4. In any of the above instances, the referring physician should be advised of other available regional facilities and of interim measures of support. Offering to contact another NICU/neonatologist to arrange transport for the referring hospital is good support for the referral region and is encouraged.

K. Air vs. ground transport

1. Most transports are done by ambulance with the exception of areas where vast distances separate facilities.

2. Decisions to use helicopter or fixed-wing aircraft are based on the following:
   a. Activity. Is the infant so critically ill that he/she needs to be in the NICU as soon as possible?
   b. Time. Is there a substantial time difference between the two modes?
   c. Stability. What are the capabilities of the referring hospital? Will a delay in arrival of the transport team jeopardize patient well being?
   d. Luxury vs. necessity. Will an unnecessary flight tie up the aircraft, preventing a subsequent emergency response?
   e. Staff. Are all personnel oriented to the helicopter and able to participate?
   f. Combination air and ground transport. Is it imperative for the team to get to the referring hospital *fast*? Consider a "fly-drive," where team is flown to referring hospital, ambulance follows with equipment and incubator, and team/baby drive back to NICU.
   g. Transports in which airborne vehicles are used for round trips should make every effort to minimize time spent at the referring hospital, thus shortening vehicle down time.
   h. Accessibility. Access to the patient may be severely limited in aircraft.

       i. Traffic. Helicopter transport may be much more efficient in reaching urban hospitals at rush hour.

L. Medical aspects

  1. Interim advice to requesting physician

    a. The NICU physician taking the phone call from the referring physician should, in addition to the basic information about the infant, ascertain what is currently being done with the infant.

      i. Whether the infant is in an *incubator* and what the respective *temperatures* of the incubator and the infant are should be recorded. If no servocontrolled incubator is available in the referring hospital, it should be suggested to the physician that the incubator be kept at 94°F for any premature infant.

      ii. If the infant receives *oxygen,* ascertain whether he/she is getting enough to keep from being cyanotic, what percentage oxygen is being given and, if this information is not available, what the flow rate of oxygen is (most incubators will achieve an oxygen concentration of 40% or above with flow rates of about 5 L/min).

      iii. The administration of *sodium bicarbonate* through the umbilical vein is an entirely acceptable emergency measure and the referring physician should not be discouraged from utilizing this route of bicarbonate administration if metabolic acidosis is present or suspected and adequate ventilation is assured.

    b. *Vitamin K* (1.0 mg IM or IV) should be given as soon as possible. *Orogastric tubes* should be placed in all infants with respiratory distress.

    c. Any infant in respiratory distress might benefit from a *chest radiograph* performed while the transport team is en route to the hospital. This might be another suggestion to the referring physician. Similarly, depending on the individual circumstances, *laboratory studies* might be performed during this time period and ordered by the referring physician, such as blood counts, electrolytes, blood gases, or blood sugar and calcium determinations. The interval could also be used to photocopy records and obtain radiography films for loan.

  2. Treatment of the infant at the referring hospital

    a. The infant should be put into a state such that an emergency would be unlikely to occur during the transport. This requires that, prior to the departure, the infant's temperature is normal or at least rising, that hypoglycemia is being corrected, and that there is unlikely to be any airway problem. This often necessitates a precautionary intubation for airway maintenance during the transport. It is possible to connect an intubated infant to the CPAP apparatus and this could be utilized in spontaneously breathing RDS patients of mild severity.

b. A blood glucose screening should be carried out and dextrose administered if needed. Most hospitals now have a good microchemistry facility so that full use should be made of the local hospital's facilities, particularly for pH determination.

c. The infant should be evaluated for any evidence of shock, and the hemodynamic state should be corrected as much as possible. Many infants do not need to be on a continuous infusion during the transport, and heparin locks can be used.

d. Procedures should be deferred whenever possible, though the infant's condition may warrant intervention. For instance, an obviously septic baby should have a sepsis work-up and initiation of antibiotics. However, a stable infant would probably be better off just stabilized, with lumbar puncture deferred until after arrival in the NICU.

e. It is a matter of judgment whether or not to insert a UAC. The principal purpose of a UAC is to obtain blood samples for blood gas monitoring and blood pressure monitoring. If the infant is primarily in need of infusion of fluids and medications, a peripheral intravenous line is preferable.

f. Before departure, the stomach should be aspirated. An orogastric tube should be left in place to ventilate.

g. At all times, the members of the transport team should remain aware that they are advisors to the referring physician who carries the primary responsibility for the patient. In his/her absence, they are entitled to use their own judgment regarding emergency treatment.

h. All initiations of treatment at the local hospital should also be considered related to how quickly the infant can be transported to the NICU. For instance, it is often not necessary to start major diagnostic procedures at a nearby hospital since the infant can be transported rapidly; on the other hand, this would be inappropriate for a 100-mile transport.

i. Before leaving the referring hospital, the infant must be connected to the portable ECG monitor.

3. Treatment during the transport

a. The portable monitor is one means of informing the team about the infant's state, but continuous visual observation is paramount. Periodic suctioning should be carried out as needed, and if the need for bagging arises in an infant that has not been intubated prior to the initiation of transport, bagging should first be attempted with a mask. If this is not successful, the ambulance should be stopped and intubation carried out. Infant status may be accurately assessed by non-invasive means such as pulse oximetry or transcutaneous monitoring.

   b. The ambulance attendants should be advised to keep the rear compartment heated to 80°F. In very cold weather, a sheet or blanket should be draped over the incubator to minimize radiant heat loss. A chemically heated mattress (Porta-Warm) is also available.

   c. Glucose screening should be done regularly. A portable infusion device (Auto Syringe) is available for careful fluid administration.

   d. During long transports, the infant's rectal temperature should be carefully checked regularly and the incubator and ambulance temperatures adjusted accordingly. Regular checks of delivered oxygen concentration and oxygen supply are to be made by the respiratory therapist.

   e. If special situations arise during the transport, the NICU should be advised by radio or telephone so that appropriate treatment can be readied or consultations arranged (e.g., need for respirator or surgery).

M. Addendum

   1. A bound set of road and city maps with routing instructions should be kept in the ambulance.

   2. A *Polaroid camera* should be included in the medication box so that parents can have a photograph of the infant. Their permission to photograph the infant is necessary.

N. In addition to its immediate purpose, the Newborn Transport Team is also one way of familiarizing the hospitals and physicians in the communities with the special services at the regional NICU. It is in everyone's interest to demonstrate *good will and cooperation* to all involved.

Suggested Reading

Donn SM, Faix RG, Gates MR: Neonatal transport. Curr Prob Pediatr 15:1–65, 1985.

Donn SM, Faix RG, Gates MR: Emergency transport of the critically ill newborn. In Donn SM, Faix RG (eds): Neonatal Emergencies. Mt. Kisco, NY, Futura Publishing, 1991, pp 75–86.

Gates MR, Geller S, Donn SM: Neonatal transport. In Donn SM, Fisher CW (eds): Risk Management Techniques in Perinatal and Neonatal Practice. Armonk, NY, Futura Publishing, 1996, pp 563–580.

Chapter 88

Perinatal Outreach Program

Molly R. Gates, M.S., R.N.C.

I. Purpose of the the Perinatal Outreach Program

A. Fosters linkage between the perinatal center and the community referral hospital; builds relationships to support clinical partnerships in the care of shared patients

B. Provides leadership from the perinatal center to the community referral hospital; serves as a catalyst and reference for practice change recommendations

C. Emphasizes communication and education directed toward appropriate identification, stabilization, and access to care for the high-risk perinatal patient; utilizes both obstetric and neonatal foci

D. Promotes the optimal use of the regional perinatal care system

E. Creates information networks with counterparts in other perinatal centers

II. Methods

A. Site visits
  1. Review referral hospital facilities.
  2. Meet with community hospital personnel.

B. Educational programming
  1. Tailored to the needs of individual hospitals
  2. Region-wide, to meet common needs efficiently

C. Communication liaison
  1. Follow-up referred patients' status.
  2. Share policy, procedure, and clinical updates as a resource to community hospitals.
  3. Provide easy access, central contact point for community hospital personnel.

D. Quality assurance activities
  1. Track referrals to identify trends.
  2. Medical record audits
  3. Facilities, equipment, procedure reviews
  4. Transport review
     a. At the perinatal center
        i. Periodic (scheduled) review of all transports
        ii. Attended by representatives of all services involved with

conducting transports, e.g., medicine, nursing, respiratory therapy, ambulance, and helicopter personnel
   iii. Transport evaluation forms completed for each transport serve as data source
   iv. Identification of trends as well as individual case issues or problems
    v. Focus on mutual problem solving
  b. At the community hospital
    i. Held periodically at each referral hospital
   ii. Conducted by the Perinatal Outreach Coordinator and a physician from the perinatal center in cooperation with the perinatal staff at the community hospital
   iii. Content similar to the monthly review, but includes only those cases referred by the host hospital
   iv. Didactic presentations may be offered also, as requested by the host hospital.
E. Facilitate back-transfer of convalescent patients
  1. Knowledge of the "home" hospital's resources aids in matching patient needs with available services
  2. Provides communication of patient clinical status
  3. Serves as a liaison to solve any post-transfer problems

Suggested Reading

Frank J, Rhodes T, Edwards W, et al: The New Hampshire perinatal program: Twenty years of perinatal outreach education J Perinatol 19:3–8, 1999.

Gardner SL: Perinatal outreach education: The beginning. Neonatal Netw 13:49–50, 1994.

Shenai JP: Neonatal transport: Outreach educational program. Pediatr Clin North Am 40:275–285, 1993.

Walden M: Collaborating with community hospitals for healthier babies through perinatal outreach education. J Pediatr Nurs 9:59–60, 1994.

Section XVI.   DISCHARGE AND FOLLOW-UP

Chapter 89

Discharge Planning

Charles R. Neal, Jr., M.D., Ph.D., and Mary E.A. Bozynski, M.D., M.S.

I. **Introduction**
   A. Discharge planning is an integral part of caring for the infant and family. If neglected, it could result in difficulty with home transition and rehospitalization of the infant.
      1. Such increased anxiety and confusion for the family and physician who assumes the infant's care is unnecessary.
      2. The best way to approach this process is to put yourself in the position of the parents and follow-up physician and determine what assessments, medications, teaching, community service, and communication of discharge information is needed.
   B. Discharge planning must be coordinated through the infant's attending physician and the patient care coordinator. It calls for a multidisciplinary approach.
      1. It should begin as soon as the infant is admitted to the unit, not on the day before discharge or transfer.
      2. The patient care coordinator, physical therapist, social worker, home care coordinator, and benefits coordinator may all need to be involved.
      3. Although the physician will have primary responsibility for only a portion of the planning, the physician (together with the patient care coordinator and the parents) is primarily responsible for assuring that the transition to home is safe and successful.
      4. As the infant convalesces, it is useful each day to assess conditions that will need future follow-up and to determine how near the infant is to transfer or discharge.
      5. Parents should be involved in the planning and should be approached to discuss plans as soon as the infant's survival is assured.

II. **Considerations**
   A. The infant should be feeding well orally and gaining adequate weight on a feeding regimen suitable for home care.
   B. The infant should be maintaining normal body temperature in a crib.
   C. The infant must be medically stable, not requiring day-to-day changes in management.

III. Necessary Consultations and Assessments

All of the following must be completed or arranged as applicable:

A. Review consults from medical subspecialists and arrange follow-up visits.

B. Review physical therapy evaluation and determine if a follow-up program has been provided.

C. Arrange or review results of ophthalmologic and audiologic testing.

D. Begin controlled withdrawal of medications that may not be required after discharge in an attempt to simplify home care safely.

E. Determine as soon as possible the need for a multichannel study.

F. Obtain a copy of key assessments, such as chest radiograph or cranial sonogram, if the infant will be transferred to another facility.

G. Assessment of the home, parents, and caregivers regarding willingness and ability to provide home care should be ongoing from admission. As discharge approaches, readily identified problem areas need to be addressed. Mobilize community and extended family resources for areas of weakness.

IV. Home and Community Arrangements

All of the following arrangements must be completed:

A. Verify that the parents are both emotionally and physically prepared and that the necessary equipment, transportation, and financial arrangements are complete.

1. Special considerations must be taken into account when choosing a car seat and in positioning the preterm infant in the car seat. Assess the infant in the car seat with a pulse oximeter.

2. Make sure that the parents or caregivers are prepared and that equipment appropriate for the particular infant is at hand, such as oxygen, suction, monitors, equipment for gastrostomy or nasogastric tube feedings, and stoma care.

B. Verify that all parental or caregiver teaching is complete, including CPR training if indicated.

1. In all cases, it is important to schedule a time to meet with the parents prior to discharge to assess their understanding of the hospitalization, the infant's condition, current care, need, and prognosis.

2. This is a good time to clear up misunderstandings and provide reassurance.

3. Remember that discharge is a time of crisis for parents and is both happy and frightening.

C. Identify and contact the follow-up physician.

D. A discharge summary, which includes the main problems and current status (e.g., weight, length, head circumference, blood pressure, hematocrit, medications doses, levels, immunizations), should be dictated, and a discharge form completed.

E. In complex cases, forward copies of all key assessments, such as chest radiographs or cranial sonograms, to follow-up physicians for reference.

F. An appointment in the appropriate follow-up clinic should be arranged if the infant meets the criteria.

G. A thorough review and evaluation of the infant's medication should be undertaken with the parents.

   1. Assure that discharge drug concentrations are therapeutic.

   2. Make sure that the parents have either prescriptions or medications in hand.

   3. Review with the parents why the infant requires the drug and what toxic side effects to monitor.

   4. Some prescriptions are best filled at the medical center, because outside pharmacies in the community may not carry the correct solution or concentration needed.

H. Determine whether community agencies should be or have been contacted (e.g., public health nurse, early intervention programs, respite care, home nursing care).

I. Make sure the caregivers have pertinent phone numbers in order to contact the primary physician, the NICU, or the office or beeper of the discharging physician for any questions or concerns that may arise in the immediate transition to home.

J. On the day before discharge, an order should be written on the chart that discharge is planned. This allows those involved ample preparation time for this important event.

Suggested Reading

Ballard RA (ed): Pediatric Care of the ICN Graduate. Philadelphia, W.B. Saunders, 1988.

Bernbaum JC, Hoffman-Williamson M: Primary Care of the Preterm Infant. St. Louis, Mosby, 1991.

Taeusch HW, Yogman MW: Follow-up Management of the High-Risk Infant. Boston, Little, Brown, 1987.

Chapter 90

Audiologic Screening of Infants

Mohammad A. Attar, M.D., and Robert E. Schumacher, M.D.

I. **Epidemiology**

Significant bilateral hearing loss is present in 1–3 per 1000 newborns in well-baby nursery population and in 2–4 per 100 infants in the intensive care unit population. The Universal Screening program is implemented in the University of Michigan Medical center as recommended by the American Academy of Pediatrics.

A. Factors associated with higher risk for hearing loss

1. Very low birthweight, < 800 g
2. Suspicion of perinatal asphyxia
3. Bacterial meningitis
4. Confirmed or highly suspected TORCH infection
5. Family history of hearing loss
6. Craniofacial or external ear abnormalities or syndromes known to be associated with hearing impairment
7. Hyperbilirubinemia (at level exceeding need for exchange transfusion)
8. Clinical suspicion of hearing loss
9. Prolonged treatment with (potentially) ototoxic drugs (e.g., furosemide, gentamicin)

B. Risk factors for neurologic and sensory (including auditory) abnormalities

1. Known high-risk for multiple neurologic handicaps
   a. Documented ICH—including subarachnoid, PVH, IVH
   b. Other brain pathology (e.g., PVL, ventriculomegaly, porencephaly)
   c. Severe or prolonged acidosis (pH < 7.1 persisting for hours)
   d. Seizures
   e. Abnormal neurologic examination at discharge
   f. In the absence of other neurologic sequelae, isolated sensorineural hearing loss should not be ascribed to "asphyxia."
2. Treatment with extracorporeal membrane oxygenation
3. Persistent pulmonary hypertension of the newborn
4. Apnea requiring ventilation or unresponsive to theophylline and usual management. Infants with apnea or considered at risk (e.g., on theophylline or monitor) for apnea at discharge.

5. Relative microcephaly (fronto-occipital head circumference below the third percentile for gestational age)
6. Culture-positive bacterial sepsis

II. Instrumentation and Methodology

A. Methods of physiologic screening include evoked otoacoustic emissions (EOAE) and auditory brainstem response (ABR).

B. Because ABR is regarded as a screening test, it is important to realize that there will be both false-positive and false-negative results, and a well-designed follow-up program is important.

1. ABR/BAER—the auditory brainstem response is a noninvasive electrophysiologic method for the determination of *hearing sensitivity* and *neuromaturational* status.

2. This procedure involves taping surface electrodes to the forehead and earlobes or mastoids and the presentation of acoustic clicks by means of standard earphones or small ear-canal receivers. Hearing sensitivity is determined from the presence or absence of a typical and intact waveform (wave V). Neurologic and maturational status is determined from the measurement of peak latency (e.g., neural conduction time from cochlea to upper medulla and lower midbrain). Infants preferably sleep through the 30-minute procedure.

C. EOAE measures sound waves generated in the inner ear (cochlea) in response to clicks or tone bursts emitted and recorded via miniature microphones placed in the external ear canals of the infants. EOAE screening may be affected by debris or fluid in the external and middle ear.

III. Schedule

A. All newborns:

1. Infants in the high-risk group who pass the ABR will be followed by means such as a parent questionnaire sent at 6 months of age.

2. Infants at risk for delayed onset or progressive hearing impairment (e.g., CMV, rubella, family history, ECMO, PPHN):
   a. ABR before discharge
   b. Repeat ABR at 2–4 months of age (arrange before discharge)
   c. Behavioral audiometric testing at 10, 20, and 36 months.

3. If ABR is failed, a repeat confirmatory ABR should be obtained. If follow-up ABR indicates a persistent hearing impairment, an ABR-assisted hearing aid evaluation and behavioral

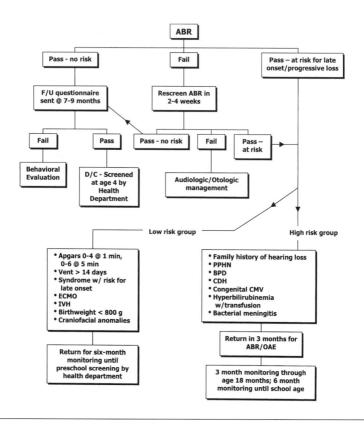

Figure 10. University of Michigan Health System early hearing detection and intervention program.

       audiologic evaluation follow-up, including otologic consultation, should be obtained.

  B. UMHS early hearing detection intervention (EHDI) program—current recommendations (Figure 10)

Suggested Reading

Erenberg A, Lemons J, Sia C, et al: Newborn and infant hearing loss: Detection and intervention. American Academy of Pediatrics. Task Force on Newborn and Infant Hearing, 1998–1999. Pediatrics, 103: 527–530, 1999.

Chapter 91

Follow-up

Mary E.A. Bozynski, M.D., M.S., and Jennifer L. Grow, M.D.

I. Goals

The goal of a neonatology follow-up clinic is to identify infants with developmental problems, ensure appropriate intervention, encourage and support parenting of the high-risk infant, and provide medical consultation to the physicians of infants with continuing medical problems. Follow-up is a multidisciplinary process involving physicians, physical and/or occupational therapists, nurses, psychologists, audiologists, speech pathologists, social workers, and dietitians.

II. Evaluation of Infants for Neonatal Follow-up

Before discharge, each infant at risk should be assigned to a risk group using criteria such as those given below. Previously, both high and moderate risk infants were scheduled for clinic follow-up. Because of higher no-show rates and a low yield in detecting developmental problems, moderate-risk infants are no longer routinely scheduled for clinic follow-up. The criteria selected for follow-up should provide low rates of missed developmental diagnoses that would need further evaluation or referral.

III. Criteria for Risk-Group Assignment

A. High-risk group criteria
1. Birthweight < 1250 g
2. Neurologic criteria
   a. Hypoxic-ischemic encephalopathy
   b. Abnormal neurologic examination at discharge
   c. IVH, grades III or IV
   d. ECMO use
   e. Periventricular leukomalacia
   f. Porencephaly or ventriculomegaly
   g. Inability to feed orally within 1–2 weeks of discharge
   h. Microcephaly
3. Respiratory criteria
   a. BPD requiring home oxygen, diuretics, or with abnormal cardiovascular examination on discharge
   b. Tracheostomy

    4. Other—team member discretion (e.g., poor social situation)
B. Moderate-risk group criteria
    1. Birthweight
        a. Birthweight 1250–1500 g
        b. IUGR
    2. Neurologic criteria
        a. Documented seizures
        b. Suspect neurologic status at discharge
        c. IVH, grades I or II
        d. Documented meningitis
        e. Congenital infection
        f. Polycythemia requiring intervention
        g. Atypical course or behavior
    3. Respiratory criteria: prolonged ventilation
        a. Term > 7 days
        b. Preterm > 14 days
    4. Other—team member discretion (e.g., suspect social situation)
    5. Infants who meet the following criteria will be under consideration for inclusion in the moderate-risk group:
        a. Hypoglycemia unresponsive to treatment
        b. Bilirubin > 20 mg/dL at term
        c. Exchange transfusion need
        d. Intrauterine fetal death of twin

IV. **Recommended Schedule of Follow-up for the First 2 Years**
A. High-risk schedule
    1. Follow-up phone call with 2–3 weeks of discharge
    2. Neonatology Clinic visit at 4, 8, 12, 18, and 24 months corrected age (may be modified based on cost and time constraints)
    3. Bayley Scales of Infant Development performed at 12 and 24 months
B. Moderate-risk schedule—when developing criteria for follow-up of moderate-risk infants, the goals of such clinic visits should be considered.
    1. If the purpose of clinic follow-up emphasizes research data collection in addition to patient care, then all moderate-risk infants should be scheduled for a visit.
    2. If the purpose of the clinic visit is to detect previously undiagnosed developmental problems either that qualify a child for services or for which effective or proven therapies are available, visits can be arranged or an additional screening performed.
    3. Specific criteria selected from lists such as in section III,B may

be useful to decide who receives follow-up. Parental questionnaires such as the Pre-screening Denver Questionnaire (PDQ) or
the Infant/Child Monitoring Questionnaire (ICMQ) may be sent
to parents as an alternative to scheduling routine clinic visits.

C. Low-risk schedule—as with most moderate-risk infants, it is suggested that parental questionnaires such as the PDQ or ICMQ be
considered to select infants for more detailed follow-up.

V.   Later Follow-up Schedule

At the end of 2 years, infants can be classified to one of three groups:
always normal, transient abnormalities or suspect exams, and abnormal. Those children who are abnormal will already be enrolled in special education services. Those who are normal and have always been
so probably do not require further follow-up. Those who have had
transient abnormalities are at higher risk for problems at school age.

VI.   Further Notes

A. Extremely preterm infants
  1. Early (first year)
     a. Developmental delay (50%)
     b. Cerebral palsy (15–20%) usually associated with major IVH
        or PVL
  2. Later (second year)
     a. Poor language development (expressive)
     b. Visual motor, perceptual, motor problems
  3. School age
     a. Physical and neurosensory sequelae, cerebral palsy most
        common (up to 25% in infants weighing < 1000 g at birth)
     b. Cognitive and behavioral difficulties, especially with mathe-
        matics, reading, and attention span (up to 50% in infants
        weighing < 1000 g at birth)
     c. Increased limitations on activities of daily living because of
        health issues
B. Term asphyxia
  1. Cerebral palsy
  2. Sensorineural hearing loss
  3. Speech and language problems
  4. Developmental delays

Suggested Reading

Ballard R (ed): Pediatric Care in the ICN Graduate. Philadelphia, W.B.
Saunders, 1986.

Bricker D, Squires J, Kaminski R, Mounts L: The validity, reliability, and cost of a parent-completed questionnaire system to evaluate at risk infants. J Pediatr Psychol 13:55–68, 1988.

Bricker D, Squires J, Potter L: Infant/Child Monitoring Questionnaires Technical Report #1. Available from Center on Human Development, Early Intervention Program, 901 East 18th Avenue, Eugene, OR 97403.

Glascoe FP, Dworkin P: The role of parents in the detection of developmental and behavioral problems. Pediatrics 95:829–836, 1995.

Hack M: Long-term developmental outcomes of low birth weight infants. Future Child 5:176–196, 1995.

Taeusch HW, Yogman MW: Follow-up Management of the High-Risk Infant. Boston, Little, Brown, 1987.

Section XVII. OTHER ROLES IN THE NICU

Chapter 92

The Role of the Neonatal Nurse Practitioner

Mary E. Linton, R.N., M.S.N., N.N.P.

I. **Introduction**

   A. Neonatal nurse practitioners (NNP) have been part of the team caring for infants in intensive care nurseries since the 1970s. The evolution of the role has been in direct response to the increasing complexity of sick and premature infants and a decline in the number of physicians available to provide care in the NICU. Research indicates that NNPs render quality care in a cost-effective manner and that they provide consistency and continuity to their patients.

   B. The educational preparation of the NNP has changed over the past several years. Initially, NNPs were given on-the-job training by neonatologists in hospital-based programs. Formal educational programs followed, and currently, new practitioners are required to have master's degree preparation. In addition to this formal education, NNPs are certified by a national certifying body and, in most states, are licensed as advanced practice nurses. They are required to provide evidence of continuing education credits to maintain certification.

   C. NNPs may be accountable to both medical and nursing departments for various components of their role. They are available as resources for staff nurses, house officers, and other support services working within the NICU.

   D. As a family-centered care provider, the NNP contributes to the education and support of parents and other family members. Early involvement in the plan of care for the infant can help the family to adapt to the stresses of the intensive care environment and help to prepare them for discharge.

II. **Responsibilities of the NNP (Including, but Not Limited to the Following)**

   A. Clinical practice

   1. Function as a member of the interdisciplinary team to meet the needs of infants and their families.

   2. Provide consistency to patients assigned to the team, following the infant from admission to discharge.

3. Perform ongoing health assessment of infants using diagnostic data, including laboratory and imaging studies, as well as physical examination.
4. Participate in daily rounds with the neonatologist, house officers, parents, and nursing staff. Validate medical diagnosis with the team and formulate a plan of care.
5. Initiate referrals for consultation with pediatric subspecialists and support services.
6. Perform diagnostic and therapeutic procedures using accepted standards and established protocols.
7. Document daily progress notes and revisions in the plan of care as part of the permanent record.
8. Provide delivery room evaluation and resuscitation for deliveries identified as high risk for which pediatric/neonatology attendance is requested.
9. Respond to medical emergencies in the NICU. Initiate interventions and notify the neonatologist and appropriate house officers.
10. Participate in family conferences, providing updates on the infant's progress and plan of care.

B. Education and professional development
1. Participate in the education and evaluation of house officers and students who are assigned to the NICU rotation.
2. Promote advanced practice nursing by providing leadership and serving as a role model.
3. Actively seek opportunities to promote professional growth.
4. Meet continuing education requirements to maintain certification as specified by National Certification Corporation for Obstetric, Gynecological, and Neonatal Specialties.
5. Participate in professional organizations.

C. Program development
1. Participate in establishing and accomplishing hospital, departmental, and unit goals and objectives.
2. Provide leadership and support to interdisciplinary work groups in the development and implementation of standards of care.

D. Research
1. Participate in and support clinical research.
2. Apply current research findings to clinical practice.
3. Participate in the development of research-based policies, procedures, and protocols for the care of neonatal patients.

Suggested Reading

American Academy of Pediatrics Conference on the Fetus and Newborn: Policy Statement: Advance Practice in Neonatal Nursing. Elk Grove Village, IL, AAP, 1992.

Bissinger RL, Allred CA, Arford PH, Bellig LL: A cost-effective analysis of neonatal nurse practitioners. Nurs Econ 15:92–99, 1997.

Farah AL, Bieda A, Shiao SPK: The history of the neonatal nurse practitioner in the United States. Neonatal Netw 15:11–21, 1996.

Ruth-Sanchez V, Lee KA, Bosque EM: A descriptive study of current neonatal nurse practitioner practice. Neonatal Netw 15:23–29, 1996.

Schultz JM, Liptak GS, Fioravanti J: Nurse practitioners' effectiveness in NICU. Nurs Manag 25:50–53, 1994.

Tschetter L, Sorenson DS: Educational preparation for the neonatal nurse clinician/practitioner: From past to future. J Perinatol Neonatol Nurs 15:61–69, 1991.

Chapter 93

The Role of Social Work in the Neonatal Intensive Care Unit

Janet C. Allen, M.S.W.

I. The Social Worker as a Team Member

A. Services should be available to:

1. Infant and family
2. NICU staff
3. Ancillary personnel

B. Goals of services

1. Alleviating stresses of hospitalization
2. Maximizing potential of optimal growth and development
3. Maintaining gains made via an effective network of services

II. Specific Services

A. Assessment of family dynamics and parental bonding process

B. Assessment of family reactions to illness or disability, including:

1. Understanding of problems
2. Levels of acceptance
3. Ability to cope
4. Available support systems
5. Other needs or problems

C. Provision of emotional support

D. Individual or family counseling in areas of:

1. Loss
2. Separation
3. Anxiety
4. Bereavement
5. Interpersonal problems

E. Coordination of hospital resources and family needs to enable effective services

F. Referral to hospital facilities or community agencies

1. Self-help parent groups
2. Business office
3. Department of Welfare (Aid to Dependent Children, Medicaid, Children's Special Health Care Services)
4. Special education

     5. Infant mental health programs
     6. Alternate placement for the baby
     7. Protective services
     8. Juvenile court petitions to allow medical intervention when parents do not consent.
G. Financial assistance (meals, transportation, lodging, personal needs)
H. Assistance to families in problem-solving: to facilitate regular visits to the NICU while maintaining other necessary obligations at home, and for the care of the child after discharge
I. Consultation with staff regarding family reactions:
     1. Adjustment
     2. Needs/strengths
     3. Demands
J. Facilitate communications
     1. Between families and medical team
     2. Between families via parent groups
K. Follow-up services after discharge or death
L. Teaching services to staff
     1. Psychosocial dynamics
     2. Bereavement issues
     3. Orientation of new staff

Chapter 94

Parents and the Neonatal Intensive Care Unit

Peter Blos, Jr., M.D.

I. **Introduction**

   A. Admission of a newborn to a NICU invariably constitutes a serious psychological crisis.

     1. Unexpected occurrence

     2. Feelings of helplessness

     3. Fears related to danger to infant

     4. Loss of expectations about baby and self

     5. Threat of greater and permanent loss(es)

   B. Best case scenario

     1. Experience is temporary and salutary.

     2. Parents and infant do well.

     3. No lasting damage

   C. Worst case scenario

     1. Significant medical problems

     2. Loss of what *might* have been

     3. Need for sufficient mourning to allow for stable attachment to the newborn, given the unexpected conditions

   D. Coping

     1. Denotes different psychological responses elicited by a perceived threat of danger

     2. Some of these mechanisms manifest as distressed states of being but may belong to a repertoire of responses that render the threat of danger emotionally manageable.

     3. Stress management styles and capacities vary considerably among individuals and over time.

     4. Couples and families operate as units within which there is a division of psychological labor and variability in coping skills and stress tolerance.

     5. Siblings of newborns perceive and react to parental stress according to their developmental phase and prior experience. Be alert for delayed reactions.

II. **Crisis**

   A. Acute phase

     1. Begins with diagnosis of a life-threatening problem for newborn

       2. Accentuated if baby is transported

  B. Intermediate phase

       1. Persists for duration of hospitalization

       2. Various events (e.g., medical set-backs, anticipated discharge) may revive intense emotions of acute phase.

  C. Concluding phase

       1. Ends with infants physical and psychological incorporation into family and home

       2. If baby dies in the hospital, crisis merges into more prolonged experience of grief and mourning.

III. Acute Phase

  A. Immediate typical reaction is perception of emergency and rapid mobilization of mastery functions.

  B. Once professionals take charge, mastery is commonly overtaken by a belated, powerful emotional upheaval.

  C. Manifestations

       1. Outward expressions of sadness, grief or intense anxiety

       2. In a contrary manner, only the defenses against these affects — denial or reversal — may be observable.

       3. These emotional expressions and defensive reactions, although not abnormal, may appear in an alternating manner. They must be closely observed, because they may interfere with parental attachment to newborn.

       4. Such intensity of affect cannot be sustained indefinitely and eventually gives way to a bearable but fragile equilibrium, usually 5–10 days after admission, though sometimes longer.

IV. Intermediate Phase

  A. Parental emotional effort of working through what has happened begins as baby stabilizes.

  B. Duration is as long as baby is hospitalized

  C. Parents begin to come to terms with events that have occurred and realize any apparent or residual sequelae and their implications.

  D. Time for critical development of attachment to newborn

  E. Parents and family begin to lead a more normal life despite knowing they have been irrevocably altered by experience. Siblings, depending on age, may begin to express their feelings through behavior and words.

  F. Anticipated discharge usually results in upsurge of the parents' anxiety, fears, and doubts about their adequacy to care for the infant at home.

1. Parents may express concerns directly.
2. Indirect expressions include delaying tactics, or raising problems that postpone discharge.
3. Denial of anticipatory anxiety is a danger signal that must be addressed.

V. Concluding Phase

A. Baby is discharged and arrives home.
B. Crisis is gradually resolved as parents claim baby as theirs and feel themselves to be competent caregivers.
C. May require weeks or months
D. Return of parental confidence and esteem may occur at different rates by mother and father.
E. Emotional support of one parent by the other remains a critically important aspect of their relationship.

VI. Manifestations of Coping with Crisis

A. Parental behavior at the onset depends not only on personality structure, prior experiences, and coping skills, but also on division of psychological labor that a couple has evolved. (If the mother is a single teenager, this division may occur between the mother and her parent[s]). Typical behaviors include:

1. Reality-oriented. Intellectual focus on issues, problems, treatments, prognosis, and sequelae. Matter-of-factness, rationality, and reasonableness are often hallmarks. Emotional components are stimulated by the experience; feared and threatened losses may be relegated to nonverbal expression (e.g., verbal intensity and tone, facial expression, posture, fatigue).
2. Denial or minimizing the severity of problems or difficulties. Conversely, an accentuation of severity and scope of the disaster may occur.
3. Strong emotional reactions and expressions with often uncontrollable anxiety and/or grief. Mothers often experience feelings of guilt, inadequacy, and loss of self-esteem. Prior abortion, miscarriage, or stillbirth may compound intensity. Self-preoccupation and guilt may interfere with onset and development of attachment.

B. None of the above are pathologic per se, but prolonged duration and intractability are signs of serious adaptational difficulty and warrant intervention. Often, a couple will adopt complementary or different reactions. The mother may be more overtly emotional, grief-stricken, or stunned, while the father may be more rational or minimizing, trying to comfort the mother through reassurance while at the same time distancing himself from his own painful emotional reactions.

C. Medical staff interventions can help during all phases of crisis by listening and talking and sometimes initiating the dialogue regarding unspoken feelings, worries, or fears. Specific ways to help include:

1. Provide facts in clear, nontechnical language.
2. Clarify diagnostic and therapeutic plans.
3. Discuss prognosis, even when uncertain.
4. Be available for questions; establish regular, planned appointment times.
5. Strongly support and encourage both parents to visit.
6. Help parents touch and hold the baby.
7. Tactfully acknowledge the emotional stresses endured by the parents, siblings, and other family members.

VII. Signs and Symptoms of Parental Deficit in Coping

A. Repetitive questions—there is a point where repetition indicates an emotional impasse that inhibits thought processes. Further factual clarification will not help. Questions and observations (in your own words) that may help include:

1. "I notice that it is hard for you to take in the answers to all your questions. Perhaps there is something else you want to know or talk about but find it hard to do so."
2. "I notice that you frequently have the same questions and do not seem satisfied with the answers. Perhaps you would like to talk about how this experience has felt."

B. Continuing or increasing manifest emotional distress, i.e., crying, disorganization, confusion, depressive mood, long and repetitive phone calls—may indicate that the parents cannot move beyond their initial emotional emergency organization because they are not in emotional touch with each other. Discussing this possibility and providing an opportunity for them to express feelings or worries may be helpful. Describing your observations may also be a way to clarify for the parents/couple the rationale for a possible referral to social work or psychiatry.

C. Withdrawal—this may be manifested in psychological or behavioral terms:

1. Decreased frequency of calls or visits, often with repeated reality explanations.
2. Continued visiting but no dialogue with staff. Commenting on one's observations in an inquiring, nonjudgmental manner may allow the parent(s) to express certain feelings or thoughts that

are felt unacceptable (e.g., the baby is too damaged and should die), protecting oneself by not getting too attached.

VIII. What the Physician Can Do

A. Provide facts clearly and nontechnically.

B. Establish a relationship that is shared with the appropriate nursing staff and NICU social worker.
1. Meet regularly.
2. Make/maintain phone contact.
3. Reflect and acknowledge affective strain and emotions (or lack thereof).
4. Let parents know you are interested in their feelings and thoughts and are aware of their fluctuations.
5. Avoid the preemptory and superficial "How are you doing?"— "Fine." level of interchange.

C. Inquire and be alert to sibling reactions to these events and their parents' preoccupation and anxiety. Provide opportunity to discuss ways of telling siblings in age-appropriate language about what has happened and what may happen.

D. Be aware of parents being "stuck" emotionally and offer opportunity for more than surface exploration of feelings. A "rational, unemotional, reality-oriented" parent may be the easiest to work with, but this stance is too often evidence of emotional distancing.

E. Consider direct consultation if caregivers are experiencing difficulties with parents, including:
1. Increasing staff irritation with parents
2. Efforts to reach parents emotionally are failing.
3. Planning with parents seems nonproductive.
4. Unusual behavior, bizarre or suicidal thoughts, or deepening depression is evident.

F. Before making a referral
1. Discuss it with appropriate staff and consultant.
2. Specifically, discuss the strategy of helping parents understand and accept the referral as being in the best interests of the *baby*.

G. Parents often experience referrals as an indication of failure and another loss. Referrals are successful only when proper preparatory emotional groundwork has been laid.

Suggested Reading

Als H, Gilkerson L: Developmentally supportive care in the neonatal intensive care unit. Zero to Three 15:1, 1995.

Boris NW, Abraham J: Psychiatric consultation to the neonatal intensive care unit: Liaison matters. J Am Acad Child Adolesc Psychiatry 38:1310–1312, 1999.

Fraiberg S: Clinical Studies in Infant Mental Health: The First Year of Life. New York, Basic Books, 1980.

Harrison H: The principles for family-centered neonatal care. Pediatrics 92:643–650, 1993.

Klaus MH, Kennell JH: Parent–Infant Bonding. St. Louis, Mosby, 1982.

Meyer EC, Coll CT, Lester BM, et al: Family-based intervention improves maternal psychological well-being and feeding interaction of preterm infants. Pediatrics 93:241–246, 1994.

Singer LT, Salvator A, Guo S, et al: Maternal psychological distress and parenting stress after the birth of a very low-birth-weight infant. JAMA 281:799–805, 1999.

Tracey N (ed): Parents of Premature Infants: Their Emotional World. Philadelphia, Whurr, 2000.

Zeanah CH (ed): Handbook of Infant Mental Health, 2nd ed. New York, Guilford Press, 2000.

Chapter 95

Grief Counseling and Palliative Care

Susan K. Gibney, R.N., M.S., L.L.P., Janet C. Allen, M.S.W., and Charles R. Neal, Jr., M.D., Ph.D.

I. Critical Issues

A. The majority of newborns are admitted to an NICU because of the existence of a life-threatening condition or diagnosis.

B. The responses of parents to these admissions involve natural grief reactions to perceived loss.

    1. There are two types of loss felt by parents.

        a. Primary loss (physical) is felt as a result of the potential death or disability of their child.

        b. Secondary loss (symbolic) is felt secondary to lifestyle changes, breastfeeding concerns, shattered dreams, and loss of the perfect birth.

    2. Grief is a psychological, behavioral, social, cultural, and physical reaction, varying between individuals.

C. Provision of grief and bereavement support is an ongoing responsibility of the health care team.

    1. Effective communication requires sensitivity to the parents' emotional state, history of past losses, social support needs, and medical conditions.

    2. Responses of caregivers generally reflect their own experiences, emotions, and education.

    3. Ability of senior staff to model compassionate caregiving and effective communication is vital.

D. Palliative care principles are used *from the outset* when any patient faces a life-threatening condition.

    1. Using these principles, palliative care begins upon admission for most NICU patients.

    2. These principles are not to be applied only when curative measures are deemed futile.

    3. The American Academy of Pediatrics (AAP) supports an *integrated model of palliative care* that begins the moment an infant is admitted to the NICU (see below).

II. Grief Support

A. Upon admission, the family is highly stressed.

1. The mother is postpartum and often has dealt with a difficult pregnancy and/or delivery.
2. Maternal–infant bonding has been interrupted.
3. The infant may have been transported from another hospital.
4. Both parents are usually sleep-deprived.
5. Talking about the experience can facilitate coping and the ability to absorb new information.
6. Eliciting the parent's emotional response can help diffuse stress and establish trust and rapport, enabling more effective communication.

B. Later, particularly during prolonged admissions, family meetings will facilitate decision making, goal setting, and the education of parents.

1. If necessary, multidisciplinary meetings enable assessment of the family's educational needs, reinforcement of information, and coordination of care with multiple services.
2. Guidelines for discussion
   a. Maintain a genuinely unhurried manner.
   b. Provide a private area for discussion.
   c. Display understanding and caring.
   d. Ensure that the mother is not alone during presentation of the infant's condition.
      i. This is especially important during the first encounter with her after the birth.
      ii. Whenever providing "bad news" to the mother regarding her baby, be sure a support person is present and will remain after you leave the room.
   e. Offer detailed, complete information *in language parents understand*.
      i. This may require such things as pictures and radiographs to describe the condition.
      ii. Translators should be present for parents whose first language is not English.
   f. Offer consultation with the Ethics Committee if points of view conflict.
   g. Designate a person to provide primary communication to the family regarding their infant during the present service month.
      i. This can becomes a serious problem if not done.
      ii. One goal of family meetings is to help define this designated person, usually the attending neonatologist.
         (a) Avoid creating an environment where the parents

obtain information regarding their infant from multiple sources.

    (b) Providing information without first consulting the treatment team (such as during rounds) often leads to the parents receiving conflicting or contradictory information.

    iii. Parents repeatedly stress that they appreciate house staff and nurses saying, "I do not know" and pursuing the answer to their inquiry with the fellow or attending.

3. Attitudinal issues

    a. Maintain *appropriate* hope for optimal outcome and relay this to the parents until it is obviously otherwise.

    b. Consider parental input in determining treatment as much as ethically possible.

    c. Take responsibility for making difficult clinical and caregiving decisions.

    d. The treatment team should do whatever it can to minimize doubt, confusion, and guilt.

4. Dealing with conflicting expectations

    a. The range of normal reactions to bad news is broad.

    b. *Disbelief and denial are adaptive natural responses* to the initial presentation of information that is overwhelming.

    c. These reactions become maladaptive only later if they interfere with making critical decisions.

    d. Open-ended questions asked empathetically by the clinician prepare the parent to face adverse news.

    e. When dealing with anger and conflicting expectations, stay calm, speak softly, and adhere to the clinical issues.

        i. Avoid reacting to the conflict.

        ii. Avoid making judgments.

C. When curative measures have been deemed futile, the goal shifts to a process of empowering parents to regain ownership of the situation and their infant.

1. Healthy mourning first requires recognition of the loss by the parents.

    a. In anticipation of death of their baby, parents focus on the infant's life and what it means to them.

    b. Understanding the course of the child's illness is a gradual process, and the concepts are difficult to absorb when one is in a highly emotional state.

    c. Repetition is often required.

2. Staff must anticipate parents' needs and guide them through the experience of their child's death.
   a. Memories are created of nurturing, comforting, and holding the baby, as well as family rituals.
   b. "They must say 'hello' before they can say 'goodbye.'"
      —Sherokee Ilse, a bereaved parent
3. Parents appreciate nonjudgmental, compassionate responses to their questions and reactions.
   a. Bereaved parents never forget the understanding, respect, and genuine warmth they received from caregivers.
   b. This can become as lasting and important as any other memories of their lost pregnancy or their baby's brief life.
4. Suggestions for comforting words:
   a. "I'm sorry."
   b. "You are very devoted parents."
   c. "I wish things could have been different for you and your baby."
5. Do not say:
   a. "You can always have another child."
   b. "There is a reason for everything."
   c. "You will get over this in time."
6. Mother/parents and the infant should be together at the time of death, using whatever means is available.
   a. Transport of the terminally ill infant back to mother may be necessary to facilitate this.
   b. The team may delay removing support as long as possible until parents can be present.

D. Loss in the neonatal period is unique.
1. Parental loss of a child is outside of the natural order of life.
   a. Parents are grateful to have some time and experiences with their baby before death.
   b. Seeing the baby's eyes open and hearing its cry are especially cherished by the parents.
2. Parents must grieve for the unattainable, dreamed-of baby and their future together.
3. It is important to remember that, until discharge or death, the NICU infant resides in the hospital. As such:
   a. Parents often do not receive the acknowledgement of their baby's existence and value.
   b. *The community and extended family may not recognize the death of a newborn as a significant loss.* This is particularly difficult for the parents.

    4. Death of one member of a multiple gestation adds another dimension to grief.
      a. Parents must deal with the conflict of grieving the child who died while celebrating the life of the surviving infant(s).
      b. There is a loss of unique status of having twins or triplets, the loss of belonging to a multiples group.
      c. The community often is not understanding of the significance of their loss.
        i. The general perception is that the parents are fortunate to have a survivor.
        ii. However, parents continue to think of their baby as a twin/triplet.
      e. Parents need to grieve the loss of the sibling, and not just concentrate on the survivor.
      f. Often, the survivor remains in the NICU for some time, a continuing stressor that challenges the parents' grief response.

III.   Palliative Care

  A. Goals and concepts of a model for palliative care for children entail "the achievement of the best quality of life for patients and their families, consistent with their values, regardless of the location of the patient" (AAP, 2000).

  B. Palliative care begins with the determination of a life-threatening or terminal condition and extends to the families of the patient.
    1. This includes most NICU admissions.
    2. Adequate implementation requires support for curative, life-prolonging, and palliative care.
      a. Pain and symptom management
      b. Effective communication with parents
      c. Support for the social, psychological, cultural, and spiritual needs of families
      d. Coordination of care within the hospital (between services and caregivers) and after discharge (home nursing and equipment, primary care physician, respite care, and hospice)
      e. Grief and bereavement support

  C. Staff issues
    1. Effective communication with parents must be stressed.
    2. Educational needs of all caregiver disciplines should be addressed regarding appropriate initiation and provision of palliative care.
    3. Stress can result from caring for patients with these conditions and their families.

    a. Senior staff must model appropriate communication styles and coping skills.

    b. Debriefing is often useful, especially in ethically and/or clinically complex cases.

    c. Expressions of condolence to the family and attendance at funerals and memorials are appropriate and healthy modes of processing caregiver grief.

D. Resource services for providing palliative care must be available to staff during hospitalization, during the discharge process, and after transferring care to either the primary care physician or hospice care.

  1. Pain management includes both pharmacologic and nonpharmacologic strategies.

    a. Music therapy, infant massage, developmentally appropriate positioning, and care interventions

    b. Pharmacologic interventions may vary from those normally used in the NICU.

    c. Consultation with the Anesthesia or Pain Control Services may be necessary in select cases.

  2. Symptom management includes therapies for signs of dyspnea, agitation, gastric reflux, feeding aversion or difficulty, wound care, and neurodevelopmental issues.

  3. Social support for families

    a. Assess parental understanding, and ability to cope with the infant's diagnosis and care needs.

    b. Facilitate transportation and housing in the vicinity of the hospital.

    c. Enable sibling and extended family attendance in the NICU.

    d. Arrange child life interventions for siblings.

    e. Provide parent support groups.

  4. Psychological support

    a. Education for parents, such as stress reduction and coping strategies

    b. Therapy for parents, such as assessment and treatment of anxiety and depression

    c. Interventions to strengthen and maintain family ties

  5. Cultural support includes accommodation for rituals and expectations unique to the family's culture.

    a. Ask the family how you can respect and accommodate their cultural traditions.

    b. Consult with the Program for Multicultural Health if necessary.

6. Spiritual support, an important area of concern for many parents and caregivers, must be provided in an open and nonjudgmental fashion.
   a. Provide pastoral care, when desired.
   b. Ask the parents how you can accommodate and respect their religious traditions.
   c. Consider the family's spiritual traditions in understanding and accepting parental decisions.
7. Coordination of care in the hospital includes anticipating and preparing the family for transfers between units.
8. Coordination of care after discharge includes anticipating, as early as possible, the needs of the patient at the time of discharge.
   a. This includes discharge to home or hospice care.
   b. Communicate this anticipation to the family, outside agencies, and potential caregivers.
   c. Document for the record, and the family, all resources available within the hospital and in the community.

E. Immediate bereavement support
1. Consistent and effective communication during the entire hospitalization
2. Timely provision of critical clinical information
   a. Both during the hospitalization and after the infant's death
   b. This is vital as the parents attempt to find meaning and closure.
3. Provide emotional and practical support to enable the parents to create comforting memories during the last hours or days of the infant's life.
4. Provide concrete mementos such as photographs, hand or footprints, hair, name tags, clothing, blankets, and memory box collections.
5. Provide written educational materials about the processes and stages of grief and guidelines for supporting the grief of siblings.
6. Extend expressions of sympathy and caring, including flowers, cards, and follow-up letters.
7. Follow-up phone calls should be provided.
   a. At approximately 1 week, 6 weeks, and 6 months after the loss.
   b. Essential to confirm a caring and trusting relationship with the parents
   c. Enables parents to ask questions and normalize their grief reactions
   d. 6–12 months of significant stress is quite normal in this scenario.

8. Screen for abnormal grief reactions to identify situations that may require prompt intervention.
   a. Suicidal ideation in either parent
   b. Inability to care for remaining children
   c. Signs of abnormal or dangerous sibling reactions
9. Provide referrals for counseling and parent support groups.

F. Follow-up bereavement support
1. Track postmortem reports and critical clinical information, such as biopsies, to enable timely provision of critical information.
2. Track anniversary dates.
3. Provide grief support contact prior to major holidays.
   a. These are critically stressful times for families who have lost children.
   b. Holiday grieving is most stressful during the first year after the loss.
4. Facilitate and attend memorial services.
   a. Memorial services relieve some of the isolation that parents say increases the pain of their loss.
   b. Since 1984, by presidential proclamation, October is Perinatal Loss Remembrance Month.
5. A system for acknowledging and managing general contributions and memorial gifts for specific patients should be in place.
   a. Name plaques for donated items
   b. Name plaques for monetary contributions
   c. Thank you notes from unit administrators and close caregivers
   d. Gift fund accounts should be active and parents assured that these funds will be used to support patients and families.

Suggested Reading

American Academy of Pediatrics Committee on Bioethics and Committee on Hospital Care: Palliative care for children. Pediatrics 106:351–357, 2000.

Bedell S, Cadenhead K, Graboys T: The doctor's letter of condolence. N Engl J Med 344:1162–1164, 2001.

Buchman R: How to Break Bad News: A Guide for the Health Care Professional. Baltimore, Johns Hopkins University Press, 1992.

Ilse S: Empty Arms: Coping with Miscarriage, Stillbirth and Infant Death. Long Lake, MN, Wintergreen Press, 1985.

Leon IG: Perinatal loss: A critique of current hospital practices. Clin Pediatr 31:366–374, 1992.

Leon IG: Perinatal loss: Understanding pregnancy loss—helping families cope. Postgrad Obstet Gynecol 19:1, 1999.

Rando TA: Grief, Dying and Death. Champaign, IL, Research Press, 1984.

Ryan R, August A: Loss in the neonatal period: Comments. In Woods JR, Woods JL (eds): Loss during Pregnancy or in the Newborn Period. Pitman, NJ, Jannetti Publications, 1997, pp 125–157.

Chapter 96

Conflict between Medical Treatment and Religious Beliefs

Steven M. Donn, M.D.

I. Taking Legal Action

    A. Cases in which a minor child requires a procedure or blood transfusion but the parents refuse permission on religious grounds necessitate a court order to allow the use of blood or medical therapy.

        1. Courts have generally not supported the right of parents to withhold medical treatment if doing so will endanger the life or welfare of the child.

        2. This is in contrast to the generally upheld right of a competent adult to refuse life-saving treatment for him- or herself.

        3. As always, in the event of a life-threatening emergency, medical treatment may be given without a court order.

    B. It is assumed that the physician has discussed the issues with the parents before legal action is begun. In order to save time in court, the representative of the hospital may suggest to the parents that they obtain an attorney. The judge may also appoint an attorney to serve as guardian ad litem for the infant.

II. Obtaining a Court Order

The actual procedure of obtaining a court order will vary, depending on the location and hospital.

    A. Involvement of social or child protective services and the hospital attorney is likely.

    B. Depending on the judge, the hearing may take place in the courtroom, the hospital, or by telephone (speaker phone).

    C. In each case, the judge will hold a hearing with testimony from a physician, acting as a witness, indicating the need for the procedure and/or blood transfusion.

    D. The following information should be included in the physician's testimony:

        1. Name, age, date of birth, and hospital registration number of patient

        2. Name(s), marital status, address(es), and phone number(s) of parents

        3. Do both parents follow the same religious beliefs prohibiting

the treatment? Has the procedure been discussed with the parents? Do the parents object to the procedure, use of blood, or other treatments?

4. Where are the parents now? It is necessary for them to be available for the court hearing.
5. Name of the physician in charge of the case and performing the procedure/transfusion who can verify that the therapy is required (this is usually the physician at the hearing).
6. The condition of the child
7. Required procedure
   a. Nature of the procedure
   b. Need for the procedure and degree of urgency
   c. Harm that will ensue if the procedure is not performed
8. If a transfusion is required, be able to answer questions such as:
   a. Why is blood needed?
   b. Can blood substitutes be used? Erythropoietin? If not, why not?
   c. What is the likely result if the transfusion is not performed? Specifically, would the child be at risk for death or serious injury?
   d. What is the child's history of blood transfusions?
   e. What is the possibility of the blood being contaminated (e.g., HIV or hepatitis) and causing other diseases or harm to the child?
   f. To what extent is the need for blood or therapy a continuing one?

III. Physician Testimony

A. When giving testimony, the physician must be clear about the *definite* need for the procedure.

B. The testimony should not, however, serve to later limit or impede the physician's care of the child, for instance by stating that "no transfusion will be given if the hematocrit is above 30%."

C. In addition, the physician should be prepared to describe in detail the need for continuing care or repeated treatment, if it is likely, to justify a broader order, allowing the continued treatment of the infant, rather than a one time order for a transfusion or procedure.

IV. The Judge

Keep in mind that although courts have been generally supportive of physicians' efforts to care for these infants, the individual philosophy of the judge is perhaps the greatest variable involved.

A. The judge must have a clear understanding of how ill the infant is. Avoid medicalese, acronyms, and jargon, because these will not further the judge's understanding on the situation.

B. A photograph of the infant, showing the ventilator and the multitude of monitors and intravenous lines may be helpful in this regard.

V.   Parental Testimony

The parents will also have an opportunity to testify and ask questions.

A. The parents will often have an attorney and/or religious advisor present.

B. Other witnesses may also testify.

VI.   If a Court Order Is Issued

A. If the judge finds that the procedure or use of blood products is necessary for the safety of the child, the court will issue an order appointing a guardian who will then allow these procedures.

B. A copy of the order should be placed in the baby's hospital chart.

Suggested Reading

Ackerman TF: The limits of beneficence: Jehovah's Witnesses and childhood cancer. Hastings Cent Rep 10:13–18, 1980.

Family Case and Medical Management for Jehovah's Witnesses. Hospital Information Services, Watch Tower, 1992.

Goldman EB: Legal aspects of emergency care. In Donn, SM, Faix RG (eds): Neonatal Emergencies. Mt. Kisco, NY, Futura Publishing, 1991, pp 645–660.

Goldman EB, Oberman HA: Legal aspects of transfusion of Jehovah's Witnesses. Transfus Med Rev 5:263–270, 1991.

Jonsen AR: Blood transfusions and Jehovah's Witnesses: The impact of the patient's unusual beliefs in critical care. Crit Care Clin 2:91–100, 1986.

Chapter 97

Infant and Child Care Review (Ethics) Committee

Eileen G. Wright, R.N., and Steven M. Donn, M.D.

I. Background

    A. The care of sick newborn infants may raise concerns about the appropriateness of the management in relation to the expected outcome. These issues may lead to disagreement between various caregivers or parents regarding decisions about the extent and duration of continuing or extending care; ethical and medical conflicts may require a forum for discussion.

    B. This is the role of the Infant and Child Care Review Committee (ICCRC). At the University of Michigan Health System, it is composed of members of the medical, nursing, social, and pastoral hospital staff and includes an attorney and an ethicist.

II. Mechanism

    A. Anyone can request that the ICCRC meet for a case review. A social worker may then start the fact-finding process and a meeting will be arranged. The family of the infant and/or support persons of their choosing are invited to participate in the presentation to the Committee.

    B. The ICCRC focuses its role on the ethical implications of the issues at hand and makes a recommendation as to the ethical appropriateness of the options under consideration. The ICCRC does not assume any prerogatives of medical decision making.

    C. The ICCRC is also available to provide educational sessions for faculty and staff and to help develop policy on ethical issues.

    D. There is no list of situations that must be reported to the ICCRC. By far, the most common conflicts result from inadequate communications pertaining to medical facts rather than true ethical controversies, and thus can be prevented by open discussions and information exchange between physicians, other staff, and parents. The ICCRC can help facilitate such discussions if necessary.

Section XIX. MEDICAL INFORMATION AND THE MEDICAL RECORD

Chapter 98

Medical Informatics

William M. Bellas, D.O.

I. Introduction

A. Doctors will need a working knowledge of technology and medical information systems in order to provide efficient and cost-effective health care.

B. Information technology can help identify and resolve physician's knowledge gaps.

C. Medical decisions can be enhanced with the use of information technologies.

D. Information increases at a rapid pace, making it nearly impossible to keep up-to-date without information tools.

II. Definition

A. Informatics encompasses the fields of information science and information technology.

   1. Information science (IS)—study of information

   2. Information technology (IT)—hardware and methods developed to store, process, analyze, transmit, and display information

B. Medical informatics is a field-specific branch of informatics encompassing the fields of medical IS and IT and is subdivided into two areas:

   1. Clinical informatics (health care provider)—study of information in a clinical environment as it affects the one-to-one situation between provider and patient

   2. Managerial informatics

      a. Historically, most funds were allocated to this segment, which dominated health care informatics (i.e., accounting)

      b. Driven by business and administration

III. Background

A. Convergence of telecommunications and informatics over the past 50 years.

B. Advanced Research Projects Agency Network (ARPANET)

   1. Internet's progenitor as a global network

495

    2. Established primarily for research purposes among top academic centers by the U.S. Department of Defense during the Cold War

    3. Email, data file transfer services evolved

  C. European Organization for Nuclear Research (CERN)

    1. World Wide Web (W3) "point and click" hyperlinks and graphical user interface (GUI)

    2. Connected library databases

      a. American National Library of Medicine

      b. Library of Congress Soviet Archives

  D. Albert Gore, U.S. Vice President

    1. Superhighway (Global Information Infrastructure or GII)

    2. International Telecommunications Union in Buenos Aires, Argentina, March 21, 1994: Advent of the "superhighway" will have profound effects on health care delivery.

IV. Basics

  A. Education and training

    1. Incidental use (e.g., word processing)

    2. Computer-assisted learning (e.g., simulations)

    3. Examinations

    4. Library searches

  B. Clinical practice

    1. Medical information

    2. Management of patients

  C. Health care task analysis will define and determine the utility of informatics in the clinical setting. This defines the characteristic of a task and focuses attention on the problem or condition at hand.

  D. Integration of medical information systems improves the learning experience by the end user, while also improving patient outcomes (i.e., simulations).

  E. Informatic tools

    1. Computers (hardware and software)

    2. Handheld devices/pen tablets

    3. Internet

    4. Networks (LAN, WAN, wireless)

    5. Storage media (CD-recordable)

    6. Multimedia

    7. Telemedicine

    8. Artificial intelligence and logic systems

V. Medical Information
A. There is an explosion of information in the medical field.
B. No longer can the physician know the "whole" of medicine, even within one's own specialty.
C. Information sources for patient care can come from many sources:
1. Patient
2. Nurses
3. Colleagues
4. Laboratory
5. Pharmacy
6. References
7. Audio or video
8. Computers
D. Medical information is often imprecise.
E. Uses of information in medicine
1. Clinical purposes
2. Management of health care
3. Study of trends in health
4. Research
F. Evidence-based medicine (EBM) requires information access at point of care.
G. Evolution of an integrated clinical workstation (ICWS)
1. Clinical patient information
2. Physician orders and instructions
3. Decision support
4. Medical education
5. Communication with local and distant resources
H. Ultimately, quick access to information can improve service for patients, while maintaining the cost-effectiveness of care.

VI. Benefits of Information Technology
A. Increased efficiency
B. Decreased resource utilization
C. Reminder systems
D. Increased productivity
E. Improved revenue
F. Improved medical decisions
G. Better follow-up and preventive care
H. Expansion of clinical research

VII. Obstacles to Information Technology
A. Security and privacy (e.g., hackers, viruses)

    B. Safety-critical hardware/software
    C. Expensive enterprise solutions
    D. Training
    E. Lack of standards
    F. Lack of expertise in field of medical informatics
    G. Ethical concerns
    H. Legal implications
    I. Obsolescence
    J. Intangibility of benefits

VIII. Future

    A. Medical informatics and information systems will continue to play an intricate and increasing role in health care administration.

    B. Information technologies need to address present concerns (practical and conceptual) of the end user.
        1. Specialty specific
        2. Nonthreatening
        3. Ease of integration into current practice
        4. Timeliness and appropriateness of information
        5. Complements end user's knowledge
        6. Based on open system standards
        7. Convergence of common terminology
        8. Protection from obsolescence
        9. Safety concerns and system failure protocols
        10. Legal and ethical concerns

    C. Integration into medical education core curriculum
    D. New legislature to protect health care providers and patient information
    E. Advanced degrees in medical informatics by way of ACGME-approved fellowship training.
    F. Continued growth and development of medical informatics as a discipline via ongoing research

Suggested Reading

Brittain JM, Norris AC: Delivery of health informatics education and training. Health Libr Rev 17:117–128, 2000.

Chilton L, Berger JE, Melinkovich P, et al: American Academy of Pediatrics, Pediatric Practice Action Group and Task Force on Medical Informatics. Privacy protection and health information: Patient rights and pediatrician responsibilities. Pediatrics 104:973–977, 1999.

Collen MF: The origins of informatics. J Am Med Inform Assoc 1:91–107, 1994.

de Dombal F: Medical Informatics: The Essentials. Woburn, MA, Butterworth-Heinemann, 1996.

The Health Insurance Portability and Accountability Act of 1996 (1996). Available at http://www.hcfa.gov/hipaa/hipaahm.htm. Accessed April 9, 2002.

Patel VL, Arocha JF, Kaufman DR: A primer on aspects of cognition for medical informatics. J Am Med Inform Assoc 8:324–343, 2001.

Wong ET, Abendroth TW: Reaping the benefits of medical information systems. Acad Med 71:353–357, 1996.

Chapter 99

Documentation

Steven M. Donn, M.D.

I. The Medical Record

The medical record is a legal document that is used to chronicle the patient's course in the hospital. Accordingly, all entries must be factual, timely, and of a permanent nature.

A. *Record date and time* of all entries. The time should indicate when the note is written. If the event being described preceded the note, the time that the event occurred should be stated.

B. *Sign all entries.* If your signature is not easily discernible, print your name below it. Many institutions also require a physician identification number.

C. All medical notes written by a nonlicensed physician or a trainee must be countersigned by a licensed physician.

II. Events Requiring Documentation

A. Admission (*see* Chapter 5)

1. Includes history, physical examination, gestational age assessment, laboratory data, impression, plan, and additional documentation.

2. A consent form authorizing admission and treatment should be signed by a parent/guardian.

3. The attending physician and service should be indicated.

B. Transport note—if the infant is transported from another facility a note must be written indicating:

1. Reason for transfer

2. All diagnostic and therapeutic procedures performed by transport service

3. Consent from parents

4. Problems and complications during transport

C. Progress note

1. At least daily, more often if needed

2. Describe patient status, significant changes in condition, diagnostic and therapeutic plans, and communications with parents, consultants, referring physicians.

3. Your impressions should be reflected in the note.

D. Procedure note

1. List procedure(s) performed.
2. Give indication(s).
3. State who actually performed the procedure.
4. Describe equipment, technique, result.
5. Describe any complications.
6. State patient's tolerance of procedure.
7. Be sure to document necessary follow-up studies (e.g., radiograph after umbilical line placement).
8. Signed consent forms should be placed in the medical record.

E. Transfer note
   1. Required when patient is transferred to another service, location, or institution
   2. Summarizes course to date, active problems, and plans
   3. Facilitates assumption of care by next individual(s)

F. Interval note/summary
   1. For chronic or long-term patients, an interval summary is extremely useful when care is shifted from one provider to another.
   2. Include all items listed in transfer note (*see* E, above).

G. Discharge note or summary
   1. Required document that narratively describes hospital course
   2. Problem-oriented method is suggested
   3. Remember that this is a summary and not a biography.
   4. Items that should be included:
      a. Final diagnoses
      b. Procedures done
      c. Treatments provided
      d. Complications
      e. Active problems at discharge
      f. Medications or ongoing care, including nutrition
      g. Follow-up needs
         i. Tests
         ii. Physician and clinic visits
      h. Prognosis
      i. Discharge data—weight, head circumference, Hb/HCT, and anything else useful as baseline for future care
      j. Copies of imaging studies, social work notes, consultations, team conferences, chart material likely to be needed for continuity of care

III. Helpful Hints
A. Changes
   1. Never alter a previous entry.

    2. An error can be contemporaneously corrected.
       a. Neatly put a single line through the word(s) to be changed.
       b. Above the line write *error* and place your initials next to this.
       c. Add the correct word(s) as close as possible to the deletion.
    3. Late entries
       a. Occasionally, an entry has to be made "after the fact" (e.g., patient requires prolonged resuscitation, other entries are made before you have an opportunity to write your note).
       b. Be sure to note "Late entry" above your note. Record time of your note and briefly explain why it is out of sequence.

B. Avoid inflammatory or judgmental language
    1. Certain terms may eventually be misinterpreted and should be replaced by other words until a definitive diagnosis is reached. Examples include:
       a. Asphyxia. Was the baby truly *asphyxiated* ($\downarrow$ pH, $\downarrow$ PaO$_2$, $\uparrow$ PaCO$_2$) or merely *depressed*?
       b. Seizure vs. jittery or tremulous
       c. Distress vs. stress
    2. Do not attempt to explain events based on secondhand information.
    3. Avoid value judgments.
    4. Do not speculate.

C. Do not leave blank spaces in the chart.
    1. OFC _____
    2. BP _____
    3. |———|———| or ————————<
    4. If a parameter is thought important enough to list, its value should be present too. If it is still pending, state this.

D. Legibility—remember, this is a legal document that someone may have to interpret years later. Be sure others can read your entries; if not, consider alternatives:
    1. Print (rather than write)
    2. Type

E. Be inclusive in documenting normal findings or routine procedures because anything not mentioned explicitly may be interpreted as not having occurred.

F. Abbreviations
    1. The use of abbreviations should be minimized in medical records and documentation.
    2. Use only commonly accepted and recognized abbreviations.

Suggested Reading

Chilton JH, Shimmel TR: Inappropriate word choice in the labor and delivery and newborn medical record. In Donn SM, Fisher CW (eds): Risk Management Techniques in Perinatal and Neonatal Practice. Armonk, NY, Futura Publishing, 1996, pp 603–616.

Chapter 100

Research

Steven M. Donn, M.D.

I. Background

   A. Clinical research is an integral part of the mission of a neonatology service in an academic center.

   B. Much of our current practice is based on controlled studies conducted in NICUs, and much needs to be learned from studies yet to be done.

   C. Research is often being conducted collaboratively with investigators from other departments. Thus, NICUs are important institutional resources with a proud tradition.

II. Staff Support of Studies

   A. All members of the staff should recognize the importance of this function and support it even if they are not direct participants in a study.

   B. This support can be shown in many ways:
   1. Careful documentation in charts
   2. Communication with parents
   3. Collection of information and specimens
   4. Most importantly, notifying investigators of an eligible patient

III. Implementing Studies

   A. In addition to seeking approval from the Institutional Review Board, proposals for studies must be reviewed for logistical and patient care practicality before implementation by the medical and nursing staff. In particular, the "crowding" of too many studies should be avoided.

   B. All active protocols and consent forms should be kept available on the unit.

IV. Informed Consent by Investigators

   A. Must be obtained by one of the investigators

   B. This person will also be responsible for the logistics of specimen and data collection, but may need (and will appreciate) help with these functions.

   C. If a specific investigator is not available, the on-call faculty or fellow should be informed.

V. Patient Care

If a physician or nurse feels that the enrollment of a patient in a research protocol or the continuation of a study is inconsistent with good care, she or he must discuss this with the investigator before excluding a patient or altering the protocol.

INDEX

Page numbers in **boldface type** indicate complete chapters.